The Unstable Ankle

The Unstable Ankle

Meir Nyska, MD
Chairman, Orthopaedic Department
Hadassah Hebrew University
Medical School
Jerusalem, Israel

Meir Hospital, Kfar Saba, Israel

Gideon Mann, MD
Sports Injury Service, Orthopaedic Department
Meir Hospital, Kfar Saba, Israel

The Ribstein Center for Research
and Sport Medicine
Wingate Institute, Israel

Sackler Tel Aviv University
Medical School, Israel

Editors

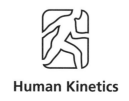

Human Kinetics

Library of Congress Cataloging-in-Publication Data

The unstable ankle / Meir Nyska and Gideon Mann, editors.
    p. cm.
   Includes bibliographical references and index.
   ISBN 0-88011-802-4
   1. Ankle--Wounds and injuries. 2. Sprains. I. Nyska, Meir, 1951- II. Mann, Gideon,
1947-

RD562 .U56 2002
617.5'84--dc21

2001039552

Acquisitions Editor: Loarn D. Robertson, PhD; **Developmental Editor:** Elaine Mustain; **Assistant Editors:** Maggie Schwarzentraub, Sandra Merz Bott, Amanda Ewing; **Copyeditor:** Kelly Winters; **Proofreader:** Julie A. Marx; **Indexer:** Craig Brown; **Permission Manager:** Dalene Reeder; **Graphic Designer:** Stuart Cartwright; **Graphic Artist:** Dawn Sills; **Photo Manager:** Leslie A. Woodrum; **Cover Designer:** Robert Reuther; **Photographer (cover):** Primal Pictures; **Art Manager:** Carl Johnson; **Illustrator:** Argosy; **Printer:** Versa Press

10 9 8 7 6 5 4 3 2 1

Human Kinetics
Web site: www.humankinetics.com

United States: Human Kinetics
P.O. Box 5076
Champaign, IL 61825-5076
800-747-4457
e-mail: humank@hkusa.com

Canada: Human Kinetics
475 Devonshire Road Unit 100
Windsor, ON N8Y 2L5
800-465-7301 (in Canada only)
e-mail: orders@hkcanada.com

Europe: Human Kinetics
Units C2/C3 Wira Business Park
West Park Ring Road
Leeds LS16 6EB, United Kingdom
+44 (0) 113 278 1708
e-mail: hk@hkeurope.com

Australia: Human Kinetics
57A Price Avenue
Lower Mitcham, South Australia 5062
08 8277 1555
e-mail: liahka@senet.com.au

New Zealand: Human Kinetics
P.O. Box 105-231, Auckland Central
09-523-3462
e-mail: hkp@ihug.co.nz

I, Meir Nyska, dedicate this book to my wife, Fruma.
I, Gideon Mann, dedicate this book to my wife, Ayala.

Contents

Contributors

Claude D. Anderson, MD
Department of Orthopaedic Surgery, The Union Memorial Hospital, Baltimore, MD

Yaakov H. Applbaum, MD
Department of Radiology, Hadassah University Hospital, Ein Kerem, Jerusalem, Israel

G. Chaimsky

Naama Constantini, MD
Ribstein Center for Sport Medicine Sciences and Research, Wingate Institute, Netanya, Israel

Deborah Mandis Cozen, PT
Foot and ankle specialist and certified Pilates instructor, Pasadena, California

George J. Davies, MEd, PT, SCS, ATC, CSCS
Professor, Graduate Physical Therapy Program, University of Wisconsin-LaCross
Director, Clinical and Research Services, Gundersen-Lutheran Sports Medicine, Onalaska, WI

Wolf-Ruediger Dingels, MD, PhD
Clinical director, Department of General Surgery, Traumatology, and Endoscopic Surgery, SANA—Krankenhaus G.m.b.H., Köln/Huerth, Germany

Richard D. Ferkel, MD
Clinical instructor, Orthopedic Surgery, UCLA School of Medicine
Southern California Orthopedic Institute, Van Nuys, CA

Alex Finsterbush, MD
Senior consultant in Sport Traumatology and Arthroscopy, Hadassah University Hospital, Jerusalem, Israel

Elisha Freund, MD
Senior orthopedic surgeon, The Zamenhof Policlinic, Tel Aviv, Israel
Fellow surgeon, The Orthopedic Department, Rabin Medical Center, Petach-Tikva, Israel

Beat Hintermann, MD
Chief of the Division of Orthopaedic Trauma and the Foot and Ankle Clinic, University of Basle, Switzerland

Jörg Jerosch, MD

Gadi Kahn, MD
Junior director, Orthopaedic Department, Soroka Medical Center, Beer-Sheva, Israel

Cobi Lidor, MD
Department of Orthopedics, Sapir Medical Center, Kfar Saba, Israel

Eli London, DPM
Department of Orthopedic Surgery, Hadassah University Hospital, Mount Scopus, Jerusalem, Israel

Joseph Lowe, MD
Department of Orthopedic Surgery, Hadassah University Hospital, Mount Scopus, Jerusalem, Israel

Scott A. Lynch, MD
Assistant professor, Department of Orthopaedics and Rehabilitation, College of Medicine, Pennsylvania State University

Gideon Mann, MD
Sackler Tel Aviv University Medical School, Israel; The Ribstein Centre of Research and Sports Medicine, Wingate Institute, Israel; Meir Hospital, Department of Orthopaedic Surgery, Jerusalem, Israel

Jeffrey A. Mann, MD

Roger A. Mann, MD
Orthopaedic surgeon, Oakland, CA
Director, Foot Fellowship Program

Marc Martens, PhD

R.K. Marti, MD, PhD
Department of Orthopaedic Surgery, Academic Medical Center, Amsterdam, The Netherlands

Y. Matan, MD
Department of Orthopedics, Hadassah University Hospital, Mount Scopus, Jerusalem, Israel

James W. Matheson, MS, PT, CSCS
Outreach coordinator/course assistant, University of Montana PT Clinic

David Mencher, DC, PhD
Chiropractor, Multidisciplinary Health Center, Jerusalem, Israel

Lyle J. Micheli, MD
Division of Sports Medicine, Children's Hospital, Boston, MA

Charles Milgrom, MD
Professor, Department of Orthopaedics, Hadassah University Hospital and Hebrew University Medical School, Jerusalem, Israel

Benno M. Nigg, PhD
Professor of Biomechanics, Engineering, Medicine and Kinesiology, The University of Calgary, Alberta, Canada
Director, Human Performance Laboratory, The University of Calgary, Alberta, Canada

Meir Nyska, MD
Hadassah-Hebrew University Hospital, Department of Orthopaedic Surgery, Jerusalem, Israel

Moira O'Brien, FRCPI
Professor of Anatomy and Head of Anatomy Department, Trinity College, Dublin, Ireland

A. Ross Outerbridge, MD, FRSC

Moshe (Perry) Pritsch, MD
Deputy Head, Department of Orthopaedic Surgery, The Chaim Sheba Medical Center, Israel

Ehud Rath, MD
Resident, instructor, Department of Orthopaedics, Soroka Hospital, Beer-Sheva, Israel

Rüdiger Reer, MD
Vice chairman, Institute of Sports Medicine, University of Hamburg, Germany

Per Renström, MD, PhD
Professor, Department of Orthopedics, Karolinska Hospital, Stockholm, Sweden

John B. Ryan, MD, FACS
Practicing orthopaedist, St. John Macomb Hospital, Orthopaedic-Sports Medicine Clinic, Warren, MI
Team physician, University of Detroit, Mercy

Moshe Salai, MD
Senior lecturer, Tel Aviv University, Israel

Lew C. Schon, MD
Attending orthopaedic surgeon, orthopaedic residency teaching staff, Dance Medicine Clinic director, The Union Memorial Hospital, Baltimore, MD
Consultant, Athletic Department, Georgetown University

Martin P. Schwellnus, MD, PhD
Associate professor, Sports Medicine, Department of Human Biology, Faculty of Health Sciences, University of Cape Town, South Africa

Ilan Shelef, MD
Department of Orthopedics, Soroka University Medical Center, Beer-Sheva, Israel

Charles C. Southerland Jr., DPM, FACFAS, FACFAOM, DABDA
Professor of Podiatric Orthopedics and Biomechanics, Barry University School, Miami Shores, FL

M. Suderer, MD
Medical Corps, Israel Border Police, Israel

Frank Spaas, MD
Foot and ankle surgeon
Head, Orthopedic Department, APRA Clinic, Antwerpen, Belgium

A.B. Stibbe, MD
Orthopaedic surgeon, the Netherlands

Steven I. Subotnick, DPM, ND, DC
Foot and ankle surgeon, Family Health Center, San Leandro, CA

Eliezer Trepman, MD

Alberto Macklin Vadell, MD
Chairman, Department of Orthopaedics, La Florida Hospital, Buenos Aires, Argentina

C. Niek van Dijk, MD, PhD
Orthopedic surgeon
Staff member, Department of Orthopaedic Surgery
Clinical director, Orthopaedic Research Center Amsterdam, The Netherlands

A. Zeev, PhD

Chaim Zinman, MD
Head, Department of Orthopedics, Rambam Medical Center, Haifa, Israel

Preface

Ankle sprains are not a benign injury. Complications are numerous, including chondral and osteochondral fractures, nerve injuries, damage to the foot and subtalar joints, osteochondritis dissecans, and, most frequently, functional instability. This leads to recurrent ankle sprains in about one-quarter of patients with ankle sprains grades II and III, and in approximately 1% of the total population.

Our knowledge of the anatomy, biomechanics, innervation and epidemiology; our acquaintance with methods of clinical scoring, staging, and evaluation; our familiarity with diagnostic measures; and our study of possible complications are all aimed at enabling us to give our patients the best treatment science can provide.

If a trend in the treatment of ankle sprains has developed during the last three decades, it would have to be described as "conservative." Although the true nature of functional instability is still not clearly understood, it is evident that, as in the knee and shoulder, simple mechanical perspectives are being replaced by the concept of combined neurological and mechanical stabilizing mechanisms. The body is not a machine, and sensation and proprioception are emerging as at least as important as the stabilizing direct effect of the intact ligament. A torn ligament is not a torn rope. It is also a torn nerve fiber, detached nerve corpuscles, and a broken reflex arc.

The result of the acceptance of this concept is the development of a conservative approach to the acute sprain, in nearly all grades of severity. Even so, this injury carries a high percentage of complications, as approximately 25% of patients with grade II and III sprains will develop recurrent ankle sprains and approximately 1% of all patients with sprains will stay disabled for life. When, eventually, a stabilizing procedure is needed, the same conservative trend has led to a gradual abandoning of the tenodesis procedure and adoption of minimal intervention procedures such as the Williams, Broström, Ahlgren, or Mann operations.

In the following chapters we will present the basic concepts and practical applications that lead the present approach to the diagnosis, treatment, and prevention of acute ankle ligament injury and acute and chronic ankle instability. Among the questions addressed include the following: Why are almost all the ankle injuries localized to the lateral ligament complex? Why do 4 of every 10 functionally unstable ankles appear stable on stress radiograph? What could be done to reduce the incidence of this injury, which is at present the most common acute injury in sport? What could be done to reduce the over 25% complication rate and the 1% chronic disability rate?

Acknowledgments

To Robin. Without her help, this book would not have come to be.

Part I

General Considerations

Health care practitioners cannot understand the pathology of ankle ligament injuries or evaluate an approach to treatment in acute or chronic situations without thoroughly understanding the anatomy of the ankle. They must also understand the ankle's rather complex biomechanics, learn the principles of joint innervation and proprioception, follow the trends in epidemiology of these all-too-common injuries, and consider the advantages and disadvantages of the various diagnostic modalities.

The ankle joint is a complex hinge joint whose motion is dictated by its bony structure and ligament restrictions. Its function cannot be fully understood apart from the concept of lower limb biomechanics, as ankle function is highly dependent on the neighboring joints—the knee joint above and the subtalar joint and foot below. The active control of this complex is totally dependent on an intact motion unit composed of the muscles and their tendons and an intact sensory network.

The following chapters will discuss the anatomy, biomechanics, innervation, and proprioception of the ankle complex.

Chapter 1

Epidemiology of Ankle Sprains

Charles Milgrom, MD

Although ankle ligamentous injuries have been said to be the most common injury in sports and recreational activities (Garrick 1977), exact incidence in the general population is unknown. Most epidemiology data are either based on studies of specific populations (Elkstrand & Tropp 1980; Gerber et al. 1998; Jackson et al. 1974; Milgrom et al. 1991) or do not include self-treated cases or those treated by the nonspecialist. These data make clear that knowing how to approach the unstable ankle is of vital importance for physicians.

■ Incidence of Ankle Sprains

According to one estimate, the incidence of injury to the ankle collateral ligaments is 37/1,000 persons per year in the general American population (Boruta et al. 1990). Broström (1964) found that 95% of the ankle collateral ligament injuries are lateral ankle sprains. The mechanism in 85% of ankle ligamentous injuries is reported to be inversion. Less frequently the mechanism is supination-internal rotation or supernation-plantarflexion (O'Donoghue 1976). More exact data about the incidence of ankle sprains are available from studies of specific populations. One-third of West Point cadets sustained ankle sprains during their 4-year program (Balduini et al. 1987). Among Israeli infantry recruits, the incidence of ankle sprains was 18% during 14 weeks of basic training (Milgrom et al. 1991). This high incidence was attributed to training on uneven terrain while fatigued. Ankle injury is reportedly the most common trauma in classical ballet and modern dance (Hardaker et al. 1985).

Holmer et al. (1994) did one of the most comprehensive prospective studies of the incidence of lateral ankle and midfoot sprain in the general population. Their study was based on admissions to the casualty ward of a Danish country hospital. By nature their data underestimate the real incidence because some sprains may have been treated elsewhere by local

physicians or may not have reached medical care at all. Overall, 4% of patients seen in the casualty ward sustained lateral ankle or midfoot sprains. Holmer et al. (1994) found the incidence of lateral ankle sprains to be 4/1,000 persons per year. Sprains of the lateral ankle were predominant in the younger population and among males, whereas midfoot sprains occurred more frequently in the older population and among women. Forty-five percent of the injuries occurred during sports activities, 20% during play, and 16% during work. The lateral ankle sprains were not divided as to severity in this study.

■ Affecting Factors

Milgrom et al. (1991) is one of several groups that have studied possible risk factors for lateral ankle sprains. They used the model of infantry recruits for their study. Risk factors can be considered to be either intrinsic or extrinsic to the subject. Examples of extrinsic factors for lateral ankle sprain are training terrain, familiarity with the terrain, shoes, lighting, weather, and the like. The study of Milgrom et al. (1991) tested the effect of two different types of shoes on the incidence of ankle sprains. Recruits were issued at random either standard infantry boots or basketball shoes and then trained for 14 weeks. No difference in the incidence of ankle sprains was found between the two shoe types. The authors observed that recruits broke the heel counter of their high-top military shoes at the level of the ankle joint, thereby negating the effect of increased ankle stability of the high-top shoe.

Before their training, recruits underwent a biomechanical examination and were questioned about their history of ankle sprains. By univariate analysis, a history of ankle sprain, height, weight, gastrocnemius circumference, leg length, and foot length and width were found to have a statistically significant relationship with the incidence of ankle sprains during the basic training. When the variables were further analyzed by multivariate analysis using stepwise logistic regression, only the variables related to the mass moment of inertia of the subjects (weight/height^2) and a history of ankle sprain were found to have statistically significant relationships to the incidence of lateral ankle sprain. Interestingly enough, these variables were not found to be related to the severity of the ankle sprain; 80% of the sprains were grade I in this study.

Although it is intuitively obvious why a history of ankle sprain increases risk for future ankle sprain, the relationship with the body's mass moment of inertia is less obvious. Milgrom et al. (1991) explained this association as follows:

The relationship between weight, height, and lateral ankle instability can be explained by their association with the inertial resistance to the human body's rotation around a horizontal axis through the ankle joint. This inertial resistance is measured by the body's moment of inertia. The computation, or measurement, of the moment of inertia is quite complex, but the product of body mass times height squared was shown to be an effective predictor of this property as well as a good scaling factor for its computation.

During the stance phase of walking, the body rotates around the ankle-subtalar joint in a complex way. The largest inertial resistance is through a transverse, or frontal, axis (figure 1.1). However, rotation through a transverse axis is controlled by powerful muscles of dorsi- and plantarflexion (gastrocnemius, soleus, and tibialis anterior). The range of the rotational component through a frontal axis is more limited and the eversion-inversion muscles are weaker; therefore the passive elements (ligaments and capsule) are more likely to be stressed during sudden rotations about this axis. This occurs clinically during sudden, unexpected movements, as when the foot bumps and stumbles. The higher the moment of inertia of the body around the ankle joint, the higher are the stresses in the tissues surrounding the joint.

It should be remembered that Milgrom et al. (1991) studied lateral ankle sprains using military recruits as a model. These recruits often carry heavy loads on their backs. This effectively increases their moment of inertia around the ankle joint, more so for taller recruits than it does for shorter recruits. The risk factor of the body's moment of inertia about the ankle joint may therefore have more importance in the military than the civilian model, because civilians usually do not carry such heavy loads on their backs.

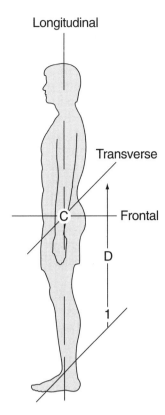

■ **Figure 1.1** Frontal, longitudinal, and transverse axes of rotation through the human body center of mass. C is the center of mass; D is the distance from center of mass to the ankle.

Baumhauer et al. (1995) studied prospectively a large number of possible intrinsic biomechanical and anatomical risk factors for lateral ankle sprain in a population of college-aged athletes. They did their initial screening of athletes participating in field hockey, lacrosse, or soccer before the sports season and excluded subjects with a history of grade II or III ankle sprains. They found that generalized joint laxity, anatomical measurements of the foot, ankle anatomical alignment, and ankle ligament stability were not risk factors for lateral ankle strain; nor was a history of grade I ankle strain. Individuals with muscle strength imbalance in ankle eversion to inversion had higher incidences of ankle sprain. The authors evaluated this by measuring peak mean torque values for eversion and inversion. The nonankle sprain group had a mean eversion-inversion ratio of 0.8 and the injured group a mean of 1.0. Analyzed as independent variables, ankle inversion and eversion peak mean torque values were not found to be related to the incidence of ankle sprain. The authors stress the importance of examining athletes for this imbalance and instituting proper exercises before the training season.

■ Outcome and Prognosis

Gerber et al. (1998), in a prospective study at the United States Military Academy (USMA), examined the disability associated with ankle sprains. Their study design was observational in that ankle sprains were diagnosed only among cadets who sought medical attention. The possibility exists that some recruits with mild ankle sprains may not have sought medical attention. They found that ankle sprains accounted for 23% of all sports injuries at the USMA: 97% were either grade I or II sprains, with 85% lateral ankle sprains, 10% syndesmosis strains, and only 5% isolated medial ankle sprains (figure 1.2). Sixty-three percent of the subjects had previously sustained ankle sprains and half of these had recurrent ankle sprains.

Treatment was given by a standard protocol and follow-up was done at 6 weeks and 6 months by patient questionnaires, physical examination, and functional tests. By 6 weeks, 95% of the subjects were participating in the schedule of regular athletic activities required by the military academy. At 6 months, all subjects had returned to high-level athletic activities, but by the criteria of the study only 60% had acceptable outcomes. The criteria for an acceptable outcome was no pain present in the ankle, no reported decrease in function, and an ability to perform functional hop tests within at least 80% of the ability of the noninjured lower extremity. Fourteen percent of subjects reported at least one recurrent ankle sprain and 29% reported episodes of the ankle giving way.

When results were analyzed for specific groups it was found that syndesmotic sprains had the poorest results with only 44% achieving acceptable outcomes. There was no statistical difference between the percentages of acceptable outcomes in grade I and grade II lateral ankle sprains. Interestingly, 54% of subjects with documented instability of the ankle still achieved acceptable outcomes. The authors state that their results are different from what one would intuitively expect, because neither a history of multiple sprains nor laxity of the ankle joint at examination were found to be strongly predictive of an unacceptable outcome. They found that even after a mild ankle sprain, a subject could continue to experience ankle dysfunction 6 months after the injury. The presence of syndesmotic sprain was a strong predictor of future likelihood of ankle dysfunction.

Jackson et al. (1974) and Bosien et al. (1955) speculated that secondary osteoarthritis of the ankle might be a long-term sequela of continued ankle instability. Harrington (1979) reported on a series of 36 cases who suffered from ankle instability for at least 10 years and who developed degenerate changes in the medial half of the tibial and talar surfaces. They reported that such changes may only be minimally apparent on plain radiographs. According to the authors, late stage stabilization of the ankle in these cases helped prevent further deterioration of the ankle joint. They reported no data as to the incidence of degenerative arthritis of the ankle secondary to long-standing lateral ligament instability, but the incidence would seem to be rare. This low incidence can be understood within the framework of Dye's (1996) envelope of function theory. According to this theory, subjects who are symptomatically unstable after ankle sprains naturally lower their envelope of function. If they restrict their activity to this safe envelope of

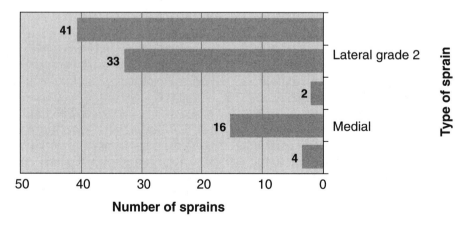

■ **Figure 1.2** The incidence, type, and grades of ankle sprains at the United States Military Academy between August 27, 1995, and October 27, 1995.

Data from Gerber et al. 1998.

function they will be unlikely to develop secondary osteoarthritis of the ankle.

■ Economic and Social Impact

In today's cost-conscious environment, the cost impact of ankle sprains has to be considered in terms of both treatment and lost time. Overall, it is estimated that ankle sprains are responsible for a quarter of time-loss injuries in basketball and football (Brand & Collins 1982). Slatyer et al. (1997) conducted a randomized controlled trial of Piroxicam in the management of acute grade I and II ankle sprains in the Australian regular army recruits. Their study also documents the economic impact of ankle sprains. The average loss of training time was 2.74 days in recruits treated with Piroxicam and 8.57 days in the control group. The direct costs of treatment in this model, with all care being given by army personnel, was $122 (US) in the Piroxicam group and $247 (US) in the control group. Although grade III ankle sprains were excluded from the treatment protocol, the authors state that recovery time for grade III ankle sprains was protracted and five out of nine of these cases required surgery. Soboroff et al., in a 1984 American study, found that the mean cost of treating severe ankle sprains was between $318 to $914 per sprain, with an annual aggregate cost of over 2 billion dollars.

■ Direction of Future Research

In spite of the multitude of articles in the literature on ankle sprains, it is surprising how little information is available about the epidemiology of ankle sprains in the general population. The best data come from the controlled environment of military studies or from specialized groups of athletes. There is a clear need for additional epidemiology studies in the general population as well as outcome studies.

■ References

Balduini BC, Vegso JJ, Torg JS, Torg E. 1987. Management and rehabilitation of ligamentous injuries to the ankle. J Sports Med 4:364-380.

Baumhauer JF, Alosa DM, Renström P, Trevino S, Beynnon B. 1995. A prospective study of ankle injury risk factors. Amer J Sports Med 23:564-570.

Boruta PM, Bishop JO, Bradley GW, Tullos HS. 1990. Acute lateral ligament injuries: A literature review. Foot Ankle 11:107-113.

Bosien WR, Staples OS, Russell SW. 1955. Residual disability following acute ankle sprains. J Bone Joint Surg Am 37:1237-1243.

Brand RL, Collins MDF. 1982. Operative management of ligamentous injuries to the ankle. Clinics Sports Med 1:117-130.

Brostrom L. 1964. Strained ankles. 1. Anatomical lesion in recent sprains. Acta Chir Scand 128:483-495.

Dye SF. 1996. The knee as a biological transmission with an envelope of function: a theory. Clin Orthop 325:10-18.

Elkstrand J, Tropp H. 1980. The incidence of ankle sprains in soccer. Foot Ankle 11:41-44.

Garrick JG. 1977. The frequency of injury, mechanism of injury, and epidemiology of ankle sprains. Am J Sports Med 5:241-242.

Gerber JP, Williams GN, Scoville CR, Arciero RA, Taylor DC. 1998. Persistent disability associated with ankle sprains: a prospective examination of an athletic population. Foot Ankle Int. 19:653-660.

Hardaker WT, Margello S, Goldner JL. 1985. Foot and ankle injuries in theatrical dancers. Foot Ankle 6:59-69.

Harrington KD. 1979. Degenerative arthritis of the ankle secondary to long-standing lateral ligament instability. J Bone Joint Surg Am 61:354-361.

Holmer P, Sondergaard L, Konradsen L, Nielsen PT, Jorgensen LN. 1994. Epidemiology of sprains in the lateral ankle and foot. Foot Ankle 15:72-764.

Jackson DW, Ashley RL, Powell JW. 1974. Ankle sprains in young athletes. Clin Orthop 101:1-15.

Milgrom C, Shlamkovitch N, Finestone A, Eldad A, Laor A, Danon Y, Lavie O, Wosk J, Simkin A. 1991. Risk factors for lateral ankle sprain: A prospective study among military recruits. Foot Ankle 12:26-30.

O'Donoghue DH. 1976. Treatment of injuries in athletes, 3rd ed. Philadelphia: Saunders. p. 707.

Slatyer MS, Hensley MJ, Lopert R. 1997. A randomized controlled trial of Piroxicam in the management of acute ankle sprain in Australian regular army recruits. The Kapooka ankle strain study. Am J Sport Med 25:544-553.

Soboroff SH, Pappius EM, Komaroff AL. 1984. Benefits, risks and cost of alternative approaches to the evaluation and treatment of severe ankle sprains. Clin Orthop 183:160-168.

Chapter 2

Anatomy of the Ankle and Talar Joints

Moira O'Brien, FRCPI, and Elisha Freund, MD

The ankle is among the most complex musculoskeletal structures in the body. Thorough familiarity with that anatomy is essential for effective treatment of the unstable ankle.

■ The Ankle Joint

The ankle joint is one of the most common joints to be injured. The ankle joint is a modified uniaxial hinge joint. It is a synovial joint. Only movements in one plane occur in a typical hinge joint, whereas some side-to-side movements take place at the ankle joint during plantarflexion.

The Bony Architecture

The bony architecture provides for the exquisitely subtle variations in movement that are necessary for locomotion on only two feet.

The Mortise

The proximal articulation is the mortise, which is made up of the lower end of the tibia, its medial malleolus, the lateral malleolus of the fibula, and the transverse tibiofibular ligament (the deep fibers of the posterior tibiofibular ligament). Its stability depends on the integrity of the syndesmosis of the inferior tibiofibular joint. All the articular surfaces are covered with hyaline cartilage (figure 2.1).

Here are further points to note about the mortise:

■ The lower articular surface of the tibia, wider in front than posteriorly, is concave anteroposteriorly and is slightly convex from side to side. It articulates with the dorsal aspect or trochlea of the body of the talus.

■ The medial malleolus is a short, stout projection on the medial aspect of the tibia. It has a comma-shaped facet that articulates with a correspondingly shaped facet on the medial aspect of the body of the talus.

■ The lateral surface of the distal tibia is triangular in outline and gives attachment to the strong interosseous tibiofibular ligament (see page 13). The lower part of this surface may articulate with the fibula as a synovial upward continuation of the ankle joint.

■ The lateral malleolus is at the distal end of the fibula, and projects more inferiorly and lies more posteriorly than the medial malleolus. There is a triangular articular facet on the medial aspect of the lateral malleolus that articulates with the corresponding triangular facet on the lateral aspect of the body of the talus. Above the facet on the fibula there is a triangular roughened area for the attachment of the interosseous tibiofibular ligament, which forms the syndesmosis with the tibia (see page 12).

■ The malleolar fossa lies posterior to the articular surface and gives attachment to the posterior tibiofibular and the posterior talofibular ligaments. The posterior talofibular ligament is the posterior band of the lateral ligament (Last 1984).

The Talus

The talus consists of a rounded head anteriorly, a neck, and a body. The body forms the lower articular surface, is cuboidal in shape, and has a dorsal or trochlear articular surface. The trochlear surface is wider anteriorly than posteriorly. It is convex from anterior to posterior and slightly concave from side to side. Other points to note about the talus:

■ The medial surface has a comma-shaped articular facet for the medial malleolus and the lateral a triangular facet for the lateral malleolus.

- The inferior surface of the body has a concave articular facet that articulates with the convex posterior articular facet on the superior surface of the calcaneus.

- The posterior surface is rough. It consists of two tubercles separated by a groove for the flexor hallucis longus. The medial tubercle is the smaller of the two (figure 2.2b). Occasionally (7% of cases), the lateral tubercle has a separate ossification center, resulting in an os trigonum (Last 1984).

The talus has no muscles attached to it and has a very extensive articular surface. As a result, fractures of the talus may result in avascular necrosis of either the body or the head.

When the ankle is dorsiflexed, the wider portion lies between the malleoli. This is the closepack, or stable position, of the ankle. During plantarflexion, the narrow posterior area is in the mortise, permitting some side-to-side movement. This is the least pack, or unstable position, of the joint.

The Joint Capsule

The ankle joint is surrounded by a fibrous capsule, which is attached just beyond the articular margins except anteriorly and inferiorly, where it attaches to the neck of the talus.

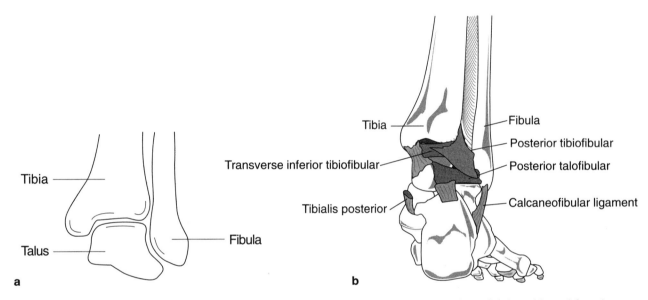

■ **Figure 2.1** (a) Posterior view of right ankle, bones of the mortise; and (b) posterior view of right ankle and foot, bones and ligaments.

Figure 2.1a reprinted from Behnke 2001; figure 2.1b adapted from Behnke 2001.

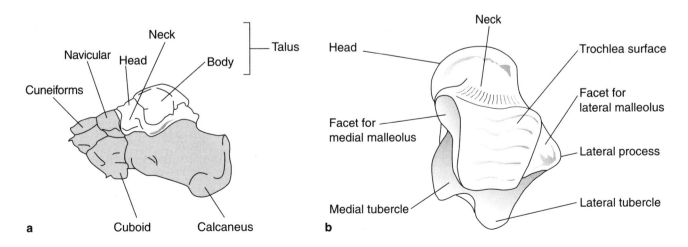

■ **Figure 2.2** (a) The lateral view of the right talus; and (b) superior aspect of the right talus.

Figure 2.2a adapted from Behnke 2001; figure 2.2b reprinted from Behnke 2001.

Posteriorly the fibers converge on the medial tubercle of the talus. Transverse fibers form the lower part of the posterior part of the capsule and blend with the transverse ligament and the posterior tibiofibular ligament. The capsule is a thin, weak structure in front and behind that allows dorsiflexion and plantarflexion.

The capsule is strengthened medially and laterally by the medial and lateral collateral ligaments.

The Ligaments

The ligaments are mainly thickenings of the capsule.

The Transverse Ligament

The transverse ligament is the deep portion of the posterior tibiofibular ligament (Sarrafian 1993). This is a strong, thick band that passes transversely across the posterior aspect of the joint from the lateral malleolus to the posterior border of the articular surface of the tibia, almost as far as the medial malleolus (See figure 2.1b) (Gray & Goss 1973).

The ligament is conoid in shape and twists along its course. It originates from the posterior fibular tubercle, which lies above the malleolar fossa, and from the proximal part of the malleolar fossa, which is behind the articular surface for the talus (Sarrafian 1993). The ligament projects below the margin of the bones, thus forming part of the articulating surface for the talus (Gray & Goss 1973).

The Deltoid (Medial Collateral) Ligament

The deltoid ligament, also called the medial collateral ligament, is a strong triangular ligament that, in conjunction with the lateral collateral ligament, strengthens the sides of the joint, adding to the medial stability of the joint and helping to maintain the medial longitudinal arch. There are many variations in the description of the deltoid ligament in the literature (Last 1984; Williams & Warwick 1980).

The deltoid ligament consists of multiple bands and is considered to be constructed of superficial and deep fibers. The superficial bands cross two joints (the ankle and the anterior portion of the clinical subtalar or talocalcaneonavicular joint). The deep bands cross only the ankle joint.

The medial ligament is attached at its apex to the anterior and posterior borders, as well as the tip, of the medial malleolus.

The base is attached anteroposteriorly to five different insertions (figure 2.3):

- The tuberosity of the navicular
- The neck of the talus

- The free edge of the spring ligament (plantar calcaneonavicular ligament)
- The sustentaculum tali
- The body of the talus

The Superficial Portions of the Deltoid Ligament

The anterior superficial portion of the deltoid ligament consists of three bundles:

- The tibionavicular fibers pass from the medial malleolus to the tuberosity of the navicular and the free edge of the spring ligament.
- The tibiocalcaneal band is almost vertical and is attached to the whole length of the sustentaculum tali.
- The posterior tibiotalar ligament passes to the medial side of the talus and to the medial tubercle of the talus, reaching the flexor hallucis longus tunnel. Occasionally it may reach anteriorly to the sustentaculum tali. Although this part of the ligament is well documented, it is not consistently present.

The Deep Portions of the Deltoid Ligament

The deep portions of the ligament are the anterior and posterior tibiotalar ligaments:

- The anterior tibiotalar is attached to the medial part of the neck of the talus and is separated anteriorly from the superficial fibers by fat (Milner and Soames 1998).
- The posterior tibiotalar portion passes to the medial side of the talus, under the tail of the comma-shaped facet. It is the strongest component of the medial ligament.

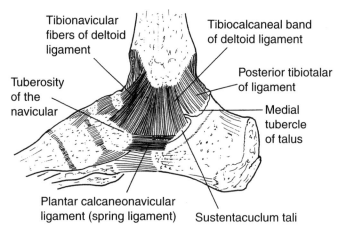

■ Figure 2.3 Deltoid (medial collateral) ligaments of the right ankle.

Reprinted from Watkins 1999.

The Lateral Collateral Ligament Complex

The lateral collateral ligament complex of the ankle attaches the lateral malleolus to the talus and calcaneus. The lateral ligament consists of three distinct parts:

- The anterior talofibular ligament (ATFL)
- The calcaneofibular ligament (CFL)
- The posterior talofibular ligament (PTFL)

The lateral ligaments are not nearly as strong as the medial ligament. This is particularly true of the ATFL, which is most frequently injured in an ankle sprain. The ligaments radiate like the spokes of a wheel. The angle between the ATFL and the CFL varies from 100° to 135° (figure 2.4) (Hamilton 1994; Peters et al. 1991.)

The Anterior Talofibular Ligament

The anterior talofibular ligament (ATFL) is part of the capsule and consists of a flat band (6-10 mm long and 2 mm thick) that extends anteromedially from the lateral malleolus to the neck of the talus, in front of the lateral articular facet. It is divided into two bands (upper and lower). The interval between the bands permits the penetration of the vascular supply.

The ligament runs parallel to the long axes of the talus when the foot is in a neutral or a dorsiflexed position, but shifts perpendicularly to the talus when the foot is in equinus as mentioned above. The ATFL is the weakest ligament in the lateral complex. The strain in the ligament increases with increasing plantarflexion and inversion.

The ATFL is a primary stabilizer against plantarflexion and inversion, and for all angles of plantarflexion (Liu & Jason 1994). The anterior drawer tests the ATFL.

The Calcaneofibular Ligament

The calcaneofibular ligament (CFL) is a long rounded cord (20-25 mm long, 6-8 mm in diameter) that passes posteroinferiorly from the tip of the lateral malleolus to a tubercle on the lateral surface of the calcaneus. The CFL is extracapsular. It is separated from the capsule by a thin fatty layer.

The CFL has the highest linear elastic modulus of the three ligaments (Siegler et al. 1988). It crosses both the ankle and subtalar joints. It is a major stabilizer of the subtalar joint (Clanton & Schon 1993). The ligament is perpendicular to the long axis of the talus if the ankle is dorsiflexed, and it is taut in dorsiflexion.

The CFL is part of the medial wall of the peroneal tendon sheath. It is crossed superficially by the tendons of the peroneus longus and peroneus brevis muscles.

The Posterior Talofibular Ligament

The posterior talofibular ligament (PTFL) is a thick structure and is the strongest part of the lateral ligament (figure 2.1b). It runs horizontally, medially, and slightly posteriorly from the lower portion of the malleolar fossa to the lateral and posterior aspects of

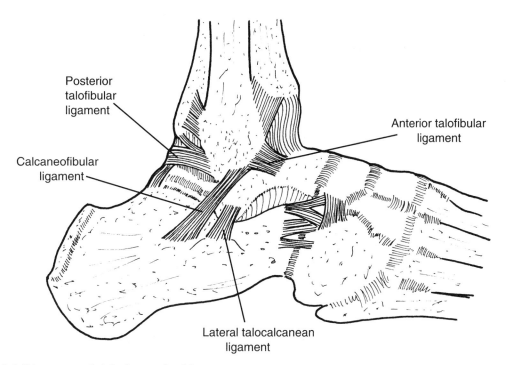

■ **Figure 2.4** Ligaments of right foot and ankle.
Reprinted from Watkins 1999.

the talus. The longer fibers reach the lateral tubercle of the posterior process or the os trigonum when present. A tibial slip passes to the medial malleolus (Williams & Warwick 1980).

The greatest strain on the ligament occurs when the foot is plantarflexed and everted. During plantarflexion, the posterior talofibular and tibiofibular are edge to edge. They separate during dorsiflexion.

The Synovial Membrane

The synovial membrane lines the inner aspect of the capsule and the other nonarticular structures of the joint. It is reflected onto the neck and the fat pads related to the anterior and posterior parts of the capsule. The synovial membrane occasionally extends up between the tibia and fibula into the inferior tibiofibular ligament.

Relations of the Ankle Joint

The anterior relations of the ankle lie posterior to the extensor retinacula. The tendons are dorsiflexors of the ankle joint.

The Anterior Aspect

Anterior to the ankle joint, from medial to lateral, from the medial malleolus, are the following structures:

- The tibialis anterior tendon in its own sheath.
- The extensor hallucis longus tendon in its own sheath.
- The anterior tibial artery and its venae committans. At the level of the ankle joint, the anterior tibial artery becomes the dorsalis pedis artery.

- The deep peroneal nerve runs parallel to these structures.
- The extensor digitorum longus and peroneus tertius run in a common sheath.

All the above mentioned structures pass beneath the superior and inferior extensor retinacula (figure 2.5). Also note that

- the medial branch of the superficial peroneal nerve is superficial to the retinacula, and
- the long saphenous vein and the saphenous nerve lie anterior to the medial malleolus.

The Medial Aspect

On the medial aspect of the ankle joint, passing under the flexor retinaculum (in the tarsal tunnel) from anterior to posterior, lie the following structures (figure 2.6):

- The tendon of the tibialis posterior.
- The flexor digitorum longus.
- The posterior tibial vessels and nerve.
- The flexor hallucis longus.
- The posterior tibial artery and the tibial nerve give off medial calcaneal branches and then divide into the medial and plantar arteries and nerves. The medial calcaneal vessels and nerve pierce the flexor retinaculum to supply the skin of the heel.

The Lateral Aspect

Lateral to the joint lie the peroneus brevis and longus (figure 2.7).

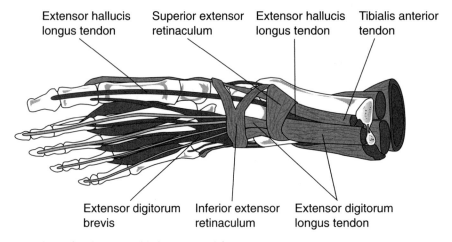

■ **Figure 2.5** Superior view of retinacula of left ankle and foot.
Adapted from Behnke 2001.

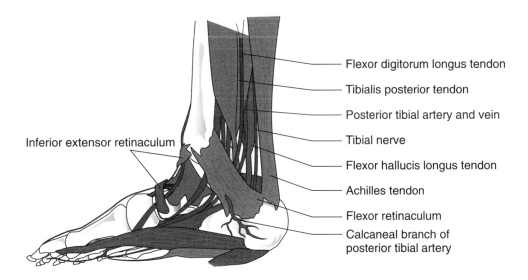

■ **Figure 2.6** Medial view of retinacula of left ankle and foot.

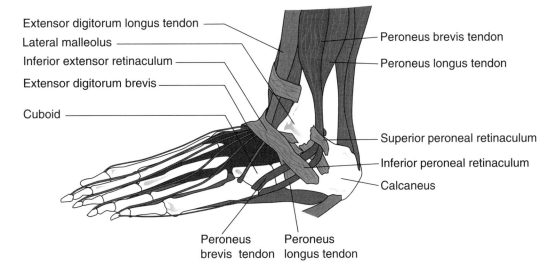

■ **Figure 2.7** Lateral view of retinacula of left ankle and foot.
Adapted from Behnke 2001.

■ The peroneus brevis lies anterior to the peroneus longus tendon in a common sheath, passing beneath the superior peroneal retinaculum, behind the lateral malleolus.

■ The two tendons then run in their own synovial sheaths. The brevis is attached to the base of the fifth metatarsal. The peroneus longus enters a groove on the inferior aspect of the cuboid and crosses the sole of the foot to be inserted into the lateral aspect of the medial cuneiform and the base of the first metatarsal. There may be a sesamoid bone in the tendon of the peroneus longus as it enters the groove in the cuboid bone.

■ The short saphenous vein and the sural nerve lie posterior to the lateral malleolus.

The Posterior Aspect

Posterior to the ankle joint, superficially, are the short saphenous vein and the sural nerve. Deeper lie

■ the retrocalcaneal fat pad and bursa, which separate the ankle joint from the Achilles tendon, and

■ the flexor hallucis longus, which enters a groove between the medial and lateral tubercles on the posterior surface of the talus and then passes medially toward the tarsal tunnel.

The Nerve and Blood Supply

Nerve supply is via the articular branches of the deep peroneal and tibial nerves from the L4 to the S2. Blood supply is from the malleolar branches of the anterior tibial, posterior tibial, and peroneal arteries.

The Joint Axis

In the anatomical position the axis of the ankle joint is horizontal but is set at 20-25° obliquely to the frontal plane, running posteriorly as it passes laterally. In dorsiflexion the foot moves upward and medially, and in plantarflexion it moves downward and laterally (Plastanga et al. 1990).

Motion at the Ankle Joint

Movements are dorsiflexion and plantarflexion. During plantarflexion, there is some side-to-side movement. Inversion and eversion take place at the subtalar joint and not at the ankle joint.

Dorsiflexion

Dorsiflexion has a range of 30°. A minimum of 10° is required for normal gait. Dorsiflexion is the closepack position: The wide part of the body of the talus is between the narrower posterior part of the tibiofibular mortise, causing increased tension in the interosseous and transverse tibiofibular ligaments.

Dorsiflexion is produced by the following muscles:

- The tibialis anterior
- The extensor hallucis longus
- The extensor digitorum longus and the peroneus tertius

Dorsiflexion is limited by tension in the Achilles tendon, the posterior part of the deltoid ligament, the posterior capsule, the calcaneofibular ligament, and the wedging of the talus between the malleoli. The inferior margin of the tibia comes in contact with the neck of the talus.

Plantarflexion

Plantarflexion is the leastpack position. During plantarflexion, the narrow portion of the talus lies between the two malleoli, permitting some side-to-side movement. During plantarflexion, the anterior capsule, the anterior fibers of the deltoid, and the anterior talofibular ligaments are under maximum tension.

Plantarflexion is caused mainly by the action of the following muscles:

- The Achilles tendon
- The tibialis posterior
- The flexor digitorum longus
- The flexor hallucis longus
- The peroneus longus and brevis

Plantarflexion is limited by the anterior muscles, the anterior portion of the deltoid, the anterior portion of the capsule, and the anterior talofibular ligament. Excessive plantarflexion may affect the posterior tubercles of the talus or os trigonum.

The ankle is most vulnerable when the ankle is plantarflexed and the foot is inverted. The anterior talofibular portion of the lateral ligament is the most frequently injured, as the ligament is stressed. The next most frequently injured is the calcaneofibular ligament. This is stressed when the foot is dorsiflexed and inverted. The deltoid ligament is much stronger than the lateral ligaments and is involved in excessive eversion injuries.

The Tibiofibular Syndesmosis

The tibiofibular syndesmosis is a fibrous joint featuring four ligaments and limited articulation.

- The interosseous ligament is the principal connection between the tibia and the fibula. It is attached to the rough triangular convex surface, above the articular facet, on the medial aspect of the lateral malleolus of the fibula and to a similar rough, triangular concave area on the lateral side of the tibia (Frazer 1933; Grant 1962; Plastanga et al. 1998; Sarrafian 1993). The interosseous ligament is a strong ligament, continuous with the interosseous membrane. It is a dense mass of short fibers intermingled with blood vessels and adipose tissue (Sarrafian 1993). It is supplemented by the anterior, posterior, and transverse tibiofibular ligaments (Frazer 1933; Grant 1962; Gray & Goss 1973). (See figure 2.1b.)

- The anterior and posterior tibiofibular ligaments are longer and more superficial than the interosseus ligament. They stretch from the borders of the fibular notch of the tibia to the anterior and posterior surfaces of the lateral malleolus of the fibula. The posterior tibiofibular ligament is thicker and wider than the anterior tibiofibular ligament (see figures 2.4 and 2.1b).

- The transverse tibiofibular ligament lies deep to the posterior ligament.

- The tibiofibular articulation, or actual contact of the fibula and the tibia, is limited to a minor crescent-shaped, cartilage-coated articular surface, which is continuous with the articular surface of the lateral malleolus and extends about 4 mm above the joint surface (Gray & Goss 1973; Morris 1879; Sarrafian 1993). A recess of the ankle joint may extend upward.

The Interosseous Membrane

The interosseous membrane is attached to the interosseous borders of the tibia and fibula. The anterior fibers are directed downward and laterally from the tibia to the fibula. The posterior fibers are nearly vertical (Sarrafian 1993).

■ The Talar Joints

The inferior surface of the talus takes part in two joints known as the clinical subtalar joint. Posteriorly the inferior aspect of the body of the talus is part of the talocalcaneal joint, while the inferior aspect of the head of the talus forms a part of the talocalcaneonavicular joint.

The Talocalcaneal Joint (The Anatomical Subtalar Joint)

The talocalcaneal or anatomical subtalar joint is a synovial plane joint, uniaxial with 1° of freedom (figure 2.8).

The Articular Surface

The articular surfaces involve two bones:

■ The concave inferior aspect of the body of the talus

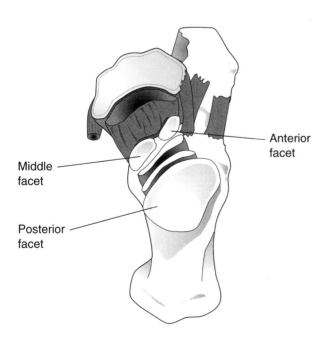

Middle facet

Posterior facet

Anterior facet

■ **Figure 2.8** The right talocalcaneal (subtalar) joint viewed from above.

■ The convex posterior facet on the superior surface of the calcaneus (Grant 1962)

Both articular surfaces are covered with articular cartilage.

The Capsule

The capsule is attached just beyond the articular margins. It is thin and loose, but it is thickened medially, laterally, and posteriorly to form the medial, lateral, and posterior talocalcaneal ligaments.

The Sinus Tarsi

The talocalcaneal joint is separated from the inferior portion of the talocalcaneonavicular joint by the sinus tarsi, which contains the interosseous ligament. The sinus is a narrow tunnel formed by the sulcus tali and the sulcus calcanei, which runs obliquely, anteriorly, and laterally (Frazer 1933; Grant 1962). Its anterolateral portion ends on the dorsum of the foot.

The Ligaments Involved in the Talocalcaneal Joint

Ligaments involved in the talocalcaneal joint are the interosseus ligament and the ligament of the neck of the talus.

The Interosseous Ligament
The interosseous ligament, or ligament of the sinus tarsi, is a portion of the united capsules of the talocalcaneonavicular and the talocalcaneal (subtalar) joints (Gray & Goss 1973). It consists of two partially united layers of fibers, each belonging to one of the joints. It is attached to the groove between the articular facets of the talus and to the corresponding area of the calcaneus along the majority of the floor of the sinus tarsi from side to side (Gray & Goss 1973). It runs from the calcaneus upward and medially before inserting into the talus, forming the roof of the sinus tarsi (figure 2.6) (Barclay-Smith 1896; Cahill 1965; Sarrafian 1993).

The Cervical Ligament
The cervical ligament is found in the lateral portion of the sinus tarsi (see figure 2.4) (Sarrafian 1993). The ligament is attached as follows:

■ To the upper surface of the calcaneus, medial to the attachment of the extensor digitorum brevis

■ The ligament passes upward, anteriorly, and medially to the neck of the talus.

The ligament is a strong ligament that is taut in inversion (Plastanga et al. 1998).

The inferior extensor retinaculum (see figure 2.6) has three roots. The medial and intermediate are attached inside the sulcus and sinus tarsi. The lateral is attached outside the sinus posterior to the ligament of the neck of the talus.

The Synovial Membrane

The synovial membrane lines the capsule and the nonarticular structures. It does not communicate with other joints.

The Talocalcaneonavicular Joint

The talocalcaneonavicular joint is a synovial ball-and-socket joint, multiaxial with 3° of freedom.

The Ball

The ball is formed by the anterior and inferior aspects of the head of the talus.

- The rounded head articulates anteriorly with the navicular.
- On the inferior surface, at the head of the talus, there are four articular areas separated by indistinct ridges, which articulate as follows from anterior to posterior:
  - With the plantar calcaneonavicular ligament (the spring ligament).
  - With the anterior facet on the superior surface of the calcaneus.
  - With the larger, middle facet on the superior aspect of the sustentaculum tali of the calcaneus.
  - With the medial part of the bifurcate ligament laterally.

The Socket

The socket is formed by the following structures:

- The posterior aspect of the navicular.
- The plantar calcaneonavicular ligament (spring ligament).
- The anterior and middle facets on the superior surface of the calcaneus.
- The lateral calcaneonavicular ligament, which is the medial limb of the bifurcate ligament. Both ligaments are covered with hyaline cartilage.

The Ligaments

Two of the ligaments involved in the talo-calcaneonavicular joint form part of the inferior articular surface.

- The plantar calcaneonavicular ligament (spring ligament) is a strong, thick, dense, fibroelastic ligament. It extends from the anterior and medial border of the sustentaculum tali to the medial surface of the navicular, posterior to the tuberosity of the navicular. The ligament articulates with, and supports, the head of the talus. The superficial fibers of the deltoid are attached to its free border. It forms the keystone, or highest point, of the medial portion of the longitudinal arch of the foot.

- The bifurcate ligament has two separate attachments to the anterior portion of the superior surface of the calcaneus. The medial limb is the lateral calcaneonavicular ligament. It is attached to the adjacent portion of the navicular. The lateral limb is the medial calcaneocuboid ligament. It has different orientations.

  - The interosseous ligament closes the posterior portion of the talocalcaneonavicular joint. It has been described on page 13.
  - The lower fibers of the deltoid ligament are attached to the free edge of the spring ligament.
  - The dorsal talonavicular ligament reinforces the capsule and runs from the neck of the talus to the navicular.
  - The synovial membrane lines the capsule and the nonarticular structures.

The Calcaneocuboid Joint

The calcaneocuboid joint is a synovial plane joint, uniaxial with 1° of freedom. It is part of the transverse tarsal joint. The articular surfaces are the anterior aspect of the calcaneus and the posterior aspect of the cuboid.

The Capsule and the Synovial Membranes

The capsule is attached just beyond the articular margin. The synovial membrane lines the capsule and the nonarticular structures inside.

The Ligaments Involved in the Calcaneocuboid Joint

The dorsal ligament is a thickening of the capsule. The main ligaments are found on the inferior surface (figure 2.9).

- The long plantar ligament is attached
  - posteriorly to just anterior to the medial and lateral tubercles of the calcaneus,
  - to the anterior tubercle of the calcaneus,
  - to the edges of the groove of the cuboid, where it acts as a retinaculum for the tendon of the peroneus longus, and
  - to the bases of the middle three metatarsals.

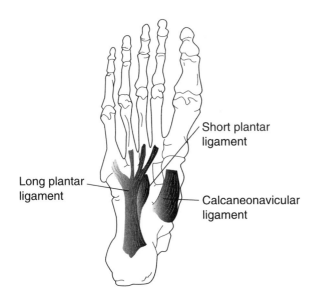

■ **Figure 2.9** Short plantar and long plantar ligament.
Adapted from Behnke 2001.

■ The lateral limb of the bifurcate ligament is the medial calcaneocuboid. It is attached to the anterior portion of the superior surface of the calcaneus and to the adjacent anteromedial angle of the cuboid. It is one of the main connections between the first and second row of tarsal bones.

■ The short plantar ligament is a broad band that passes from the area just anterior to the anterior tubercle of the calcaneus, to the area just posterior to the groove for the peroneus longus on the cuboid. A pronated or flat foot is often associated with subluxation of the cuboid, resulting in pain on the posterolateral aspect of the foot.

Motion of the Talar Joints

The joints involved in inversion and eversion enable us to walk on uneven surfaces. Inversion, or supination, is raising the medial border of the foot, so that the sole faces medially. It is usually accompanied by adduction of the forefoot. Supination is the closepack position. Eversion, or pronation, is raising the lateral border so the sole faces laterally. It is usually accompanied by abduction of the forefoot.

The Joints Involved in Inversion and Eversion

Inversion and eversion are initiated at the transverse tarsal joint. "Transverse tarsal joint" is a radiological term and consists of two joints:

■ The talonavicular (anterior) portion of the talocalcaneonavicular joint

■ The calcaneocuboid joint

The main movement occurs at the clinical subtalar joint, which also consists of two joints:

■ The talocalcaneal, (anatomical subtalar) joint

■ The inferior portion of the talocalcaneonavicular joint

The pivot structure for inversion and eversion is the cervical ligament, or the ligament of the neck of the talus (Last 1984). The axis of motion passes upward and medially through the most convex portion of the posterior facet on the superior surface of the calcaneus, to the most convex point on the anterior aspect of the head of the talus (Last 1984).

Muscles Involved in Eversion and Inversion of the Foot

The inverters are attached to the medial aspect of the foot, the everters to the lateral side.

■ Inverter and dorsiflexor: Tibialis anterior. Muscle supplied by the deep peroneal nerve.

■ Inverter and plantarflexor: Tibialis posterior. Muscle supplied by the tibial nerve.

■ Everter and dorsiflexor: Peroneus tertius. Muscle supplied by the deep peroneal nerve.

■ Everter and plantarflexor: Peroneus brevis and peroneus longus. Muscles supplied by the superficial peroneal nerve.

■ References

Barclay-Smith E. 1896. The astragalo-calcaneo-navicular joint. J Anat Physiol 30:390.

Cahill DR. 1965. The anatomy and function of the contents of the human tarsal sinus and canal. Anat Rec 153:1.

Clanton TO, Schon LC. 1993. Athletic injuries to the foot and ankle. In Mann RA, Coughlin ML, editors. Surgery of the foot and ankle. St. Louis: Mosby, p. 1095-1224.

Frazer JE. 1933. Anatomy of the human skeleton, 3rd ed. London: Churchill, p. 156-170, 177-181.

Grant JCB. 1962. Anatomy, 5th ed. London: Bailliere, Tindal & Cox, p. 303, 309, 322, 332, 336, 337, 340.

Gray H, Goss CM. 1973. Anatomy of the human body. Philadelphia: Lea & Febiger, p. 356-365.

Hamilton WG. 1994. Current concepts in the treatment of acute and chronic lateral ankle instabilities. Sports Med Arthroscopy Rev 2:2264-2266.

Last RJ. 1984. Anatomy, regional and applied, 7th ed. London: Churchill Livingstone, p. 182-189.

Liu SH, Jason WJ. 1994. Lateral ankle sprains and instability problems. Clin Sports Med 13(4):793-809.

Milner CE, Soames RW. 1998. The medial collateral ligaments of the ankle joint: Anatomical variations. Foot Ankle Int 19(5):289-292.

Morris HL. 1879. The anatomy of the joints of man. London: Churchill, p. 384.

Peters W, Trevono SG, Renstrom PA. 1991. Chronic lateral ankle insta-
    bility. Foot Ankle 12(3):182-191.

Plastanga N, Field D, Soames R. 1990. Anatomy and human movement,
    2nd ed. Woburn, MA: Butterworth Heinemann, p. 524-562.

Plastanga N, Field D, Soames R. 1998. Anatomy and human movement,
    3rd ed. Woburn, MA: Butterworth Heinemann, p. 488-531.

Sarrafian SK. 1993. Foot and ankle-topographic, functional. Philadel-
    phia: Lippincott, p. 37-65, 159-162, 192-199.

Siegler S, Block J, Schneck CD. 1988. The mechanical characteristics of
    the collateral ligaments of the human ankle joint. Foot Ankle 8:234-
    242.

Williams PL, Warwick. 1980. Gray's anatomy, 36th ed. London: Churchill
    Livingstone, p. 491-495.

Chapter 3

Biomechanics of the Ankle Joint Complex and the Shoe

Benno M. Nigg, PhD, and Beat Hintermann, MD

Humans use shoes to protect the foot during various activities and to support foot function and mobility. To understand foot function and the effects shoes can have on it, one must analyze

- the movement of foot and leg during typical activities,

- the coupling mechanism between foot and leg, and

- the forces acting on and in the human foot and ankle joint.

This chapter will explain these three aspects of foot and shoe biomechanics and discuss how shoes may affect movement, movement transfer, and forces acting on and in the foot and the ankle joint. To follow the discussion, one must understand a number of definitions in kinematics and kinetics. See pages 17–18 for these definitions.

Definitions

To follow the discussion in this chapter, one must understand a number of definitions in both kinematics and kinetics.

Kinematics

- **Ab-adduction** angle of the foot is the angular position of the foot relative to the leg about an axis determined by the intersection of the frontal and the sagittal planes of the leg. Comments: The terms **abduction** and **adduction** are used to describe an angular position or a rotation of the foot with respect to the leg. Abduction represents a rotation in which the tip of the foot points or moves toward the outside. Adduction represents a rotation toward the inside of the foot.

- **Ankle joint in-eversion** angle is the angular position of the foot relative to the leg about an axis

determined by the intersection of the transverse and sagittal planes of the foot. Comments: The terms **inversion** and **eversion** are used to describe an angular position or movement of the foot with respect to the leg. Inversion represents an angular position or a rotation of the foot sole toward the inside, eversion toward the outside. The terms in- and eversion are sometimes defined with respect to the ground. To distinguish between these two definitions, the following terms are used:

- **Foot in-eversion** is the movement of the foot with respect to the ground.

- **Ankle joint in-eversion** is the movement of the foot with respect to the leg.

- **Dorsiflexion-plantarflexion** angle is the angular position of the foot relative to the leg about an axis determined by the intersection of the frontal and transverse planes of the leg. Comments: The terms **dorsiflexion** and **plantarflexion** are used to describe an angular position or movement of the foot with respect to the leg. **Dorsiflexion** represents an extension position or movement of the foot-leg segments.

- **Plantarflexion** represents a position or movement of the foot-leg segments in which the foot is extended at the ankle and the plantar surface of the foot is flexed. It is the movement understood when a dancer is told, "Point your toe." Although the term **dorsalextension** is considered by some to be the more accurate term for this position (Perry 1992), it differs from the nomenclature most commonly accepted in the field, and thus will not be used here.

- **Tibial rotation** angle is the angular position of the tibia relative to the foot about a longitudinal axis of the tibia. The term **tibial rotation** is used to describe an angular position or movement of the leg with respect to the foot. **Internal tibial rotation** represents an angular position or rotation of the anterior part of the tibia toward the inside. **External tibial rotation** refers to a position or rotation toward the outside.

- **Pronation-supination** angle is the angular position of the foot relative to the talus about the talocalcaneal axis (subtalar joint axis). This motion is to a large extent parallel with eversion and inversion but includes the subtalar joints. Comments: The terms **pronation** and **supination** are used to describe an angular position or movement of the calcaneus with respect to the talus. **Pronation** represents an angular position or rotation in which the foot sole moves toward the outside. The term **supination** refers to a movement in which the foot sole moves toward the inside. Pronation and supination are a combination of ab-adduction, in-eversion, and plantarflexion-dorsalextension (Engsberg 1987).

- **Ankle joint complex** (AJC) is the combination of the talocrural and the talocalcaneal joints (ankle and subtalar joints), which provide the angular rotation between the leg and the foot.

- **Clinical axes** are axes that are typically used in clinical assessment. For the foot, the clinical axes are the anterior-posterior axis, the mediolateral axis, and the inferior-superior axis.

- **Functional axes** are axes about which the actual rotation between two segments occurs. For the AJC, the two functional axes are the talocrural and the talocalcaneal joint axes (the ankle joint and the subtalar joint axes).

Kinetics

- **Ground reaction forces** are forces acting from the ground onto the object being in contact with the ground. Ground reaction forces are typically subdivided into three orthogonal components. These are the vertical, anterior-posterior, and mediolateral components.

- **Impact forces** in human locomotion are forces that result from a collision of two objects. Impact forces reach their maximum earlier than 50 milliseconds after the first contact of the two objects (Nigg 1994).

- **Active forces** in human locomotion are forces generated by movement that is entirely controlled by muscular activity (Nigg 1994).

■ Movement

The AJC allows for relative movement between the foot and the leg. The following paragraphs will con-

centrate on the possibilities of assessing this movement, specifically addressing the following aspects:

- Clinical and functional variables
- Three-dimensional assessment
- Examples of foot movement variables for one specific case

Clinical and Functional Variables

Rotational movement between two segments occurs around a momentary axis of rotation, which is determined primarily by the shape, the ligamentous structures, and the muscle tendon units of the joint. Rotations attempting to describe the functional movement of two adjacent segments are rotations about functional axes. The AJC is a peculiar joint in the sense that one can estimate during locomotion the location of two of the three bones that make up the joint—the tibia and the calcaneus.

However, it is practically impossible to estimate during locomotion the location of the talus. Additionally, it is extremely difficult to determine the ankle joint axes (van den Bogert et al., 1994) around which the actual rotational movements occur. Consequently, it is difficult to describe the movement of the AJC using functional axes. The movement of the foot, however, can be determined much more easily in a clinical environment by defining foot axes such as the anterior-posterior, the mediolateral, and the inferior-superior axes.

Movement of the foot can be defined with respect to the direction of locomotion (Perry 1992), the position of the foot with respect to a laboratory coordinate system, or the position of the foot with respect to the leg. Specific descriptions of foot movement may be advantageous in answering specific questions. The foot movement with respect to the direction of movement of the center of mass may be appropriate for energy considerations. The foot movement relative to the leg may be appropriate for local loading aspects. In any case, it is crucial to define the system of reference clearly because, depending on the system of reference, the results are different. The following discussions use variables that have been defined as movement between the foot and the leg (see definitions, pages 17–18).

It is obvious that functional variables would be ideal in discussing functional aspects of the foot-leg complex. However, for practical reasons, functional variables are rarely available for research or clinical applications. Expressions such as "pronation" or "supination" are often used incorrectly because they are often used to represent "eversion" or "inversion," respectively. Clinical variables are used in the majority of clinical and research applications.

Three-Dimensional Assessment

The rapid development of technology provides gait analysis systems that offer the possibility for three-dimensional movement analysis. This development is not without concern. Two concerns will be discussed:

- The use of two-dimensional analysis
- The sequence of the angle determination

For many questions, a two-dimensional approach is appropriate, and the errors resulting from this approach are minimal. It is, therefore, appropriate to check first whether a three-dimensional analysis is really necessary and what errors are introduced by changing to a two-dimensional analysis.

A three-dimensional rotational movement, subdivided into its three rotational components, will provide different results depending on the sequence of the rotations chosen (Areblad et al. 1990; Cole et al. 1993). One can easily verify this by moving the arm from an "initial position," in which the arm is along the body with the palm facing the side of the body, to a "final position," in which the arm points horizontally at an angle of 45° from the sagittal plane and the palm faces to the side. The angular components used are extension (EX), abduction (AB), and axial rotation (AR). One may reach the final position by first moving the arm upward and second by abducting it

45°. This would correspond to a sequence of FL-AB-AR with the values 90-45-0°. However, one may reach the same final position by first axially rotating the arm by 45° and second by extending the arm by 90°. This corresponds to a sequence of AR-FL-AB with the values 45-90-0°. Both movement sequences include 90° of extension.

However, the first movement sequence includes 45° of abduction and no axial rotation, whereas the second movement sequence includes no abduction but 45° of axial rotation. It is, therefore, important to understand for which movement analyses the sequence of the angular components is crucial. This concern is illustrated for the foot in table 3.1.

Many authors have argued about the appropriateness of one or the other sequences (Areblad et al. 1990; Grood & Suntay 1993; Mann 1982). However, logical arguments that have been described earlier (Nigg & Cole 1994) using the anatomical definitions of flexion-extension, ab-adduction, and axial rotation indicate that the appropriate sequence that agrees with the definition of these movements for all human joints is

- in general,
  1. flexion-extension,
  2. abduction-adduction, and
  3. axial rotation.

Table 3.1 Comparison for the Three Components of Angular Positions for the Ankle Joint Complex

Activity	Component	Sequence of determination of rotation	
		PL-DO	PL-DO
		AD-AB	IN-EV
		IN-EV	AD-AB
Running	Dorsiflexion	25.0	21.4
	Abduction	10.0	10.6
	Eversion	20.0	19.7
Side-shuffle	Dorsiflexion	20.0	30.3
	Abduction	15.0	18.1
	Inversion	35.0	33.6
ROM	Plantarflexion	40.0	26.8
	Abduction	40.0	41.8
	Inversion	20.0	15.2

From Nigg et al. 1994.

- For the AJC, the sequence is
  1. plantarflexion-dorsiflexion (PD),
  2. abduction-adduction (AA), and
  3. inversion-eversion (IE).

In any case, the results in table 3.1 indicate that caution is necessary when using three-dimensional analysis for mediolateral movements and for the assessment of range of motion. However, the sequence of angular component determination is not critical for movements such as walking and running.

Examples of Foot Movement Variables

Several authors have quantified foot movement variables for walking and running (Eberhart et al. 1968; Mann 1982; Murray et al. 1964; Perry 1992; Winter et al. 1974). Lower extremity locomotion has been subdivided into many different phases. For the purpose of a functional analysis of foot movement, in this section the gait cycle is subdivided into two phases, a stance phase and a swing phase. The forces acting on and in the various structures of the AJC are typically much higher in the stance than in the swing phase. Consequently, the following illustrations and discussions concentrate on the stance phase.

The stance phase is subdivided functionally into two parts, an impact phase and an active phase. The impact phase includes approximately the initial 50 milliseconds of ground contact. The active phase includes the rest of ground contact. There is a fuzzy boundary between the impact and active phase.

During the impact phase, the subject cannot react to sudden changes and change strategies in muscle response. Typically, the system is preprogrammed for a given situation. However, if sudden changes occur, the system reacts with the "old" pattern response. During the impact phase, the human leg behaves like a passive structure with certain mechanical properties. In contrast, the movement during the active phase is controlled fully by muscular activation and the system acts as an active structure.

The variables ab-adduction, plantarflexion-dorsiflexion, ankle joint in-eversion, and tibial rotation are illustrated in figure 3.1 for 10 subjects running heel-toe. The angular variables were determined using the sequence PD-AA-IE.

Even though such mean curves are published in many textbooks, they may not be typical for understanding the loading situation in a subject-specific case. Figure 3.1b illustrates a subject who has movement variables for the AJC that are substantially different from the mean curves. Careful study of such graphs may provide insight into subject-specific problems or advantages.

■ Movement Transfer Between Foot and Leg

Let us consider the calcaneus, the tibia, the femur, and the pelvis during one ground contact in running. The calcaneus touches the ground and everts until about midstance (at about 150 to 250 ms). The calcaneus eversion movement is associated (through the talus) with an internal rotation of the tibia. At the same time (from initial contact to midstance) the pelvis rotates externally with respect to the supporting leg, initiating an external rotation of the femur. The two movements are, however, in opposite directions, and somewhere between the calcaneus and the pelvis, the movement transfer between neighboring segments cannot be direct (Allinger & Engsberg 1993). A high transfer of the eversion movement of the calcaneus to the tibia may, however, be associated with potential overloading problems at the knee level. It is, therefore, important to understand the transfer mechanism between calcaneus and tibia. The following paragraphs address this transfer mechanism, discussing an in vitro and an in vivo experiment.

Movement Transfer in Vitro

The mechanical coupling between calcaneal and tibial movement can be studied by mounting a cadaveric foot-leg specimen in a 6-DOF fixture (Allinger & Engsberg 1993; Hintermann & Nigg 1994), inserting bone pins with markers into the calcaneus and the tibia, and quantifying the movement of calcaneus and tibia kinematically. The relationship between calcaneal and tibial movement using movement of the calcaneus as input and movement of the tibia as output is illustrated in figure 3.2.

The initial calcaneal inversion of about 20° resulted in an external tibial rotation of about 5°. The maximal calcaneal inversion of about 32° resulted in an external tibial rotation of about 14°. The transfer in the initial phase corresponded to about 25%, and the transfer in the final inversion movement (27 to 32°) corresponded to a transfer of about 100%. The return of the foot to the neutral position followed a different tibial rotation-inversion path than the onset of the inversion movement. The subsequent eversion movement of the calcaneus produced an internal rotation of the tibia. The transfer for this part of the movement corresponds to about 18%. The cutting of the anterior talofibular and the calcaneofibular ligaments changes the transfer mechanism.

Based on both the results illustrated in figure 3.2 and previously published results (Hintermann & Nigg 1994; Hintermann, Nigg, & Cole 1994; Hintermann, Nigg, & Sommer 1994), one must conclude that the

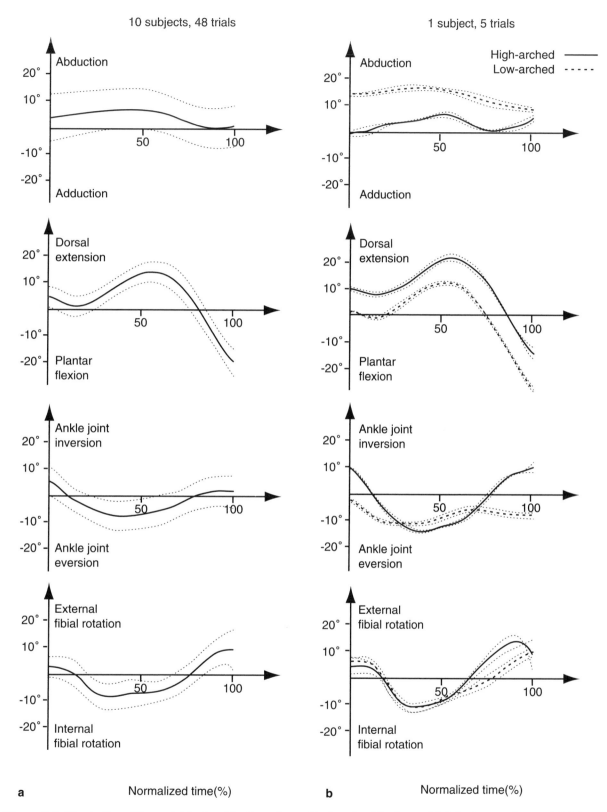

■ **Figure 3.1** Illustration of the variable ab-adduction, plantarflexion-dorsiflexion, ankle joint in-eversion, and tibial rotation during ground contact for running toe-heel with a running speed of 4 m/s. *(a)* is the mean and standard deviation for 10 subjects (48 trials) and *(b)* is for one subject (5 trials). The illustration for one subject *(b)* indicates the rather substantial variability that a single subject-shoe combination may produce.

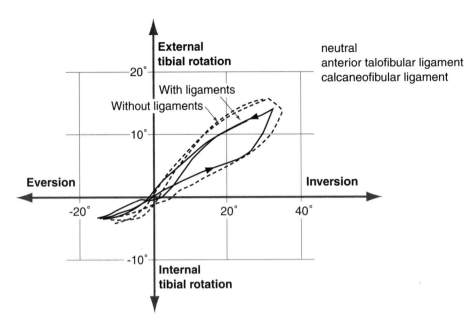

■ Figure 3.2 Movement transfer between calcaneus and tibia for one cadaveric foot-leg specimen with and without intact ligaments mounted in a 6-DOF fixture with calcaneal in-eversion as input and tibial rotation as output. The curve without ligaments illustrates the increased laxity of the AJC.

transfer of movement from calcaneus to tibia is not constant. It depends on various factors, such as the type of the input movement, the plantarflexion-dorsiflexion position of the foot (Hintermann & Nigg 1994; Hintermann, Nigg, & Sommer 1994), the loading of the AJC (Hintermann & Nigg 1994), the fusion of selected joints (Hintermann, Nigg, & Cole 1994), and the integrity of the ligaments (Hintermann & Nigg 1994; Hintermann, Nigg, & Sommer 1994). Consequently, the talocrural (ankle) and the talocalcaneal (subtalar) joints are not universal joints as had been suggested earlier (Inman 1976; Stauffer et al. 1977).

Movement Transfer in Vivo

The quantification of the mechanical coupling of calcaneus and tibia is technically much more difficult in vivo than in vitro. Markers must be placed at the skin of the heel or at the heel of the shoe and on the skin of the leg, and movement of the skin markers relative to the bone is possible. Several techniques are currently being developed and should be available clinically in the near future. The following examples stress the basic possibilities rather than the measuring technique. An illustration of a movement transfer characteristic (in-eversion vs tibial rotation characteristic) is illustrated in figure 3.3.

The illustrated curve is typical for the movement analyzed, the footwear, and the anatomical specifics of the tested subject. Changes in one of these parameters, for instance changes in footwear, will change

the characteristics of the curve. Such analyses, therefore, have potential use in assessments of the appropriateness of an intervention.

It is, for instance, possible to assess whether a foot orthotic changes the maximal eversion of the rearfoot or the transfer of movement from the calcaneus to the tibia. Depending on the problem at hand, interventions can be assessed and accepted or rejected. Consequently, this approach allows one to understand functional connections in the lower extremities.

■ Forces

Whenever the foot is in contact with the ground, forces act from the ground onto the foot and vice versa. These forces are called **ground reaction forces**. Ground reaction forces are resultant forces that correspond to the movement of the center of mass and gravity. Ground reaction forces are typically subdivided into **impact** and **active forces**. Examples of the magnitude of external forces, summarized in table 3.2, illustrate that ground reaction forces are different for various activities and can easily exceed several times body weight.

Typical ground reaction force components for heel-toe running are illustrated in figure 3.4 for a group of subjects and for one individual.

The external forces acting on the human foot, the geometrical alignment of the foot and the leg, the muscle forces, and the segmental inertia forces are

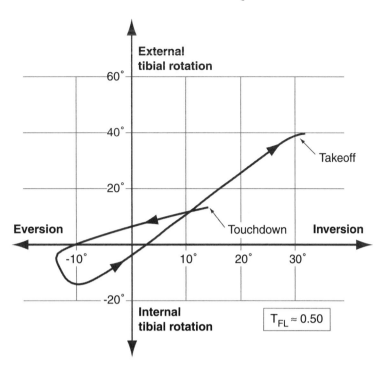

■ **Figure 3.3** Illustration of an ankle joint movement transfer characteristic for one subject running heel-toe barefoot (mean for 6 trials). The subject has medium arch height and a third degree sprain. The transfer coefficient (T_{FL}) describes the percentage of movement that is transferred from one segment to another segment. A transfer coefficient of 0.50, for instance, indicates that 50% of the movement is transferred.

Table 3.2 Summary of the Magnitude of External and Internal Forces of the Ankle Joint Complex in the Unit Body Weight (BW) From Different Sources

Type	Location	Magnitude [BW]	Description of activity
External	Heel	0.55	Impact forces during heel strike while walking barefoot
	Heel	0.37	Impact forces during heel strike while walking in army boots
	Heel	0.27	Impact forces during heel strike while walking in street shoes
	Forefoot	~1	Active forces during take-off in walking
	Heel	1-4	Impact forces during heel strike in heel-toe running for running speeds between 3 to 6 m/s
	Forefoot	3	Active forces during take-off in running at about 3 to 6 m/s
Internal	Ankle joint	1	Standing on one leg
	Ankle joint	0	Heel strike for walking and heel-toe running
Running	Ankle joint	2-5	Stand phase and take-off in walking
	Ankle joint	3-8	Stand phase and take-off for jogging
	Ankle joint	5-10	Take-off in sprinting

responsible for the internal forces acting in joints, ligaments, and tendons. Mathematical models are used to estimate the magnitude of forces in internal structures such as joints, tendons, and ligaments. These estimations use several (sometimes different) assumptions, which are still being discussed. However, the order of magnitude of the estimated forces is assumed to be correct.

Typically, the geometry of the acting forces (i.e., the distance of the line of action of an acting force to

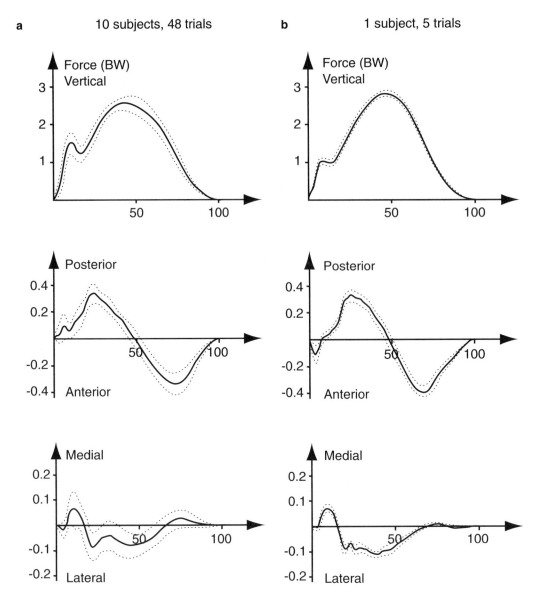

■ **Figure 3.4** Mean and standard deviation of ground reaction force components for heel-toe running for *(a)* 10 subjects and *(b)* one subject, illustrating the typical mean values and also possibilities deviating substantially from the "typical" mean curves.

a joint of interest) is the most important factor that determines the internal forces.

Ground reaction forces are resultant forces that are determined by the movement of the various segments involved in the locomotion process. They are integral quantities and are limited in providing information on local phenomena, especially on phenomena specific for the foot. Ground reaction forces for high-arched and flat-footed people can easily look similar. Pressure distribution sensors are useful in providing more local information. A pressure distribution sensor is a summation of many hundreds of small force plates, which measure the force perpendicular to the surface (Cavanagh

et al. 1983; Hennig et al. 1981; Nicol & Hennig 1976).

Pressure distribution sensors are often used in the form of insoles to assess foot-specific problems. In addition to the direct measurement of pressure distribution in footwear, pressure distribution sensors have been used to estimate internal forces in the anatomical structures of the human foot (Cole et al. 1995; van den Bogert et al. 1994). Results from pressure distribution measurements have been used as localized input into the different foot structures, making it possible to quantify internal forces in joints, ligaments, and tendons of the foot, an estimation which cannot be made using the ground reaction force as force input.

■ Shoes

The literature on the biomechanics of shoes includes a substantial majority of reports concentrating primarily on sport shoes, specifically running shoes. However, some of the general findings may find applications in everyday situations. The most important findings that have general significance are the following:

1. Impact forces

   ■ Impact forces in structures of the lower extremities (internal impact forces) during activities such as walking and running are much smaller than internal active forces (Scott & Winter 1990; Cole et al. 1995).

   ■ Epidemiological evidence of a possible association between external or internal impact forces during walking and running and related injuries is not conclusive. Some sources speculate that impact forces are associated with the development of injuries. Others speculate that they are not.

   ■ It has been proposed that impact forces may be related more to comfort than to injuries (Cole et al. 1995). It may be possible that "good cushioning" influences energy and fatigue in locomotion.

2. Ankle joint eversion

   ■ Excessive ankle joint eversion has been typically associated with the development of overuse injuries in locomotion (Clancy 1982; Clement et al. 1981; Leach 1982). Subjects with injuries typically have a foot eversion movement that is about 2° to 4° bigger than that of subjects with no injuries. However, between 40% and 50% of runners with excessive ankle joint eversion do not have overuse injuries (Hintermann & Nigg 1994; Nigg et al. 1993; Bahlsen 1988). It has been suggested that a combination of excessive ankle joint eversion and a high movement transfer of foot eversion into internal tibial rotation is a better predictor for the development of (especially knee) overuse injuries (Hintermann & Nigg 1994; Nigg et al. 1993; Bahlsen 1988).

   ■ It has been proposed that the movement transfer between foot eversion and tibial rotation is small for subjects with low arches and high for subjects with high arches (Nigg et al. 1993). Consequently, subjects with high arches are more susceptible to overuse injuries than subjects with low arches if they show excessive ankle joint eversion.

   ■ Ankle joint eversion is strongly influenced by the shoe. Differences in ankle joint eversion for a subject using different running shoes are substantial. It is easily possible that the maximal ankle joint eversion movement is 31° for one running shoe and 12° for another running shoe (Nigg et al. 1986) (figure 3.5).

   ■ A medial support in a shoe may provide increased stability to the foot and leg and may reduce the maximal ankle joint eversion. However, it may at the same time increase the internal rotation of the tibia. It is assumed that this change is associated with an increased inclination of the subtalar joint axis (Nigg et al. 1993).

3. Torsion

   ■ Without shoes, the foot has the natural ability to allow for a torsional motion between the rear- and the forefoot. Shoes often have a torsional stiffness that is too high, and don't allow this movement. It is proposed that a low torsional stiffness is advantageous, especially for movements with landing on the forefoot, as are typical in volleyball or basketball (Stacoff et al. 1989; Stussi & Stacoff 1993).

4. Shoe inserts and arch supports

   ■ Shoe inserts and foot arch supports are often used successfully in treatment and prevention of occupational and sports injuries. They are used to limit the overuse of foot structures, to increase foot-leg stability, and to change foot function. The application of these aids is typically based on the expertise of the orthotist and podiatrist, and many problems are successfully treated employing these strategies. However, in most applications the mechanical functioning of such orthoses is not well understood, and further

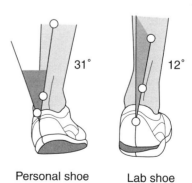

Personal shoe   Lab shoe

■ **Figure 3.5** Illustration of a shoe-induced difference in maximal ankle joint eversion for two subjects running heel-toe at 4 m/s with two different pairs of running shoes, a "personal shoe" and a "lab shoe."

research is needed to improve the functional-mechanical understanding of such orthoses.

■ References

Allinger TL, Engsberg JR. 1993. A method to determine the range of motion of the ankle joint complex in vivo. J Biomech 26:69-76.

Areblad M, Nigg BM, Ekstrand J, Olsson KO, Edström H. 1990. Three-dimensional measurement of rearfoot motion during running. J Biomech 23:933-940.

Bahlsen A. 1988. The etiology of running injuries: a longitudinal prospective study. PhD thesis. Calgary, Canada: The University of Calgary.

Cavanagh PR, Hennig EM, Bunch RP, Macmillian NH. 1983. A new device for the measurement of pressure distribution inside the shoe. In Matsui, H. and Kobayashi, K, editors. Biomechanics VIII-B. Champaign, IL: Human Kinetics, p. 1089-1096.

Clancy WG. 1982. Tendonitis and plantar fasciitis in runners. In: d'Ambrosia R, Drez D, editors. Prevention and treatment of running injuries. Thorofare, NJ: Slack Inc., p. 77-87.

Clement DB, Taunton JE, Smart GW, McNicol KL. 1981. A survey of overuse injuries. Physician and Sportsmedicine 9:47-58.

Cole GK, Nigg BM, Fick GH, Morlock MM. 1995. Internal loading of the foot and ankle during impact in running. J Appl Biomech 11:25-46.

Cole GK, Nigg BM, Ronsky JL, Yeadon MR. 1993. Application of the joint coordinate system to three-dimensional joint attitude and movement representation: A standardization proposal. J Biomech Eng 115:344-349.

Eberhart HD, Inman VT, Bressler B. 1968. The principal elements in human locomotion. In Klopsteg PE, Wilson PD, editors. Human limbs and their substitutes. New York: Hafner Publishing, p. 437-471.

Engsberg JR. 1987. A biomechanical analysis of the talocalcaneal joint in vitro. J Biomech 20:429-442.

Frederick EC, Hagy JL, Mann R. 1981. A prediction of vertical impact forces during running. J Biomech 14:498.

Grood ES, Suntay WJ. 1933. A joint coordinate system for the clinical description of three-dimensional motions: Application to the knee. J Biomech Eng 105:136-144.

Hennig EM, Cavanagh PR, Albert HT, Macmillian NH. 1981. A piezo-electric method of measuring the vertical contact stress beneath the human foot. J Biomed Eng 4:213-222.

Hintermann B, Nigg BM. 1994. Die Bewegungsubertragung zwischen Fuss und Unterschenkel in vitro (movement transfer between foot and leg in vitro). Sportverletwng-Sportschaden 2:60-66.

Hintermann B, Nigg BM, Cole GK. 1994. Influence of selective arthrodesis on the movement transfer between calcaneus and tibia in vitro. Clin Biomech 9(6):356-361.

Hintermann B, Nigg BM, Sommer C. 1994. Foot movement and tendon excursion: An in vitro study. Foot and Ankle 15:386-395.

Inman VT. 1976. The joints of the ankle. Baltimore: Williams & Wilkins.

Leach R. 1982. Running injuries of the knee. In d'Ambrosia R, Drez D, editors. Prevention and treatment of running injuries. Thorofare, NJ: Slack Inc., p. 55-75.

Mann RA. 1982. Biomechanics of running. In Mack RP, editor. Symposium on the foot and leg in running sports. St. Louis: Mosby. p. 1-29.

Murray MP, Drought AB, Kory RC. 1964. Walking pattern of normal men. J Bone Joint Surg Am 46:335-360.

Nicol K, Hennig EM. 1976. Time dependent method for measuring force distribution using a flexible mat as a capacitor. In Komi PV, editor. Biomechanics V-B. Baltimore, MD: University Park Press, p. 433-440.

Nigg BM. 1994. Force. In Nigg BM, Herzog W, editors. Biomechanics of the musculo-skeletal system. Chichester, UK: Wiley and Sons, p. 200-224.

Nigg BM, Bahlsen AH, Denoth J, Luthi, SM, Stacoff A. 1986. Factors influencing kinetic and kinematic variables in running. In Nigg BM, editor. Biomechanics of running shoes. Champaign, IL: Human Kinetics, p. 139-159.

Nigg BM, Cole GK. 1994. Optical methods. In Nigg BM, Herzog W, editors. Biomechanics of the musculo-skeletal system. Chichester, UK: Wiley and Sons, p. 254-286.

Nigg BM, Cole GK, Nachbauer W. 1993. Effects of arch height of the foot on angular motion of the lower extremities in running. J Biomech 26:909-916.

Perry, J. 1992. Gait analysis: normal and pathological function. Thorofare, NJ: Slack, Inc.

Scott SH, Winter DA. 1990. Internal forces at chronic running sites. Med Sci Sports Exerc 22:357-369.

Stacoff A, Kalin X, Stussi E, Segesser B. 1989. The torsion of the foot in running. Int J Sports Biomech 5:375-389.

Stauffer JE, Chao EY, Brewster RC. 1977. Force and motion analysis of the normal, diseased and prosthetic ankle joint. Clin Orthop 127:189-196.

Stussi E, Stacoff, A. 1993. Biomechanische und orthopadische Probleme des Tennis-und Hallenschuh (biomechanical and orthopaedic problems in tennis and indoor shoes). Sportverletzung-Sportschaden 7:187-190.

van den Bogert AJ, Smith GD, Nigg BM. 1994. In vivo determination of the anatomical axes of the ankle joint complex: An optimization approach. J Biomech 27(12): 1477-1488.

Winter DA, Quanbury AO, Hobson DA, Sidwall HG, Reimer G, Trenholm BC, Steinkle T, Shiosser H. 1974. Kinematics of normal locomotion: a statistical study based on TV data. J Biomech 6:479-486.

Chapter 4

Biomechanics of Ligaments in Ankle Instability

Beat Hintermann, MD

Fundamental information about the mechanical characteristics of the ankle ligaments may contribute to a better understanding of the normal function of the ankle ligaments, the pathomechanics of injury and resulting ankle instability, and the optimal treatment of injured ankle ligaments. In the first part of this chapter, basic data on the structure and biomechanics of ligaments are reviewed, and mechanisms of injury to the ligaments and their repair response are discussed. In the second part, biomechanical data relevant to the function of the ankle ligaments in relation to joint stability and joint mechanics are reviewed, and mechanisms of injury to the ankle ligaments and their pathomechanical response to the ankle joint complex are discussed.

■ Morphological Aspects of Ligaments, Ligament Injury, and Ligament Healing

The collateral ligaments of the ankle have characteristic morphology and structure that explain their response to loading as well as the injury pattern when they become acutely overloaded. Knowledge of their morphology and structure may help one to understand the healing response to injury and treatment.

Structure of Ligaments

Mature adult ligaments are composed of large diameter type I collagen fibrils (>150 nm in diameter) tightly packed together with a small amount of type III collagen and dispersed in an aqueous gel containing small amounts of proteoglycan and elastic fibers. The outstanding feature of these unique load-bearing tissues is the collagen "crimp," which is a planar wave pattern found extending in phase across the width of

all ligaments. The crimp appears to be built into the tertiary structure of the collagen molecule and is probably maintained in vivo by inter- and intramolecular collagen cross-links as well as by a strategically placed elastic fiber network.

Mechanical Properties of Ligaments

Various factors that may affect the mechanical properties of ligaments have been studied in detail. Some of the most consistent results of these studies indicate that

- older, diseased, or immobilized ligaments demonstrate increased linear stiffness and modulus of elasticity, decreased ultimate load and strain, and higher frequency of bone avulsion failures compared to ligament tears (Siegler et al. 1988);
- freezing and thawing do not significantly alter the mechanical properties of the ligaments (Siegler et al. 1988);
- the mechanical properties of ligaments are insensitive to a wide range of temperatures (23-45°C) (Dorlot et al. 1980); and
- testing at low strain results in a higher frequency of bone avulsion failures, whereas testing at high strain rates results in a higher frequency of ligament tears (Siegler et al. 1988).

Ligament Trauma

Ligament injury can be closely correlated with the load-deformation curve (Butler et al. 1983; Oakes 1981). The load-strain curve can be divided into three regions (figure 4.1):

- **Toe region:** The "toe" or initial concave region represents the normal physiological range of ligament strain up to about 3% to 4% of initial length and

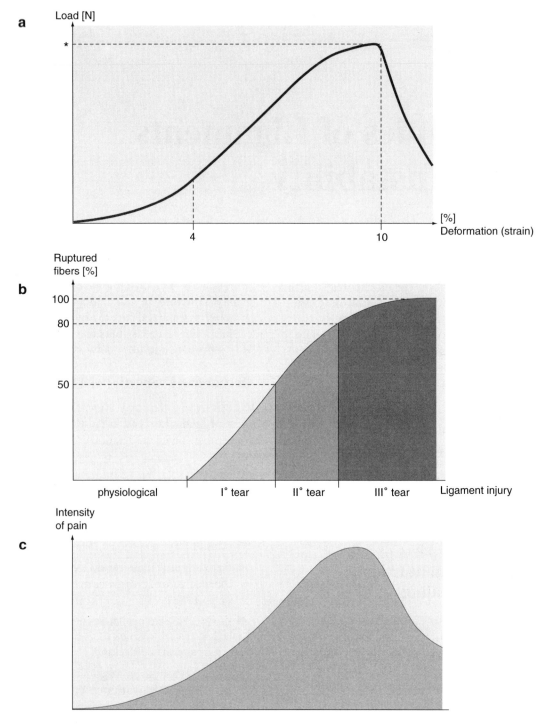

■ **Figure 4.1** *(a)* The load-deformation (strain) curve for ligaments, *(b)* the clinical correlation with the grading of the injury, and *(c)* the pain. Note the "toe" region of the curve is entirely within the normal physiological range and that greater than approximately 4% strain causes tissue damage (* indicates load to failure [strength] of the ankle ligament: ATFL, 130 ± 50 N, PTFL 260 ± 50 N, CFL 325 ± 60 N, and Ldelt 240 ± 70 N).

is due to flattening of the collagen crimp. Repeated cycling within the toe region or physiological strain in the range of 3% to 4% can normally occur without irreversible macroscopic or molecular damage to the tissue.

■ **Linear region:** The second part of the load-deformation curve is the linear region, where pathological irreversible ligament elongation occurs as a result of partial rupture of intermolecular cross-links. As the load is increased further, intra- and intermolecular cross-links are disrupted until macroscopic failure is clinically evident. The early part of the linear region corresponds to mild or grade I ligament tears (0-50% fiber disruption), and the second part corresponds to grade II tears (50-80% fiber disruption), where there is obvious clinical laxity on stress testing.

■ **Rupture region:** In the third region the curve flattens and the yield of failure point is reached at 10% to 20% strain depending on the macro-organization of the ligament fiber bundle. In this region, complete ligament rupture occurs at the maximum breaking load; this is the dangerous grade III ligament rupture on clinical testing.

There is always some pain associated with grade I and II injuries after the initial trauma, and an athlete with a grade II injury usually cannot continue sport. Because complete ligament rupture occurs in grade III injuries, pain usually decreases. Thus, although the severity of pain provides a rough guide to the clinical severity of degree I and II injuries, pain may not correspond to the severity of ligament injury in grade III injuries (figure 4.1).

Ligament Healing

In the first few days following injury, vascular granulation tissue proliferates through hemorrhagic tissues. This is followed by progressive fibrosis for 2 to 3 weeks. At about 1 month, scar formation and maturation begins. Contraction and remodeling of this scar is sufficiently advanced at 6 weeks for some to note "complete healing" (Frank, Schachar et al. 1983). However, months or years may be required to approach normality. Tensile tests of healing ligaments suggest that the return to normal strength and elastic stiffness in ligaments is slow (Frank, Woo et al. 1983). The rate of return to normal of structural and mechanical properties in a healing ligament is probably dependent on stress and may therefore be controlled to some extent by levels of physical activity (Cabaud et al. 1980; Clayton et al. 1968; Vailas et al. 1981).

With surgical repair, there may be alterations in the healing process. There is evidence of an early improvement in biomechanical properties of repaired ligaments compared to nonrepaired ligaments (Clayton et al. 1968; Clayton & Weir 1959; O'Donoghue et al. 1961). This advantage, however, may not be sustained, as after one year, sutured and unsutured ligaments have nearly equal length when measured at rest, and have comparable failure strength when subjected to exercise (Clayton et al. 1968; Frank, Woo et al. 1983; Woo et al. 1987).

Because each structure has an anticipated healing time, one cannot accelerate the normal recuperative abilities of the tissues. Therefore therapy is aimed at optimizing healing conditions. With extra-articular collagenous structures, ligamentous strength after tearing is in the region of 60% to 70% of normal 6 weeks after injury. More specifically, there is often a revascularization phase during healing that is usually accompanied by a dramatic reduction of tensile strength. It requires considerable knowledge and skill to balance exercise progression with protection of the vulnerable tissue. It may take up to 3 months before 80% of the original strength is acquired. Although little is known of the effects of ligament tears on the neural protective mechanism of joints, it is likely that after significant tears there is distorted or decreased biofeedback. This may particularly be true for the major weightbearing joints, such as the knee and the ankle.

■ Mechanical Characteristics of the Ankle Ligaments

The ankle joint and its surrounding ligaments represent a complex mechanical structure whose mechanical properties have received only limited attention. The ligaments that have been studied most extensively include the ligaments of the knee in animals (Alm et al. 1974; Butler et al. 1983; Dorlot et al. 1980; Hefti et al. 1991; Kennedy et al. 1976; Nigg et al. 1991; Noyes et al. 1974), the cruciate ligaments of the knee in humans (Noyes et al. 1974), and the human intervertebral ligaments (Nachemson & Evans 1968; Tencer et al. 1982; Tkaczuk 1968). The information available about the collateral ligaments in the human ankle, however, appears to be limited, including data on the mechanical properties of the anterior talofibular ligament (Attarian et al. 1985; Colville et al. 1990; Nigg et al. 1991; Renström et al. 1988; St. Pierre et al. 1983; Siegler et al. 1988), the calcaneofibular ligament (Attarian et al. 1985; Colville et al. 1990; Nigg et al. 1991; Renström et al. 1988; Siegler et al. 1988), the posterior talofibular ligament (Attarian et al. 1985; Colville et al. 1990; Nigg et al. 1991; Siegler et al. 1988), and the deltoid ligament (Nigg et al. 1991; Rasmussen et al. 1983; Siegler et al. 1988).

Anatomical Aspects

Table 4.1 lists the length, width, and thickness of the ankle ligaments. Further anatomical characteristics are discussed.

■ **The anterior talofibular ligament.** The anterior talofibular ligament, which blends with the anterior capsule of the ankle, spans the anterior lateral ankle joint. The ligament originates at the distal anterior tip of the fibula and inserts on the body of the talus just anterior to the articular facet.

Table 4.1 Morphology of the Ankle Ligaments (mm)

	ATFL	PTFL	CFL	Ldelt
Length	15-20	30	20-30	10-45
Width	6-8	5	4-8	5-16
Thickness	2	5-8	3-5	2-10

■ **The posterior talofibular ligament.** The posterior talofibular ligament takes origin from the medial surface of the lateral malleolus and courses medially in a horizontal fashion to the posterior aspect of the talus. The ligament is confluent with the joint capsule and is well vascularized by vessels going to the talus and the fibula via the digital fossa (Sarrafian 1994).

■ **The calcaneofibular ligament.** The calcaneofibular ligament originates from the anterior border of the distal lateral malleolus just below the origin of the anterior talofibular ligament. Contrary to popular belief, it does not originate from the apex of the tip of the lateral malleolus. The ligament courses medially, posteriorly, and inferiorly from its fibular origin to the calcaneal insertion. The calcaneofibular ligament effectively spans the ankle and subtalar joints, which have markedly different axes of rotation (Close 1956; Hintermann et al. 1994; Inman 1991; Manter 1941). Thus, this ligament must be attached such that it does not restrict motion in either joint, whether the joints move independently or simultaneously. When projected onto the sagittal plane of the subtalar joint axis, the ligament parallels this axis. When projected onto a vertical transverse plane, the ligament diverges from the subtalar axis at an acute angle (Inman 1991). The angle between the calcaneofibular ligament and anterior talofibular ligament was measured on 50 cadavers. In the sagittal plane, the average angle was 105° and varied from 70 to 140°. In the coronal plane the average angle was 100° and varied from 60 to 140° (Inman 1991).

■ **The deltoid ligament.** Wide variations have been noted in the anatomic description of the deltoid ligament. This ligament is divided into four parts. The tibiocalcaneal ligament constitutes the superficial layer of the deltoid and spans the medial malleolus to the medial aspect of the calcaneus. The other three divisions, the anterior tibiotalar ligament, intermediate tibiotalar ligament, and posterior tibiotalar ligament, attach the medial malleolus to the talus. Although the tibiocalcaneal ligament is very thin and supports only negligible forces prior to failing, the tibiotalar ligaments are very strong (Siegler et al. 1988).

Stabilizing Function

Each of the collateral ligaments has a characteristic role in stabilizing the ankle and subtalar joint, depending on the position of the foot.

Lateral Ligaments of the Ankle

Each of the lateral ligaments has a role in stabilizing the ankle or subtalar joint, depending on the position of the foot. In dorsiflexion, the posterior talofibular ligament is maximally stressed and the calcaneofibular ligament is taut, while the anterior talofibular ligament is loose. In plantarflexion, the anterior talofibular ligament is taut, and the calcaneofibular and posterior talofibular ligaments become loose (Colville et al. 1990; Renström et al. 1988; Sarrafian 1994). Some variation to this is allowed by the different patterns of divergence between the anterior talofibular and calcaneofibular ligaments.

It has to be emphasized that the calcaneofibular ligament retains its parallel to the axis of the subtalar joint as the ankle passes from plantarflexion to dorsiflexion. In plantarflexion, both the ligament and the subtalar joint axis become horizontal, while in dorsiflexion, they approach a more vertical position. Thus, in dorsiflexion, the calcaneofibular ligament can act as a true collateral ligament and prevent talar tilt. As the ankle joint passes from dorsiflexion to plantarflexion, the calcaneofibular ligament is less able to resist talar tilt, and reciprocally, the anterior talofibular ligament is more able to resist talar tilt.

Sequential sectioning of the lateral ligaments has demonstrated the function of these ligaments in different positions and under various loading conditions. Johnson and Markolf (1993) studied the laxity after sectioning the anterior talofibular ligament and found the most changes to occur in plantarflexion. They found a smaller change in laxity in dorsiflexion, suggesting that the anterior talofibular ligament limits talar tilt throughout motion but has the greatest advantage in plantarflexion. Rasmussen and Tovberg-Jensen (1982) further confirmed these findings, stating that talar tilt is limited in plantarflexion and in the neutral position by the anterior talofibular ligament, and in dorsiflexion by the calcaneofibular ligament plus the posterior talofibular ligament.

The cutting studies of Kjaersgaard-Andersen et al. (Kjaersgaard-Andersen, Wethelund, & Helmig 1987; Kjaersgaard-Andersen, Wethelund, & Nielsen 1987) showed a 20% increase in rotation of the subtalar (talocalcaneal) joint and a 61% to 77% increase in talocalcaneal adduction after release of the calcaneofibular ligament. Heilman et al. (1990) performed a similar cutting study with sequential release of the calcaneofibular ligament, the lateral capsule, and the interosseous talocalcaneal ligament. They documented a 5-mm opening between the posterior facets of the talus and calcaneus with a stress radiograph after the calcaneofibular ligament was released and an increase of 7 mm when sectioning of the talocalcaneal ligament was added.

Deltoid Ligament

Close (1956) found the deltoid ligament to be a strong restraint limiting talar abduction. With all lateral structures removed, he found that the intact deltoid ligament allowed only 2 mm of separation between the talus and medial malleolus. When the deep deltoid ligament was released, the talus could be separated from the medial malleolus by a distance of 3.7 mm. Grath (1960) confirmed these findings in a similar experiment. Rasmussen et al. (Rasmussen 1985; Rasmussen & Tovberg-Jensen 1982) investigated the function of various parts of the deltoid ligament and stated that the tibiocalcaneal ligament or "superficial" deltoid ligament specifically limited talar abduction or negative talar tilt. On the other hand, the deep layers of the deltoid ligament ruptured by external rotation of the leg without the superficial portion being involved.

Kinematics of Ankle Instability

Motion between the tibia and the foot is a complex combination of ankle and subtalar motion limited by osseous shape and soft tissue interaction (Anderson & Lecocq 1956; Inman 1991; Renström et al. 1988) (figure 4.2). It has been recognized that ankle motion does not occur about one axis alone (Barnett & Napier 1952; Hicks 1953; Hintermann et al. 1994; Lundberg 1989). Rather, ankle motion combines dorsiflexion and plantarflexion with slight internal and external rotation and some anterior/posterior translation of the talus on the tibia (Close 1956; Hicks 1953; Hintermann

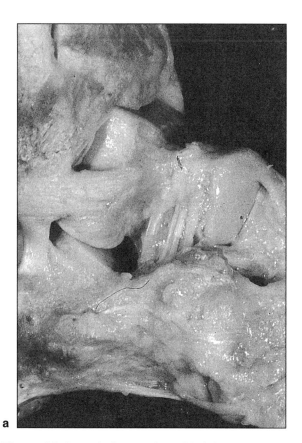
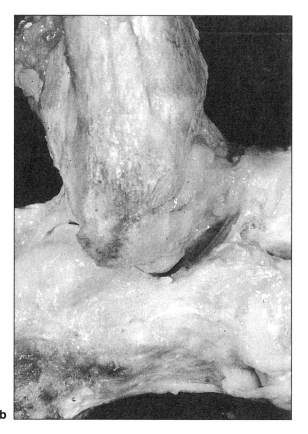

a   b

■ **Figure 4.2** Lateral view on the ankle joint complex in *(a)* supination and *(b)* pronation position showing the complex combination of ankle and subtalar motion..

et al. 1994; Lundberg 1989). Many studies have tried to elucidate how the ligaments contribute to this functional interplay with the bone structures (Cass & Settles 1994; Fraser & Ahmed 1983; McCullough & Burge 1980; Michelson et al. 1990; Nigg et al. 1993; Parlasca et al. 1979; Stormont et al. 1985). However, most reports have focused on the lateral ligaments and the role they play in maintaining lateral ankle stability (Boruta et al. 1990; Larsen 1986; Laurin et al. 1995; Rasmussen 1985; Renström et al. 1988) (figure 4.3). Some have tried to determine the amount of tilting that occurs after selective release of the anterior talofibular, calcaneofibular, posterior talofibular, and deltoid ligaments (Cass & Settles 1994; Larsen 1986; Laurin et al. 1995; Stormont et al. 1985). Although the magnitude of tilt has been shown to vary significantly (Cass & Settles 1994; Rasmussen 1985), there is a consensus that some tilt occurs with the loss of these ligaments (Boruta et al. 1990; Larsen 1986; Renström et al. 1988). These measurements of talar tilt, however, do not provide information about the rotational instability that is created by the ligament release. Thus, despite the vast amount of literature (Boruta et al. 1990; Cass et al. 1984; Cass & Settles 1994; Peters et al. 1991), the debate continues over the instability being one of tilting the talus in the mortise, or one of axial rotation, or both.

Coupling Mechanism Between Foot and Leg

Hintermann et al. (1995) studied, in vitro, the role of the ankle ligaments in the coupling mechanism between foot and leg, especially in transferring movement between calcaneal and tibial rotation. They found that transection of the lateral ligaments did not significantly affect the tibial rotation and foot eversion-inversion for a given dorsi-plantarflexion. Further cutting of the deltoid ligament, however, highly changed the movement transfer, especially during plantarflexion. From this, the authors concluded that the transfer mechanism at the ankle joint complex does depend markedly on the integrity of the deltoid ligament (Hintermann et al. 1995). One explanation may relate to the inconstant axis of rotation of the talus in the mortise, as the talus rotates about a variable axis in all three planes as a result of the trochlea having a conical rather than cylindrical shape (Barnett & Napier 1952; Hicks 1953; Inman 1991; Sammarco 1977). It could be that the rotation of the talus with respect to the tibia depends significantly on the integrity of the deltoid ligament. The strong del-

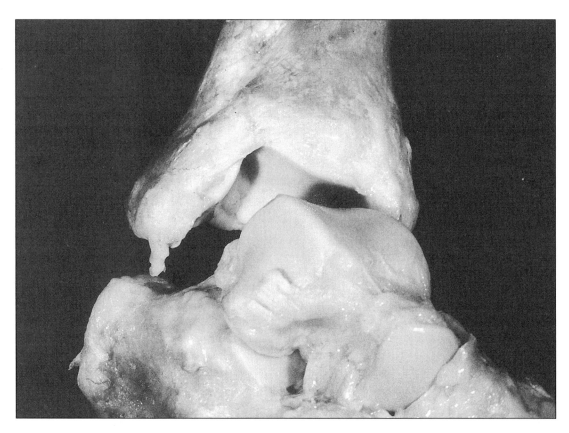

■ **Figure 4.3** Anterolateral view on the unstable ankle after release of the lateral ligaments (ATFL, PTFL, CFL, and Ldelt), analogous to table 4.1.

toid ligament, therefore, may not be only an important stabilizer of the medial side (Close 1956), but may also be a crucial structure in the movement transfer of the ankle joint complex.

Rotational Stability

Fraser and Ahmed (1983) studied the passive rotational stability of the loaded ankle and found that with increasing load, rotation decreased. McCullough and Burge (1980) looked at the internal/external rotation of the ankle with application of an axial load. They also found that increasing the axial load decreased the axial rotation in both conditions, that of the ankle with intact ligaments as well as that of the ankle after ligament release. Stormont et al. (1985) evaluated the effects of lateral ligament sectioning in a preloaded model and found that the articular surfaces supplied 30% of the stability in rotation and 100% of the stability in inversion testing. However, in the two latter studies, rotation was allowed only about one axis: either leg rotation was allowed and eversion/inversion was constrained, or vice versa. The data from these two studies should, therefore, be cautiously applied to the in vivo situation of ankle instability. This becomes more evident, as one considers Inman's (1991) emphasis that both ankle and subtalar motion required rotation about all three reference axes, and Laurin et al.'s (1995) statement that if external rotation is restricted, talar tilt will likewise be limited.

Cass and Settles (1994) studied the kinematics of ankle instability after lateral ligament sectioning in a model in which axial rotation was not constrained. They found no tilting of the talus in the mortise to occur with isolated release of the anterior talofibular or calcaneofibular ligament. After both ligaments were released, an average talar tilt of 20.6° occurred. External rotation of the leg occurred with inversion averaging 11.1° in the intact specimen. The leg averaged a further external rotation of 4.9° after anterior talofibular ligament release and 12.8° further than the intact inverted specimen when the calcaneofibular ligament had also been released. The authors concluded that the anterior talofibular and calcaneofibular ligaments work in tandem to prevent tilting of the talus, and that the articular surfaces do not seem to prevent tilting of the talus in the mortise.

Obviously, talar tilt does occur with inversion, even in the presence of an axial load (Cass & Settles 1994; Lundberg 1989). Inversion is accompanied by a mandatory external rotation of the leg (Hintermann et al. 1994; Inman 1991; Laurin et al. 1995; Lundberg 1989). In the intact specimen, this external rotation occurs at the subtalar joint (Cass & Settles 1994; Lundberg 1989). After loss of ligamentous support,

the external rotation increases, but not at the subtalar joint (Cass & Settles 1994; Hintermann et al. 1995). Rather, this increase occurs between the tibia and the talus. One may thus speculate that ankle instability in at least one form is an axial rotational quality.

This rotational concept may be used to explain why symptoms of ankle instability occur in the absence of radiographically demonstrable talar tilt. Another factor that may be taken into account is the role of the subtalar joint in ankle instability (Clanton 1989).

Hintermann et al. (1995) studied the effect of selective ligament release on calcaneal and tibial rotation when the foot was axially loaded. When loading the foot by 600 N, they found an average 0.6° of calcaneal eversion and an average 3.8° of internal rotation to occur in the intact specimen. The calcaneus averaged a further eversion of 2.3° and the tibia averaged a further internal rotation of 2.3° after anterior talofibular ligament release. There was no further calcaneal eversion or further internal tibial rotation noted when the calcaneofibular ligament had also been released. Obviously, under axial load, the talus rotated internally and plantarflected while the talar head glided medially and distally. The authors concluded that the anterior talofibular ligament essentially stabilizes the talus in the ankle mortise.

■ Conclusions and Clinical Implications

There is general agreement that motion between the tibia and the foot is a complex combination of ankle and subtalar joint motion limited by osseous shape and soft tissue interaction. How the ligaments contribute to this functional interplay with the bone structures, however, is still not clarified in detail. Recent in vitro studies have supported the hypothesis that, in addition to maintaining lateral ankle stability, the lateral ankle ligaments play a significant role in maintaining rotational ankle stability. It has been shown that loss of the anterior talofibular or calcaneofibular ligaments leads to a measurable increase in inversion without any tilting of the talus or subtalar gapping. It has also been shown that loss of the anterior talofibular ligament does allow an increase in external rotation of the leg to occur. The loss of anterior talofibular restraint, in fact, unlocks the subtalar joint, allowing further inversion. It is this increase in inversion that may lead to symptomatic instability. Under this hypothesis, no tilting is necessary at either ankle or subtalar levels to prove functional instability.

These rotational concepts may explain why repair of the anterior talofibular ligament alone can provide successful clinical results for treatment of ankle instability (Broström 1966). It may also explain why reconstructions that simply tenodese the fifth metatarsal to the fibula, thereby preventing external rotation, cure ankle instability (Cass et al. 1985). Most of the common tenodesis procedures (Chrisman & Snook 1969; Evans 1953; Lee 1957; Nilsonne 1932; Watson-Jones 1940), however, do significantly restrict subtalar motion and thus alter the physiological interplay of ankle and subtalar motion. As they interfere with the hindfoot mechanics, these tenodesis procedures should be avoided (Colville et al. 1992). When surgical repair of the calcaneofibular ligament is directed to stabilize the subtalar joint, this ligament must be attached in such a way as not to restrict motion in either joint, whether the joints move independently or simultaneously. To do this, the calcaneofibular ligament retains its parallelism to the axis of the subtalar joint as the ankle passes from plantarflexion to dorsiflexion.

■ References

Alm A, Ekstrom H, Stromberg B. 1974. Tensile strength of the anterior cruciate ligaments in the dog. Acta Chir Scand 445:15-23.

Anderson KJ, Lecocq JK. 1956. Operative treatment of injury to the fibular collateral ligament of the ankle. J Bone Joint Surg Am 36:825-832.

Attarian DE, McCrackin HJ, DeVito DP. 1985. Biomechanical characteristics of human ankle ligaments. Foot Ankle 6:54-58.

Barnett CH, Napier JR. 1952. The axis of rotation at the ankle joint in man. Its influence upon the form of the talus and mobility of the fibula. J Anatomy 86:1-9.

Boruta PM, Bishop JO, Braly WG, Tullos HS. 1990. Acute ankle ligament injuries: a literature review. Foot Ankle 12:107-112.

Broström L. 1966. Sprained ankle V—treatment and prognosis. Acta Chir Scand 132:537-550.

Butler DL, Hulse DA, Kay MD, Grood ES, Shires PK, D'Ambrosia R, Shoji H. 1983. Biomechanics of cranial cruciate ligament reconstruction in the dog. II. Mechanical properties. Vet Surg 12:113-118.

Cabaud HE, Feagin JF, Rodkey WG. 1980. Acute anterior cruciate ligament injury and augmented repair: experimental studies. Am J Sports Med 8:79-86.

Cass JR, Morrey BF, Chao EY. 1984. Three-dimensional kinematics of ankle instability following serial sectioning of lateral collateral ligaments. Foot Ankle 5(3):142-149.

Cass JR, Morrey BF, Katoh Y, Chao EY. 1985. Ankle instability: comparison of primary repair and delayed reconstruction after long-term follow-up study. Clin Orthop 198:110-117.

Cass JR, Settles H. 1994. Ankle instability: in vitro kinematics in response to axial load. Foot Ankle Int 15(3):134-140.

Chrisman OD, Snook GA. 1969. Reconstruction of lateral ligament tears of the ankle. An experimental study and clinical evaluation of seven patients treated by a new modification of the Elmslie procedure. J Bone Joint Surg Am 51:904-912.

Clanton TO. 1989. Instability of the subtalar joint. Orthop Clin North Am 20:583-592.

Clayton ML, Miles JS, Abdulla M. 1968. Experimental investigations of ligamentous healing. Clin Orthop 61:146-153.

Clayton ML, Weir GJ. 1959. Experimental investigations of ligamentous healing. Am J Surg 98:373-378.

Close JR. 1956. Some applications of the functional anatomy of the ankle joint. J Bone Joint Surg Am 38:761-781.

Colville MR, Marder RA, Boyle JJ, Zarins B. 1990. Strain measurement in lateral ankle ligaments. Am J Sports Med 18(2):196-200.

Colville MR, Marder RA, Zarins B. 1992. Reconstruction of the lateral ankle ligaments. A biomechanical analysis. Am J Sports Med 20(5):594-600.

Dorlot JM, Ait Ba Sidi M, Trembley GM, Drouin G. 1980. Load-elongation behavior of the canine anterior cruciate ligament. ASME Trans Biomech Eng 102:191-193.

Evans DL. 1953. Recurrent instability of the ankle: a method of surgical treatment. Proc R Soc Med 46:343-344.

Frank CB, Schachar N, Dittrich D. 1983. The natural history of healing in the repaired medial collateral ligament: a morphological assessment in rabbits. J Orthop Res 1:179-88.

Frank CB, Woo SLY, Amiel D, Gomez MA, Harwood KFL, Akeson WH. 1983. Medial collateral ligament healing. A multidisciplinary assessment in rabbits. Am J Sports Med 11:379-389.

Fraser GA, Ahmed AM. 1983. Passive rotational stability of the weight-bearing talocrural joint: an in vitro biomechanical study (abstract). Orthop Trans 7:248.

Grath G. 1960. Widening of the ankle mortise. A clinical and experimental study. Acta Chir Scand 263:1-88.

Hefti F, Kress A, Fasel J, Morscher EW. 1991. Healing of the transected anterior cruciate ligament in the rabbit. J Bone Joint Surg Am 73:373-383.

Heilman AE, Braly WG, Bishop JO. 1990. An anatomic study of subtalar instability. Foot Ankle 10:224-228.

Hicks JH. 1953. The mechanics of the foot. 1. The joints. J Anatomy 87:345-357.

Hintermann B, Nigg BM, Sommer C, Cole GK. 1994. Transfer of movement between calcaneus and tibia in vitro. Clin Biomech 9:349-355.

Hintermann B, Sommer C, Nigg BM. 1995. The influence of ligament transection on tibial and calcaneal rotation with loading and dorsi-plantarflexion. Foot Ankle 16:567-571.

Inman VT. 1991. The joints of the ankle. Baltimore: Williams & Wilkins, p. 31-74.

Johnson EE, Markolf KL. 1983. The contribution of the anterior talofibular ligament to the ankle laxity. J Bone Joint Surg Am 65:81-88.

Kennedy JC, Hawkins RJ, Willis RJ, Donylchuk KD. 1976. Tension studies of human knee ligaments. Yield point, ultimate failure, and disruptions of the cruciate and tibial ligaments. J Bone Joint Surg Am 58:350-355.

Kjaersgaard-Andersen PL, Wethelund J, Helmig P. 1987. Effect of the calcaneofibular ligament on hindfoot rotation in amoutation specimens. Acta Orthop Scand 58:135-138.

Kjaersgaard-Andersen PL, Wethelund J, Nielsen S. 1987. Lateral talocalcaneal instability following section of the calcaneofibular ligament: a kinesiologic study. Foot Ankle 7:355-361.

Larsen E. 1986. Experimental instability of the ankle. Clin Orthop 204:193-200.

Laurin CA, Quellet R, Jacques R. 1995. Talar and subtalar tilt. Can J Surg 11:270-278.

Lee HG. 1957. Surgical repair in recurrent dislocation of the ankle joint. J Bone Joint Surg Am 39:828-834.

Lundberg A. 1989. Kinematics of the ankle and foot. In vitro stereophotogrammetry. Acta Orthop Scand 60 (Suppl 233):1-24.

Manter JT. 1941. Movements of the subtalar and transverse tarsal joints. Anat Rec 80:397-400.

McCullough CJ, Burge PD. 1980. Rotatory stability of the load-bearing ankle. An experimental study. J Bone Joint Surg Br 62:460-464.

Michelson JD, Clarke HJ, Jinnah RH. 1990. The effect of loading on tibiotalar alignment in cadaver ankles. Foot Ankle 10:280-284.

Nachemson AL, Evans JH. 1968. Some mechanical properties of the third interlaminar ligament (ligament flavum). J Biomech 1:211-220.

Nigg BM, Cole GK, Nachbauer W. 1993. Effects of arch height of the foot on angular motion of the lower extremities in running. J Biomech 26(8):909-916.

Nigg BM, Skarvan G, Frank CB, Yeadon MR. 1991. Elongation and forces of ankle ligaments in a physiological range of motion. Foot Ankle 11:30-40.

Nilsonne H. 1932. Making a new ligament in ankle sprain. J Bone Joint Surg 14:380-381.

Noyes FR, DeLucas JL, Torvick PJ. 1974. Biomechanics of anterior cruciate ligament failure: an analysis of strain-rate sensitivity and mechanisms of failure in primates. J Bone Joint Surg Am 56:236-253.

Oakes BW. 1981. Acute soft tissue injuries - Nature and management. Austral Fam Phys 10:1-16.

O'Donoghue DH, Rockwood C, Zarecnyj B. 1961. Repair of knee ligaments in dogs. 1. The lateral collateral ligament. J Bone Joint Surg Am 43:1167-1178.

Parlasca R, Shoji H, D'Ambrosia RD. 1979. Effects of ligamentous injury on ankle and subtalar joints: a kinematic study. Clin Orthop 140:266-272.

Peters JW, Trevino SG, Renström PA. 1991. Chronic lateral ankle instability: a review. Foot Ankle 12:182-191.

Rasmussen O. 1985. Stability of the ankle joint. Acta Orthop Scand 211(Suppl):56-78.

Rasmussen O, Kroman-Andersen C, Boe S. 1983. Deltoid ligament: functional analysis of the medial collateral ligamentous apparatus of the ankle joint. Acta Orthop Scand 54:36-44.

Rasmussen O, Tovberg-Jensen I. 1982. Mobility of the ankle joint: recording of rotatory movements in the talocrural joint in vitro with and without the lateral collateral ligaments of the ankle. Acta Orthop Scand 53:155-160.

Renström PA, Wertz M, Incavo S, Pope M, Ostgaard HC, Arms S, Haugh L. 1988. Strain in the lateral ligaments of the ankle. Foot Ankle 9:59-63.

St. Pierre RK, Rosen J, Whitesides TE, Szczukowski M, Fleming LL, Hutton WC. 1983. The tensile strength of the anterior talofibular ligament. Foot Ankle 4(2):83-5.

Sammarco J. 1977. Biomechanics of the ankle: Surface velocity and instant center of rotation in the sagittal plane. Am J Sports Med 5:231-223.

Sarrafian SK. 1994. Anatomy of foot and ankle. Philadelphia: Lippincott, p. 239-240.

Siegler S, Block J, Schneck CD. 1988. The mechanical characteristics of the collateral ligaments of the human ankle joint. Foot Ankle 8:234-42.

Stormont DM, Morrey BF, An KN, Cass JR. 1985. Stability of the loaded ankle. Relation between articular restraint and primary and secondary static restraints. Am J Sports Med 13(5):295-300.

Tencer AF, Ahmed AM, Burke DL. 1982. Some static mechanical properties of the lumbar intervertebral joint, intact and injured. J Biomech Eng 104:193-20.

Tkaczuk H. 1968. Tensile properties of human lumbar longitudinal ligaments. Acta Orthop Scand 115:30-6.

Vailas AC, Tipton CM, Matthes RD, Gart M. 1981. Physical activity and its influence on the repair process of medial collateral ligaments. Connective Tissue Research 9:25-31.

Watson-Jones R. 1940. Fractures and other bone joint injuries. Edinburgh: Livingstone, p. 1-55.

Woo SLY, Inoue M, McGurk-Burlson M, Gomez MA. 1987. Treatment of the medial collateral ligament injury: structure and function of canine knees in response to differing treatment regimens. Am J Sports Med 15:22-29.

Chapter 5

Proprioception of the Ankle Joint

Rüdiger Reer, MD, and Jörg Jerosch, MD

Proprioception plays an important role in the prevention and rehabilitation of injuries of different joints. Studies in recent years mainly focused on the knee (Fischer-Rasmussen & Jensen 2000; Pap et al. 1999), the shoulder (Brindle et al. 1999; Jerosch, Thorwesten et al. 1996; Zuckerman et al. 1999), and the ankle joint (Lephart et al. 1998; Refshauge et al. 2000). Because of the high trauma rate—the ligamentous rupture of the ankle joint after supination trauma has the highest incidence among all ligamentous lesions—the ankle joint and its proprioceptive ability is of great importance.

■ Basic Knowledge

First, mechanical instability received a great deal of attention as a cause of ankle injuries. Over the following years, functional instability was considered to play an important role as well. It could be demonstrated that the functional instability resulted from a proprioceptive deficit.

Injuries of the Ankle Joint and the Importance of Proprioception

Ligamentous injury of the ankle joint, especially of the ligament–capsule area, is the most common injury occurring during sports and leisure time. According to studies by Renström and Thies (1993), the incidence of ankle joint traumas in the United States is approximately 23,000 cases per year (Garrick & Requa 1988; Renström et al. 1997). An especially high risk could be demonstrated in jump-accentuated sports such as volleyball, handball, badminton, and squash (Garrick & Requa 1988; Godolias & Dustmann 1985).

Because of the high incidence of ankle injuries, mechanically effective external stabilizing devices have now achieved great importance in the field of prevention and rehabilitation of ankle traumas. In several scientific studies, the effective prophylactic role of ankle braces could be proven (Garrick 1977; Glencross & Thornton 1981; Litt 1992; Miller & Hergenroeder 1990; Sitler et al. 1994; Surve et al. 1994; Tropp et al. 1985). Over the last several years it has become obvious that, as in other joints, the stabilization of the ankle joint depends to a great extent on coordinative and proprioceptive capabilities. Therefore, there is an increasing interest in neurophysiological interrelations and their role in the field of sports practice and therapy (Feuerbach et al. 1994; Freemann et al. 1965; Greene & Hillman 1990; Jerosch, Hoffstetter et al. 1995; Jerosch & Prymka 1996; Jerosch, Thorwesten et al. 1996; Jerosch, Thorwesten, & Frebel 1997; Jerosch, Thorwesten, Frebel, & Linnebecker 1997; Karlsson & Andreasson 1992; Kimura et al. 1987; Klein et al. 1991; Konradsen & Ravn 1990; Konradsen et al. 1993; Lephart et al. 1997; Meeuwsen et al. 1993; Stuessi et al. 1987; Takebayashi et al. 1997).

General Overview of Proprioception

The term **proprioception** was introduced by Sir Charles Sherrington in 1906 and describes the awareness of position and orientation of the body segments. Its roots are the Latin words *(re)ception* (the act of receiving) and *propius* (one's own). Proprioception is the result of the synthesis of afferent signals of different mechanoreceptors (Jerosch & Prymka 1996; Skoglund 1973; Takebayashi et al. 1997). General opinion holds that it is a combination of position sense, motion sense, and force sense and facilitates the perception of positions and motions of joints and limbs (kinaesthesia) as well as the estimation of the muscle force that is necessary for keeping or altering a joint position. The sensors of proprioception are located in joint structures, participating muscles, ligaments, tendons, and the skin above the joint. They belong to the type of mechanoreceptors that perceive mechanical inputs and convert them into nerve conductions (figure 5.1).

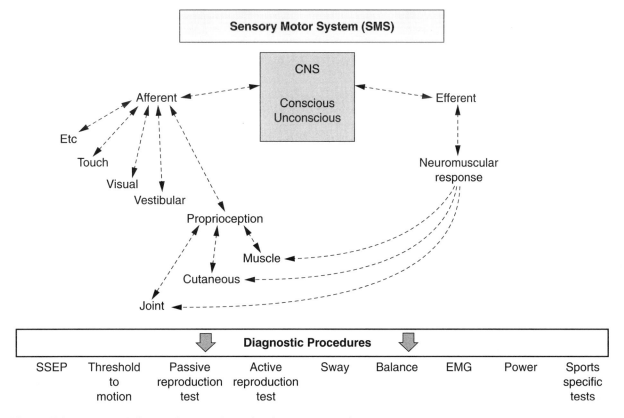

■ **Figure 5.1** Set-up and diagnostic procedures for the sensomotoric system.

Today, several authors rank the role of the joint receptors highest (Coiton et al. 1991; Cordo et al. 1994). Craske (1977), however, considers the muscle spindles, and Moberg (1985) the skin receptors, to be the most important receptors for proprioception. The issue, however, is not a simple one. Because a single narrow point of view is not adequate to describe the complex interaction of afferent and efferent pathways of proprioception, approaches from different areas are necessary: *anatomic* studies with preparation of selected articular structures from cadavers (Schultz et al. 1984; Schutte et al. 1987); *clinical* studies (Baker et al. 1990; Hovelius et al. 1983; Rowe & Zarins 1981) with description of the intra-articular pathology; and *biomechanical* studies (Hammon et al. 1987; Howell et al. 1988; Jerosch, Moersler, & Castro 1990; Schwartz et al. 1987; Turkel et al. 1981) on selected sections of cadaveric ligaments or direct measurements of the strain on the ligaments in different positions.

In a light-, scanning electron-, and transmission study, Haus et al. (1990) classified three types of nerve endings with proprioceptive qualities:

1. **Pacini's corpuscles** transferring fast alterations of forces. They show a fast adaptation and low stimulation threshold.

2. **Ruffini's corpuscles** signaling slowly changing dimensions of effecting forces. They are characterized by a slow adaptation and a low stimulation threshold.

3. **Free nerve endings** reacting as nociceptors. They indicate pain. They may also indicate mechanical and thermal stimuli.

Intraoperative electrical stimulation tests of specific mechanoreceptors demonstrated clearly that the definition of proprioception as a direct muscle reflex cannot be supported any longer. The long latency of the EMG response measured in these tests was between 100 msec to 516 msec (Jerosch, Steinbeck et al. 1997). This response was substantially longer than the time measured for monosynaptic or polysynaptic reflexes (Dewhurst 1967).

Proprioceptive Deficit Caused by Ankle Injuries

The importance of proprioceptive control mechanisms for functional joint stability and the influence of supination traumas on the proprioceptive capability is quite controversial.

Freeman et al. (1965) examined the influence of injuries of the capsular-ligamentous apparatus on the proprioception of the ankle joints. Damage to the receptors, caused by supination traumas, can lead to a partial disturbance of the afferent pathways and therefore to a functional instability of the ankle joint. Glencross and Thornton (1981) analyzed the position sense of athletes. With reference to the injured ankle joints, they found a significantly greater angle reproduction error as well as a correlation between the extent of movement and the reproduction error. The accuracy of angle reproduction rose in a linear manner with increasing degree of plantar flexion of the foot. Konradsen and Ravn (1990) as well as Gleitz et al. (1993) came to the conclusion that a post-traumatic proprioceptive deficit may be the cause for the functional instability of the ankle joint. The delay in time of the reflex response of the long peroneal muscle with a sudden inversion of the injured ankle joints was put down to a disturbed proprioception of these ankles (Konradsen & Ravn 1990). This post-traumatic delay of the reflex response was also described by Van Linge (1988). Gleitz et al. (1993) compared the stability of injured and noninjured ankle joints by applying a single-limb stance test. They demonstrated a diminished proprioceptive ability of the injured ankle joints in the form of a decreased stability. Jerosch et al. (1995) demonstrated the reduced proprioceptive capability of functionally unstable ankle joints by means of an angle

reproduction test (figure 5.2), a single-leg stance test, and a single-leg jump test. The attempt to correlate the results of the different tests with each other showed only very little or no correlation (figures 5.3-5.5), indicating that there are completely different proprioceptive qualities. Therefore, it is not very useful to practice proprioceptive abilities with a so-called proprioceptive trainer using a standardized program within the framework of rehabilitation. It can therefore be seen that proprioceptive training must be designed for each individual with that person's unique requirements in mind.

However, there are some authors who did not find any proprioceptive deficits after ankle joint injuries. Using the reproduction accuracy of inversion angles and the reflex response of the long peroneal muscle to sudden inversions, Konradsen et al. (1993) examined the effect of an anesthetic blockade of the receptors of the lateral ligaments on the proprioceptive ability of the ankle joint. Although the passive position sense diminished, thereby making a precise angle reproduction impossible, the active position sense (motion sense) was not affected by the blockade. The authors concluded that the afferent pathway of intact receptors of the lateral ligaments is important for a correct position sense of the ankle joint. However, a missing afferent pathway of these receptors can be replaced by information from receptors of the crural muscles.

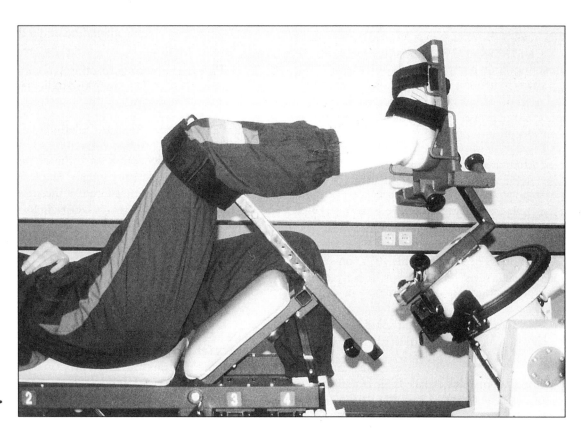

■ **Figure 5.2** Set-up of the angle reproduction test at a Cybex-6000 unit.

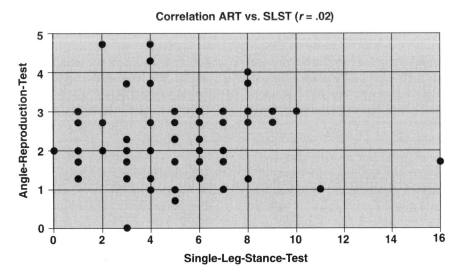

■ **Figure 5.3** Correlation between angle reproduction test (ART) and single-leg standing test (SLST).

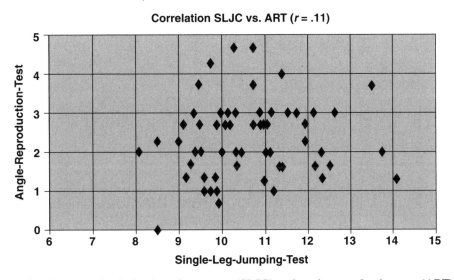

■ **Figure 5.4** Correlation between single-leg jumping course (SLJC) and angle reproduction test (ART).

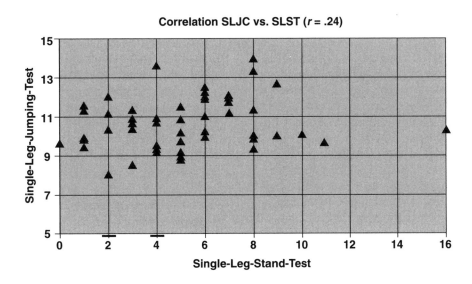

■ **Figure 5.5** Correlation between single-leg jumping course (SLJC) and single-leg standing test (SLST).

These results suggest that the proprioceptive perceptions of these muscle receptors may be responsible for a dynamic protection against sudden inversions. Gross (1987) came to a similar conclusion when testing the proprioception of subjects with and without supination traumas. The accuracy of reproducing inversion and eversion angles did not differ between injured and noninjured ankle joints.

Unanimously, all authors concluded that apart from proprioceptors of the joint capsule and ligaments, skin and muscle receptors also provide information regarding the joint position and motion. Current knowledge cannot answer the question of which receptors are responsible for which proprioceptive perceptions. It is likely that a complex interaction of different receptors is responsible for a precise proprioception of the ankle joints. The trauma-induced failure of some joint receptors cannot be completely compensated for by other proprio- or exteroreceptors. A proprioceptive deficit as a result of an ankle joint injury may be the cause for the functional instability of ankle joints.

■ Prophylaxis and Rehabilitation

External stabilizing devices are often used for prophylaxis and rehabilitation of ankle traumas. They are effective because of mechanical or functional stabilization.

Influence of Bandages, Braces, and Tapes on Proprioception

The most widely used external stabilizing devices are bandages, braces, and tapes. These three types of stabilizing devices influence proprioception to a different degree.

Prophylactic Effect of External Stabilizing Devices

Different studies demonstrated the prophylactic effect of ankle orthoses during physical activity. Garrick and Requa (1973) followed up on basketball players from the University of Washington over a period of 2 years. The players were divided into four groups according to the type of prophylactic orthotic care (high top/not taped, high top/taped, low top/not taped, low top/ taped). At 2,562 games, 55 ankle injuries were documented. The highest injury rate (33.4 injuries per 1,000 games) was found with the low top/not taped combination. The combination of high top/untaped (30.4/1,000) and low top/taped (17.4/1,000) showed a lower injury rate. The best result (6.5/1,000) could be demonstrated with the combination high top/taped.

In a retrospective study Rovere et al. (1988) tested a lace-on brace and a tape bandage as stabilizing devices. All college football players of Wake Forest University participated in the study over a period of 6 years. In the first 1.5 years, all players were taped. In the following 4.5 years, the players had the option to choose between a lace-on brace and a tape bandage. During the observation period, 224 ankle joint injuries occurred; 195 were supination traumas. With a tape bandage, 182 injuries in 38,658 games were documented, whereas with a lace-on brace, only 38 injuries in 13,273 games were documented. By this, it can be concluded that subjects with lace-on braces have only half the injury risk in comparison to subjects with tape bandages.

Sitler et al. (1994) documented basketball injuries of 1,601 cadets from the United States Military Academy over a period of 2 years. The subjects participated in 13,430 games during this period. Six thousand six hundred and eighty-two subjects wore an Aircast brace and 6,748 subjects played without any brace. In this 2-year period, 46 injuries of the ankle joint occurred: 35 of them had not used any stabilizing devices, while 11 had worn an Aircast brace on their ankle joint. According to the results of this study the injury rate of the subjects without any stabilizing devices was approximately three times higher.

Surve et al. (1994) investigated the incidence of ankle joint injuries over a period of 1 year among 504 soccer players. In this study, a group of 258 players with a former ankle joint injury were compared to a group of 246 players without any former ankle trauma. These two test groups were divided into two subgroups—the first with and the second without bracing. The groups with an ankle brace showed a significant reduction in the incidence of ankle injuries (injuries/1,000 game hours). The injury incidence of subjects with former trauma and bracing (0.14) was significantly lower compared to the group without any bracing (0.86). In the group without former ankle joint injury and without a brace, a lower incidence rate (0.46) was documented. Compared to the group without a former injury, the risk of an ankle trauma was approximately double that of the group with a positive past history of ankle trauma. The prophylactic bracing reduced this high risk for an already traumatized ankle to get traumatized again by almost five times.

Mechanical Stabilization by External Stabilizing Devices

The majority of previous studies did not deal with functional stabilization, investigating only mechanical stabilization. Vaes et al. (1985) as well as Löfvenberg and Kärrholm (1993) used a stress radiograph to study the lateral instability of the upper ankle joint in supination. Vaes et al. (1985) demonstrated a significantly reduced lateral instability for all ankle joints by applying a tape bandage. Exercises such as zigzag and curve runs, as well as jumping, reduced the stabilizing effect of the tape bandage. Löfvenberg and Kärrholm (1993) examined the mechanical support of a thermoplastic brace, which demonstrated a significant reduction in the lateral instability of unstable ankle joints.

Bunch et al. (1985) documented the secondary support effect by means of tape bandages, elastic bandages, and five different lace-on braces using a foot model made out of polyurethane, which was adapted from human anatomy. All stabilizing devices were tested directly after application and after an exercise of 350 motion cycles. Before exercise, the tape bandage showed better support by 25% compared to the best lace-on brace, and a better effect by 70% compared to the elastic bandage. The stabilizing loss of the tape bandage was highest after exercise (by 21%) compared to the lace-on brace (4.5-8.5%). These findings are in contrast to the study by Rovere et al. (1988), who found a better stabilizing result of braces compared to bandages. But the study by Bunch et al. (1985) documents the decreasing stabilizing effect of tape with increasing time between application and measurement due to the lower adhesion forces.

Gross et al. (1987), as well as Greene and Hillman (1990), analyzed the influence of stabilizing devices on the passive mobility of the ankle joints. With a Cybex unit, Gross et al. (1987) examined the maximal passive degree of motion without stabilization, with an Aircast Stirrup brace, and with a tape bandage before and after exercise. The Aircast brace, as well as the tape bandage, decreased mobility in inversion and eversion. The stabilization effect after exercise, however, was decreased by applying the tape bandage, while the values of the Aircast brace remained basically the same.

Greene and Hillman (1990) also showed that braces produce a significant reduction in mobility, which is not influenced by physical exercise. With the tape bandage, a significant limitation of the mobility was also achieved. But the tape bandage showed a loss in stabilization after only 20 minutes of physical exercise. After 1 hour no significant reduction in mobility was detected beyond that which resulted from the initial application of the tape bandage. Kimura et al. (1987) investigated the reaction of the ankle joints to sudden inversion stress. The inversion degree resulting from the sudden force was documented by means of a high-speed camera system,

which showed that the Aircast brace reduced the maximal inversion degree by an average 9.8°.

Independent of the method used, the efficiency and the stabilizing effect of single-use bandages and of reusable braces could be proven. In opposition to the good mechanical stabilization by tape bandages right after the application, is the loss in stability during physical exercise. The reusable braces showed no loss, or only a little loss of the stabilizing effect.

Influence of External Stabilizing Devices on Proprioception

Whereas in former times only the ability of functional stabilizing braces to provide passive stabilization was measured, interest today is increasingly focused on their capacity to support proprioceptive abilities. One can demonstrate that there are afferent receptors in the skin, muscles, ligaments, tendons, and joint capsules, and that these receptors contribute to the proprioceptive input of both the knee and ankle (Clark et al. 1985; Horch et al. 1975; Kennedy et al. 1982; Miyatsu et al. 1993). The primary position sense or movement receptors located in the joint capsule and ligaments are located deep within the soft tissues. These deep-set receptors may not be affected by an external ankle or knee support that is too superficial (for example, an elastic bandage or tape with full contact of the skin). In this case, the most likely receptors to be involved include free nerve endings and hair end organs that react strongly to new stimuli and adapt quickly (Perlau et al. 1995). In deeper subcutaneous areas, Ruffini's organs show tonic and slow adapting responses that can provide dynamic and static input (Guyton 1986).

The influence of braces on proprioceptive capabilities of the upper ankle joint has been investigated with different purposes and different methods. Kimura et al. (1987) suggested that the air bag of the Aircast brace stimulated additional skin receptors and could therefore even out a possible proprioceptive deficit. This would be a great advantage for persons with former injuries. Stuessi et al. (1987) examined the EMG activity of the long peroneal muscle, the main inhibitor of supination. The authors assumed that the tension developing in the muscle is proportional to the electrical activity. Their sample group consisted of 11 subjects with unstable ankle joints with and without Aircast braces. However, they could not demonstrate lower EMG values for the group with stabilized ankle joints. The peroneal muscles showed a similar degree of activity for both groups.

Scheuffelen et al. (1995) analyzed three stabilizing devices (Aircast, Ligafix, and stabilized shoe) and a normal running shoe under functional conditions.

To include the plantar flexion and rotation component during the injury mechanism, they applied a three-dimensional sprain mechanism under functional conditions. Additionally, surface EMG results were documented for detecting neuromuscular parameters. On this occasion, the temporal course as well as the extent of the neuromuscular activities of the long peroneal muscle, the anterior tibial muscle, the gastrocnemius muscle, and the vastus medialis muscle were examined. The results showed that the EMG signals were mostly reduced, but the typical innervation characteristics remained the same. High angle velocities during the sprain movements caused a substantial reflex response, and vice versa. In this study the reduction of the reflex response of the applied Aircast and Ligafix brace was lower compared to what had been expected due to the reduced angle velocity. The authors understood this phenom-

enon to be due to the different stimulation of proprioreceptors (e.g., those of the skin) by braces and interpreted this as a positive effect of the braces.

In their studies, Jerosch et al. (1995) demonstrated by means of different functional tests (angle reproduction test, one-leg stand test, single-leg jumping test) that the proprioceptive deficits of functionally unstable ankle joints could be significantly improved by reusable braces. All three tests documented an improvement of the proprioceptive capabilities when either of two commonly used braces (Mikros, Aircast) were applied to the subjects with stable and unstable ankle joints. In contrast, tape bandages achieved worse results than the braces in all three tests, and it was only in the single-leg jumping test and the angle reproduction test that a better range was seen for tape bandages than for subjects without any stabilizing devices (figures 5.6-5.8).

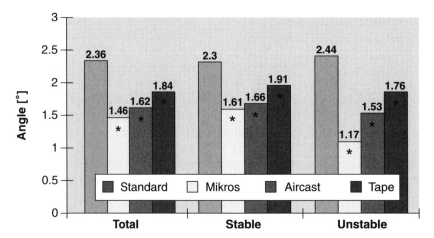

■ **Figure 5.6** Results (angle deviation in degrees) of subjects with stable and unstable ankle joints in the angle reproduction test when applying no brace (Standard), brace (Mikros, Aircast), and tape (* indicates a significant deviation from the "Standard").

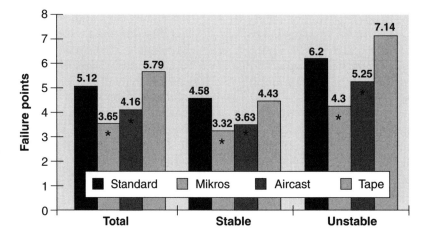

■ **Figure 5.7** Results (number of failure points) of subjects with stable and unstable ankle joints in the single-leg standing test when applying no brace (Standard), brace (Mikros, Aircast), and tape (* indicates a significant deviation from the "Standard").

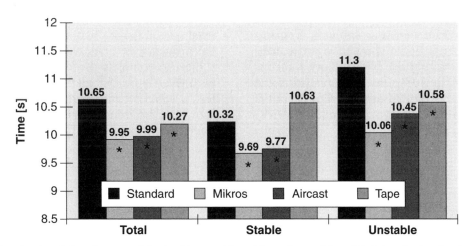

■ **Figure 5.8** Results (total time in seconds) of subjects with stable and unstable ankle joints in the single-leg jumping test when applying no brace (Standard), brace (Mikros, Aircast), and tape (* indicates a significant deviation from the "Standard").

One of the most important questions is by which mechanisms stabilizing devices show their effects. Little objective evidence demonstrates that any brace design has the ability to protect joint ligaments mechanically from harmful strain or loads of the magnitude seen in injury situations (Beynnon 1991). Therefore, it has been suggested that the true benefit of functional bracing may not be biomechanical reinforcement, but rather proprioceptive enhancement. Feuerbach et al. (1994) examined the effects of a brace as well as anesthesia on one or two lateral ligaments (anterior fibulotalar ligament or anterior fibulocalcanear ligament) on the proprioceptive capability of the ankle joints. In their investigation the anesthesia of the collateral ligaments did not prove any effects on angle reproduction ability. According to the authors' opinion, the feedback of the skin, muscles, and other receptors was more important because the angle reproduction error was lower with than without the brace.

It can be concluded that the positive prophylactic effects of ankle braces were proven several times and that these effects may possibly be caused by neurophysiological mechanisms. However, there is data proving that not all uninjured subjects will show an enhanced proprioception with the application of an external support. An effect may only be present in a subgroup of individuals who present an inherent suboptimal level of proprioception or neuromuscular control. The application of a brace may then normalize their proprioceptive values (Perlau et al. 1995).

Influence of External Stabilizing Devices on Physical Performance

Apart from the effect of external stabilizing devices on mechanical and functional stabilization, their in-fluence on physical performance is important for athletes. A preventive application of ankle braces will only be accepted by the athlete or coach if the physical performance will not be negatively affected. Different findings described in the literature often refer only to short-term effects (Burks et al. 1991; Cottman & Mize 1989; Jerosch & Prymka 1996; Jerosch, Thorwesten, & Frebel 1997; MacKean et al. 1995; Mayhew 1972; Pienkowski et al. 1995; Robinson et al. 1986; Thomas & Cotten 1977; Wiley & Nigg 1996).

Among six subjects, Robinson et al. (1986) investigated the influence of external stabilization of the ankle joint on physical performance. They applied a high-top basketball shoe without stabilizing effect and three other high-top basketball shoes that showed an increasing degree of stabilization by means of different support stripes. The subjects then completed an obstacle course on a basketball court, and completion time was used as a measure for performance. The data suggested that the subjects with stabilized shoes achieved worse results than those wearing the shoe without stabilization. The time loss correlated with the degree of stabilization.

Burks et al. (1991) examined the influence of tape, Swede-O braces, and Kallassy braces on physical performance. Thirty students performed four different tests. The tape bandage and Swede-O brace significantly reduced the physical performance in three tests, while the Kallassy brace showed a reduction only in one. According to the opinion of Burks et al., the reduction in physical performance is too low to reject the prophylactic stabilization of ankle joints.

Cottman and Mize (1989) tested the Aircast brace and a tape bandage on four basketball players and four students. They designed a sprint test and a jump test and carried them out both with a stabilizing device and without any stabilization. In the sprint test, the subjects wearing tape and an Aircast brace showed significantly worse test times than those without any stabilizing device. For the jump test, the results were different: only the tape showed a significantly worse value compared to the examinations without any support.

Jerosch, Thorwesten, and Frebel (1997) developed special Japan and one-leg jump tests to describe the influence of braces on how long it takes each subject to complete the "mini-course" presented in each test (figures 5.9 and 5.10). In the one-leg jump test, a deficit of the sports-specific ability could be shown for the group with functionally unstable ankle joints. The test results of subjects with functionally

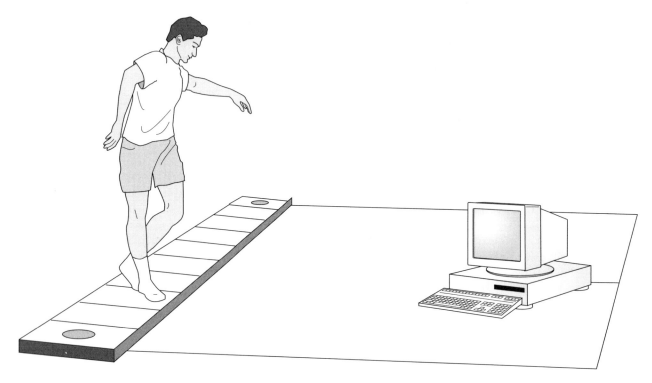

■ **Figure 5.9** Set-up of the Japan test with electronic measuring system.

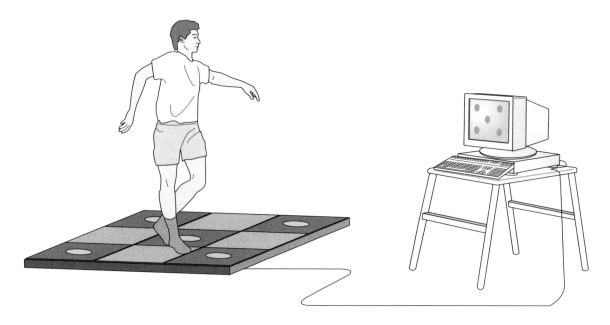

■ **Figure 5.10** Set-up of the jumping course with the KOMET measuring system.

unstable ankle joints showed that the application of different braces, as well as the tape bandage, led to significantly shorter stabilization times than the tests without any support (figure 5.11). The test subjects wearing braces spent less time on the ground than those who were not wearing braces. This shorter ground time indicates a faster stabilization of the ankle joint, which is an indicator for a better neuro-physiological influence by means of improved proprioceptive feedback mechanisms of the muscles. The improvement was especially substantial among the patients with unstable ankle joints. Simultaneously, no negative effects of the applied stabilizing devices could be detected for the physical performance in the jump test among the uninjured subjects (figure 5.12).

Furthermore, it could be demonstrated that the tested stabilizing devices did not show any negative effect on the physical performance in the Japan test among the healthy subjects (figure 5.13). Among the injured persons, the Japan test revealed a significant improvement when applying a brace (figure 5.14). To conclude, in sports disciplines that are based on movement patterns similar to those tested with the Japan test (e.g., volleyball), according to the present test results and the well-known prophylactic effect, stabilizing devices seem to be recommendable without fear of a loss in physical performance.

In another study MacKean et al. (1995) dealt with the influence of braces on the physical performance of 11 basketball players. Every ankle joint in the study

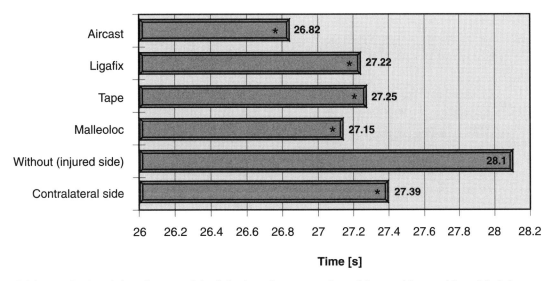

■ **Figure 5.11** Results (total time in seconds) of the jumping course for subjects with unstable ankle joint: contralateral uninjured ankle without brace or tape, injured ankle without brace, with Malleoloc, Tape, Ligafix, and Aircast (* indicates a significant deviation to the injured ankle without brace).

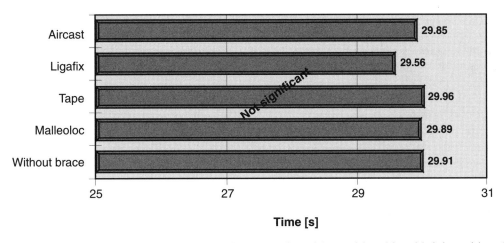

■ **Figure 5.12** Results (total time in seconds) of the jumping course for subjects with stable ankle joint: without brace or tape, with Malleoloc, Tape, Ligafix, and Aircast (n.s. = not significant).

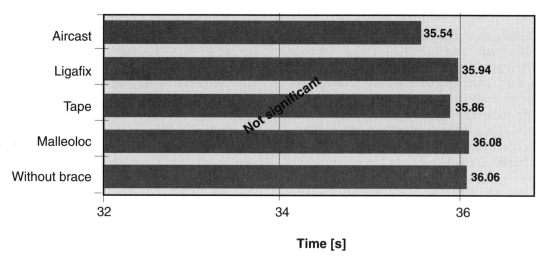

■ **Figure 5.13** Results (total time in seconds) of the Japan test for volunteers with stable ankle joints in relation to the applied external stabilizing device (n.s. = not significant).

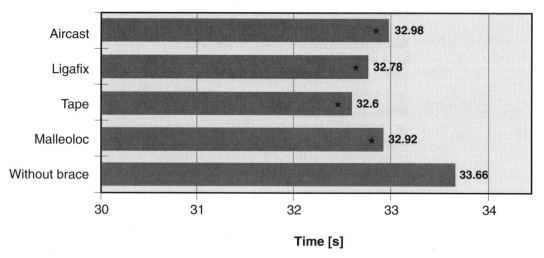

■ **Figure 5.14** Results (total time in seconds) of the Japan test for volunteers with unstable ankle joints in relation to the applied external stabilizing device (* indicates a significant deviation to the injured ankle without brace).

was supplied with one of four different stabilizing devices (tape bandage, Swede-O-Universal brace, Active Ankle brace, Aircast brace). The braces influenced the physical performance in standing jumps, as well as in the jump throw parcours, in a negative manner. However, with reference to the sprint test, no negative effects could be detected. Thomas and Cotten (1977), as well as Mayhew (1972), found a marginally negative effect of the tape on the standing jump in comparable studies but they could not show any negative effect on sprints and skill runs.

Pienkowski et al. (1995) examined the influence of three stabilizing devices (Universal, Kallassy, Air-stirrup) on physical activity among 12 basketball players. In the interval of 1 week, four basketball-related tests were performed with and without a brace. The results did not reveal any significant effects of the three braces on physical performance. In accordance with the data of this study, the prophylactic bracing can be supported. Wiley and Nigg (1996) found no influence of the Malleoloc brace on the figure-of-eight run or the jump test.

It can be concluded that there are, dependent on the experimental design, slightly different results regarding the effects of braces on sports-specific abilities. However, most authors agree that if there is any impairment, this is very little compared to the prophylactic advantage. Therefore, prophylactic bracing of the ankle joint can be considered to be useful.

■ Diagnostics

According to our findings, the following principal methods exist for objectively quantifying proprioception (figure 5.1):

1. Passive and active joint position reproduction tests as a measure for the evaluation of the joint position sense.

2. Threshold to motion as a measure for joint kinaesthesia.

3. EMG, Muscle Reflex Reaction Time.

4. Single-limb postural stability (postural sway amplitude and sway frequency).

5. SSEP: Somatosensory evoked potential.

6. Sense of force (power).

7. Functional sports-specific tests.

1. **Passive and active joint position reproduction tests.** This method involves quantifying joint position sense, or the accuracy and reliability with which a particular joint angle can be reproduced, either by the ipsilateral (Barrack et al. 1984) or by the contralateral joint (Horch et al. 1975). Although of importance for the control of movement, measurement of this angular reproduction ability would seem to have little relevance for understanding the causes of ankle injury in time-critical situations such as landing after a jump.

2. **Threshold to motion.** By definition, the threshold to motion is the ability to detect a change in joint position (Barrack et al. 1983). This important measure was already introduced by Goldschneider in 1889. He performed 4,000 measurements made at a constant velocity (0.3°/sec). According to his results, he found the ankle to be the joint with the largest threshold (1.2°), while the shoulder was the joint with the smallest threshold (0.2°) of the joints studied. Two different estimates of the detection threshold were defined. The lower threshold was the smallest foot rotation (THmin) required by a subject to discriminate correctly the direction of an inversion or eversion rotation. Another threshold with a higher degree of reliability is the TH75 (i.e., the threshold with at least a 75% probability of a subject detecting it). A Rotation Success Rate (SRR) was defined with regard to whether or not the occurrence of any rotation was correctly detected. A Direction Success Rate (SRD) was correspondingly defined as the ratio of trials in which the direction of the rotation was correctly identified to the number of nonzero angle trials (Gilsing et al. 1995). The detection of motion itself is known to have a lower threshold (Laidlaw & Hamilton 1937) than that for specification of direction (Goldschneider 1889) and probably depends on muscle spindles, tendon organs, and cutaneous pressure receptors.

3. **EMG.** For the diagnostic evaluation of proprioception, the electromyogram (EMG) is of importance. Several studies described a short to medium delay of the EMG response between 49 to 90 msec. This signal is followed by a cortical signal of substantial size and length, which can be voluntarily suppressed as a first reaction to a sudden inversion of the ankle joint. According to strength measurements of the ankle joint by means of a strength measurement plate, it could be demonstrated that eversion forces begin approximately 150 msec after the start of a sudden inversion and that 75% of the maximal torque was achieved after a period of 250 to 300 msec (Isakov et al. 1986; Johnson & Johnson 1993; Karlsson & Andreasson 1992; Konradsen & Ravn 1990; Konradsen et al. 1997; Löfvenberg et al. 1995; Nawoczenski et al. 1985).

Peroneal muscle reaction time. By definition, the time from a sudden inversion of the ankle to a measurable EMG reaction in the peroneal muscles is usually measured as the peroneal reaction time. The first EMG signal is a medium latency loop response. However, on the basis of the results of several studies (Isakov et al. 1986; Johnson & Johnson 1993; Karlsson & Andreasson 1992; Konradsen & Ravn 1990; Löfvenberg et al. 1995) it seems unclear whether or not an increased peroneal reaction time to sudden inversion exists in functional instability or not. The reaction of the peroneal muscles is the first dynamic response to sudden ankle inversion (Konradsen et al. 1997). In several studies, subjects with unstable ankles achieved peroneal reaction latencies of 85 msec, while healthy subjects had lower latencies of 70 msec (Karlsson & Andreasson 1992; Sprigings et al. 1981).

4. **Single-limb postural stability (postural sway amplitude and sway frequency).** The single-leg stand test with closed eyes allows the study of proprioceptive capabilities (figure 5.15). However, a problem with this technique is that it measures complex proprioceptive functions, including afferent information from the vestibular system and from vision, as well as motor skills. Tropp et al. (1985) found a 27% increase of postural sway among 29 soccer players with a former ankle joint instability compared to the control group. Leanderson et al. (1993) tested the balance of 38 basketball players on a computer-assisted strength measurement plate. Players with a previous ankle joint trauma had a significantly different impairment compared to the control group. Freeman et al. (1965) found worse results for postural sway among subjects with repeated ankle inversion traumas. In a study by Lentell et al. (1990) examining subjects with unilateral ankle trauma, the results of the injured ankle joint were proven worse in comparison to the uninjured ankle joint. Garn and Newton (1988) demonstrated that among 20 subjects with repeated inversion traumas, 67% had a postural sway. Jerosch and Bischoff (1996) used the number of touchdowns of the contralateral foot as an indicator of instability. They found a statistically significant

difference between stable and unstable ankle joints compared to healthy subjects (figure 5.16).

5. **Somatosensory evoked potentials (SSEP).** To describe proprioceptive capabilities, so-called somatosensory evoked potentials (SSEP) can be employed. They are a response created in the spine (spinal SSEP) and the cortex (cortical SSEP) to an electrical stimu-

lation of sensory or mixed nerves. This response can be derived in the lower back, the nuchal area, and the sensory cortex respectively. In particular, the posterior funiculus of the spinal cord is of importance because this system is functionally associated with the mechanoreceptors of the skin and with proprioceptive capabilities (Guyton & Hall 1996). In contrast to other measurement methods, the afferent part of the somatosensory system can be selectively measured by means of the somatosensory potentials.

6. **Sense of force.** The ability to distinguish the extent of muscle force is necessary to carry out a movement and to maintain joint position (e.g., during changing gravitational strains). If we compare two loads by means of simultaneously lifting them in our hands, a load difference of between 3% and 10% can be differentiated. However, if we measure weights lying on top of both hands, when the hands are positioned on a surface, the weight assessment is much more inaccurate—probably as a result of the limitation on the afferent information of the skin sensors. The point at which we can begin to distinguish differences in weights is called the *discrimination threshold*.

7. **Functional tests (sports-specific tests).** Functional tests can measure proprioceptive abilities under dynamic sports-specific conditions. Jerosch and Bischof (1996) applied a single-limb hopping course test (figure 5.17). The test was performed according to Chambers et al. (1982), who used it to test ankle

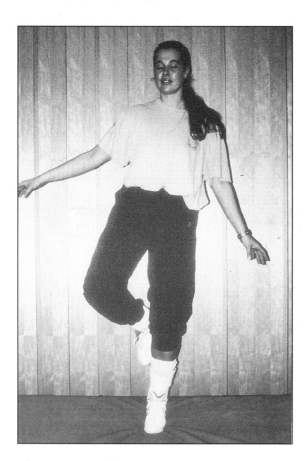

■ **Figure 5.15** Set-up of the single-leg standing test.

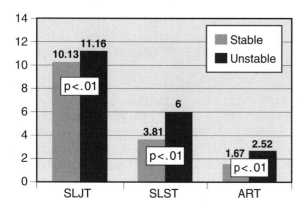

■ **Figure 5.16** Results of the single-leg jump test (SLJT) (total time in seconds), the single-leg standing test (SLST) (number of failure points), and the angle reproduction test (ART) (angle deviation in degrees) for noninjured stable ankle joints and for unstable ankle joints.

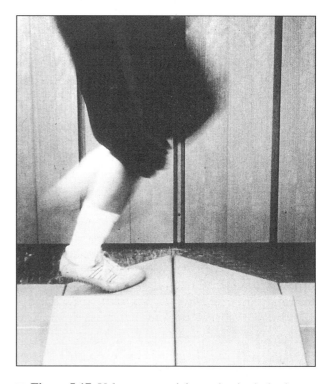

■ **Figure 5.17** Volunteer practicing at the single-leg jumping course.

function following surgery. The jumping course covers an area of 140 × 70 cm and consists of eight squares (35 × 35 cm each square). Four of these squares are even, one square has a 15° inclination, another square a 15° decline, and two squares showed a 15° lateral inclination. The volunteers were asked to jump across this hopping course with one leg by touching each area once, and to do this as quickly as possible without leaving the course. This test was considered to measure the functional ability of the ankle and of the proprioceptive co-activity of the foot, knee, hip, and upper extremity as well as the ability of the visual and vestibular systems. The results showed a significant ($p < .01$) increase of 10% in the time used for the hopping course for the injured leg (see figure 5.5).

■ Summary

In summary, it can be concluded that according to the results of many studies, a proprioceptive deficit as a consequence of an injury of the ankle joint can be demonstrated. It could be shown that there are different proprioceptive qualities. The proprioceptive deficit can be seen as reason for a functional instability of the ankle joints. Braces improve the proprioceptive capabilities of injured ankle joints. Among subjects with healthy ankle joints, the stabilizing devices tested by us did not reveal any negative influence on sports-specific abilities, but led to an improvement of sports-specific characteristics of subjects with functionally unstable ankle joints.

Regarding the presented results and those in the literature, brace applications can be considered to be an efficient preventive measure to avoid sports injuries as well as to improve the proprioceptive function of functionally unstable ankle joints. Furthermore, there are indications that specific preventive and rehabilitative proprioceptive-coordinative exercise therapy improves the proprioceptive abilities of the ankle joint and therefore can contribute to a great extent to a decrease in the injury incidence of the ankle joint. For a detailed discussion of this latter point, with suggested exercises, see "Further Thoughts on Proprioceptive Training As a Therapeutic Measure" (pages 195-199 in chapter 22).

■ References

Alves JW, Alday RV, Ketcham DL, Lentell GL. 1992. A comparison of the passive support provided by various ankle braces. J Orthop Sports Phys Ther 15:10-18.

Baker CL, Uribe JW, Whitman C. 1990. Arthroscopic evaluation of acute initial anterior shoulder dislocation. Am J Sports Med 18:25-28.

Barrack RL, Skinner HB, Brunel ME, Haddad RJ. 1983. Functional performance of the knee after intraarticular anesthesia. Am J Sports Med 11:258-261.

Barrack RL, Whitecloud TS, Burke SW, Cook SD, Harding AF. 1984. Proprioception in idiopathic scoliosis. Spine 9:681-685.

Beynnon BRP. 1991. The effect of bracing and taping in sports. Ann Chir Gyn 80:230-238.

Brindle TJ, Nyland J, Shapiro R, Caborn DN, Stine R. 1999. Shoulder proprioception: latent muscle reaction times. Med Sci Sports Exerc 31:1394-1398.

Bruns B, Staerk H. 1990. Muskuläre Stabilisation des oberen Sprunggelenkes bei lateraler Instabilität. Orthop Traumatol 37:597-604.

Bunch RP, Bednarski K, Holland D, Mancinanti R. 1985. Ankle joint support: a comparison of reusable Lace-on-Braces with taping and wrapping. Phys Sports Med 13:59-62.

Burks RT, Bean BG, Marcus R, Barker HB. 1991. Analysis of athletic performance with prophylactic ankle devices. Am J Sports Med 19:104-106.

Chambers RB, Cook TM, Cowell HR. 1982. Surgical reconstruction for calcaneonavicular coalition. J Bone Joint Surg Am 64:829-836.

Clark FJ, Burgess RC, Chapin JW, Lipscomb WT. 1985. Role of intramuscular receptors in the awareness of limb position. J Neurophysiol 54:1529-1540.

Coiton Y, Gilhodes JC, Velay JL, Roll JP. 1991. A neural network model for the intersensory coordination involved in goal directed movements. Biol Cybern 66:167-176.

Cordo P, Carlton L, Beveau L, Carlton M, Kerr GK. 1994. Proprioceptive coordination of movement sequences: role of velocity and position information. J Neurophysiol 71:1848-861.

Coffman JL, Mize NL. 1989. A comparison of ankle taping and the Aircast-Sport-Stirrup on athletic performance. Athl Train 24:123.

Craske B. 1977. Perception of impossible limb positions induced by tendon vibrations. Science 196:71-73.

Dewhurst DJ. 1967. Neuromuscular control system. IEEE Trans Biomed Engin 14:167-171.

Feuerbach JW, Grabiner MD, Koh TJ, Weiker GG. 1994. Effect of an ankle orthosis and ankle ligament anesthesia on ankle joint proprioception. Am J Sports Med 22:223-229.

Fischer-Rasmussen T, Jensen PE. 2000. Proprioceptive sensitivity and performance in anterior cruciate ligament-deficient knee joints. Scand J Med Sci Sports 10:85-89.

Freemann MAR, Dean MRE, Hanham IWF. 1965. The etiology and prevention of functional instability of the foot. J Bone Joint Surg Br 47:678-685.

Garn SN, Newton RA. 1988. Kinesthetic awareness in subjects with multiple ankle sprains. Phys Ther 68:1667-1671.

Garrick JG. 1977. The frequency of injury, mechanisms of injury, and epidemiology of ankle sprains. Am J Sports Med 5:241-242.

Garrick JG, Requa RK. 1973. Role of external support in the prevention of ankle sprains. Med Sci Sports 5:200-203.

Garrick JG, Requa RK. 1988. The epidemiology of foot and ankle injuries in sports. Clin Sports Med 7:29-36.

Gilsing MC, Van den Bosch SG, Lee SG, Ashton-Miller JA, Alexander NB, Schultz AB, Ericson WA. 1995. Association of age with the threshold for detecting ankle inversion and eversion in upright stance. Age and Ageing 24:58-66.

Gleitz M, Rupp T, Hess T, Hopf T. 1993. Bei instabilen Sprunggelenken: Reflextraining und Stabilisierung. Orthopädie und Schuhtechnik 5:65-68.

Glencross D, Thornton E. 1981. Position sense following joint injury. J Sports Med Phys Fitness 21:23-27.

Godolias G, Dustmann HO. 1985. Häufigkeit und Ursachen von Bandverletzungen des Sprunggelenkes bei verschiedenen Sportarten. Orthop Praxis 9:697-702.

Goldschneider A. 1889. Untersuchungen über den Muskelsinn. Arch Anat Physiol 3:369-502.

Greene TA, Hillman SK. 1990. Comparison of support provided by a semirigid orthosis and adhesive ankle taping before, during, and after exercise. Am J Sports Med 18:498-506.

Greene TA, Wright CR. 1990. A comparative support evaluation of three ankle orthoses before, during, and after exercise. J Orthop Sports Phys Ther 11:453-466.

Gross MT. 1987. Effects of recurrent lateral ankle sprains on active and passive judgement of joint position. Phys Ther 67:1505-1509.

Gross MT, Ballard CL, Mears HG, Watkins EJ. 1992. Comparison of DonJoy ankle ligament protector and Aircast Sport-Stirrup orthoses in restricting foot and ankle motion before and after exercise. J Orthop Sports Phys Ther 16:60-67.

Gross MT, Bradshaw MK, Ventry LC, Weller KH. 1987. Comparison of support provided by ankle taping and semirigid orthosis. J Orthop Sports Phys Ther 9:33-39.

Gross MT, Lapp AK, Davis JM. 1991. Comparison of Swede-O-Universal ankle support and Aircast Sport Stirrup orthoses and ankle tape in restricting eversion-inversion before and after exercise. J Orthop Sports Phys Ther 13:11-19.

Guyton AC, Hall JE. 1996. Textbook of medical physiology. 9th ed. Philadelphia: Saunders.

Guyton AC. 1986. Somatic sensations: the mechanoreceptive sensations. In: Textbook of medical physiology. 7th ed. Philadelphia: Saunders. p. 588-589.

Hammon DJ, France EP, Terry GC. 1987. Stabilizing function of passive shoulder restraints. Trans Orthop Res Soc 12:77.

Haus J, Halata Z, Refior HJ. 1990. Propriozeption im vorderen Kreuzband des menschlichen Kniegelenkes: morphologische Grundlagen. Z Orthop 130:484-494.

Horch KW, Clark FJ, Burgess PR. 1975. Awareness of knee joint angle under static conditions. J Neurophys 38:1436-447.

Hovelius L, Eriksson K, Fredin H, Hagberg G, Hussenius A, Lind B, Thorling J, Weckström J. 1983. Recurrences after initial dislocation of the shoulder. J Bone Joint Surg Am 65:343-348.

Howell SM, Galinat BJ, Renzi AJ, Marone PJ. 1988. Normal and abnormal mechanics of the glenohumeral joint in the horizontal plane. J Bone Joint Surg Am 70:227-232.

Isakov E, Mizrahi J, Solzi P, Susak Z, Lotem M. 1986. Response of the peroneal muscles to sudden inversion of the ankle during standing. Int J Sports Biomech 2:100-109.

Jerosch J, Bischof M. 1996. Proprioceptive capabilities of the ankle in stable and unstable joints. Sports Exerc Injury 2:167-171.

Jerosch J, Hoffstetter I, Bork H, Bischoff M. 1995. The influence of orthoses on the proprioception of the ankle joint. Knee Surg Sports Traumatol Arthroscopy 3:39-46.

Jerosch J, Moersler M, Castro WHM. 1990. Über die Funktion der passiven Stabilisatoren des glenohumeralen Gelenkes: eine biomechanische Untersuchung. Z Orthop 128:206-212.

Jerosch J, Prymka M. 1996. Proprioception and joint stability. Knee Surg Sports Traumatol Arthroscopy 4:171-179.

Jerosch J, Steinbeck J, Schröder M, Westhues M, Reer R. 1997. Intraoperative EMG response of the musculature after stimulation of the glenohumeral joint capsule. Acta Orthopaedica Belgica 63:8-14.

Jerosch J, Thorwesten L, Bork H, Bischof M. 1996. Is prophylactic bracing of the ankle cost effective? Orthopedics 19:405-414.

Jerosch J, Thorwesten L, Frebel T. 1997. Einfluß von externen Stabilisierungshilfen am Sprunggelenk auf sportmotorische Fähigkeiten beim Einbeinsprung. Sportverl Sportschad 11:27-32.

Jerosch J, Thorwesten L, Frebel T, Linnebecker S. 1997. Influence of external stabilizing devices of the ankle on sport-specific capabilities. Knee Surg Sports Traumatol Arthroscopy 5:50-57.

Jerosch J, Thorwesten L, Steinbeck J, Reer R. 1996. Proprioceptive function of the shoulder girdle in healthy volunteers. Knee Surg Sports Traumatol Arthrosc 3:219-225.

Johnson MB, Johnson CL. 1993. Electromyographic response of peroneal muscles in surgical and nonsurgical injured ankles during sudden inversion. J Orthop Sports Phys Ther 18:497-501.

Karlsson L, Andreasson GO. 1992. The effect of external ankle support in chronic lateral ankle joint instability: an electromyographic study. Am J Sports Med 20:257-261.

Kennedy JC, Alexander IJ, Hayes KC. 1982. Nerve supply of the human knee and its functional importance. Am J Sports Med 10:329-335.

Kimura IF, Nawocenski DA, Epler M, Owen MG. 1987. Effect of the Air-Stirrup in controlling ankle inversion stress. J Orthop Sports Phys Ther 9:190-193.

Klein J, Rixen D, Albring T, Tiling T. 1991. Funktionelle versus Gipsbehandlung bei der frischen Außenbandruptur des oberen Sprunggelenkes: eine randomisierte klinische Studie. Unfallchir 94:99-104.

Konradsen L, Ravn JB. 1990. Ankle instability caused by prolonged peroneal reaction time. Acta Orthop Scand 61:388-390.

Konradsen L, Ravn JB, Sorenson AI. 1993. Proprioception at the ankle: the effect of anesthetic blockade of ligament receptors. J Bone Joint Surg Br 75:433-436.

Konradsen L, Voigt M, Hojsgaard C. 1997. Ankle inversion injuries: the role of the dynamic defense mechanism. Am J Sports Med 25:54-58.

Laidlaw RW, Hamilton MA. 1937. A study of thresholds in apperception of passive movement among normal control subjects. Bull Neurol Inst NY 6:268-273.

Leanderson J, Wykman A, Eriksson E. 1993. Ankle sprain and postural sway in basketball players. Knee Surg Sports Traumatol Arthroscopy 1:203-205.

Lentell G, Baas B, Lopez D, McGuire L, Sarrels M, Snyder P. 1995. The contributions of proprioceptive deficits, muscle function, and anatomic laxity to functional instability of the ankle. J Orthop Sports Phys Ther 21:206-215.

Lentell GL, Katzman LL, Walters MR. 1990. The relationship between muscle function and ankle stability. J Orthop Sports Phys Ther 11:605-611.

Lephart SM, Pincivero DM, Giraldo JL, Fuu FF. 1997. The role of proprioception in the management and rehabilitation of athletic injuries. Am J Sports Med 25:130-137.

Lephart SM, Pincivero DM, Rozzi SL. 1998. Proprioception of the ankle and knee. Sports Med 25:149-155.

Litt KC. 1992. The sprained ankle: diagnosis and management of the lateral ligament injuries. Aust Fam Physician 21:452-456.

Löfvenberg R, Kärrholm J. 1993. The influence of an ankle orthosis on the talar and calcaneal motions in chronic lateral instability of the ankle. Am J Sport Med 21:224-230.

Löfvenberg R, Kärrholm J, Sundelin G. 1995. Prolonged reaction time in patients with chronic lateral instability of the ankle. Am J Sports Med 23:414-417.

MacKean LC, Bell G, Burnham RS. 1995. Prophylactic ankle bracing vs. taping: effects on functional performance in female basketball players. J Orthop Sports Phys Ther 22:77-81.

Mayhew JL. 1972. Effects on ankle taping on motor performance. J Athl Train 7:10-11.

Meeuwsen HJ, Sawicki TM, Stelmach GE. 1993. Improved foot position sense as a result of repetitions in older adults. J Gerontol 48:137-141.

Miller EA, Hergenroeder AC. 1990. Prophylactic ankle bracing. Pediatr Clin North Am 37:1175-1185.

Miyatsu M, Atsuta Y, Watakabe M. 1993. The physiology of mechanoreceptors in the anterior cruciate ligament. J Bone Joint Surg Br 75:653-657.

Moberg E. 1985. New facts about hand control kinaesthesia. Am Chir Main 4:64-66.

Nawoczenski DA, Owen MG, Ecker ML, Altman B, Epler M. 1985. Objective evaluation of peroneal response to sudden inversion stress. J Orthop Sports Phys Ther 7:107-109.

Pap G, Machner A, Nebelung W, Awiscus F. 1999. Detailed analysis of proprioception in normal and ACL-deficient knees. J Bone Joint Surg Br 81:764-768.

Perlau R, Frank C, Fick G. 1995. The effect of elastic bandages on human knee proprioception in the uninjured population. Am J Sports Med 23:251-255.

Pienkowski D, McMorrow M, Shapiro R, Caborn DNM, Stoyton J. 1995. The effect of ankle stabilizers on athletic performance: a randomized prospective study. Am J Sports Med 23:757-762.

Refshauge KM, Kilbreath SL, Raymond J. 2000. The effect of recurrent ankle inversion sprain and taping on proprioception at the ankle. Med Sci Sports Exerc 32: 10-15.

Renström PA, Beynnon B, Haugh L, MacDonald L. 1997. A prospective randomized outcome study of acute first time ankle sprains, grade I and II [abstract]. First Biennial Congress of the International Society of Arthroscopy, Knee Surgery and Orthopaedic Sports Medicine, May 11-16, 1997, Buenos Aires, Argentina.

Renström P, Thies M. 1993. Die Biomechanik der Verletzungen der Sprunggelenkbänder. Sportverl Sportschad 7:29-35.

Robinson JR, Frederick EC, Cooper LB. 1986. Systematic ankle stabilization and the effect on performance. Med Sci Sports Exerc 18:625-628.

Rovere GD, Clarke TJ, Yates CS, Burley K. 1988. Retrospective comparison of taping and ankle stabilizers in preventing ankle injuries. Am J Sports Med 16:228-233.

Rowe CR, Zarins B. 1981. Recurrent transient subluxation of the shoulder. J Bone Joint Surg Am 63: 863-872.

Scheuffelen C, Gollhofer A, Lohrer H. 1995. Sprunggelenksorthese Ligafix-Air zur Therapie der lateralen Kapselbandverletzung des oberen Sprunggelenks. Wissenschaftliches Gutachten des Instituts für Sport und Sportwissenschaft der Unitversität Freiburg 1995.

Schultz RA, Miller DC, Kerr CS, Micheli L. 1984. Mechanoreceptors in human cruciate ligaments: a histologic study. J Bone Joint Surg Am 66:1072-1076.

Schutte MJ, Dabezies EJ, Zimny ML, Happel LT. 1987. Neural anatomy of the human anterior cruciate ligament. J Bone Joint Surg Am 69: 243-247.

Schwartz RE, Torzilli PA, Warren RF. 1987. Capsular restraints to anterior-posterior motion of the shoulder. Trans Orthop Res Soc 12:78.

Shapiro MS, Kabo JM, Mitchell PW, Loren G, Tsender M. 1994. Ankle sprain prophylaxis: an analysis of the stabilizing effects of braces and tape. Am J Sports Med 22:78-82.

Sitler M, Ryan J, Wheeler B, McBride J, Arciero R, Anderson J, Horodyski M. 1994. The efficacy of a semirigid ankle stabilizer to reduce acute ankle injuries in basketball. Am J Sports Med 22:454-461.

Skoglund ST. 1973. Joint receptors and kinesthetics. In: Handbook of sensory physiology. Vol. 2. p. 111-136.

Sprigings EJ, Pelton JD, Brandell BR. 1981. An EMG analysis of the effectiveness of external ankle support during sudden ankle inversion. Can J Sports Sci 6:72-75.

Stuessi E, Tigermann V, Gerber H, Raemy H, Stacoff A. 1987. A biomechanical study of the stabilization effect of the Aircast ankle brace. International Series on Biomechanics 6-A: 159-164.

Surve I, Schwellnus MP, Noakes T, Lombard C. 1994. A fivefold reduction in the incidence of recurrent ankle sprains in soccer players using the Sport-Stirrup orthosis. Am J Sports Med 22:601-606.

Takebayashi T, Yamashita T, Minaki Y, Ishii S. 1997. Mechanosensitive afferent units in the lateral ligament of the ankle. J Bone Joint Surg Br 79:490-493.

Thomas JR, Cotten D. 1977. Does taping slow down athletes? Coach Athlete 34:20-37.

Tropp H. 1986. Pronator muscle weakness in functional instability of the ankle joint. Int J Sports Med 7(5):291-294.

Tropp H, Askling C, Gillquist J. 1985. Prevention of ankle sprains. Am J Sports Med 13(4):259-261.

Turkel SJ, Panio MW, Marshall JL, Girgis FG. 1981. Stabilizing mechanisms preventing anterior dislocation of the glenohumeral joint. J Bone Joint Surg Am 63:1208-1217.

Vaes P, De Boeck H, Handelberg F, Opdecam P. 1985. Comparative radiologic study of the influence of joint bandages on ankle stability. Am J Sports Med 13:46-50.

Van Linge B. 1988. Activity of the peroneal muscles, the maintenance of balance, and prevention of inversion injury of the ankle: an electromyographic and kinematic study. Acta Orthop Scand 59:67-68.

Wiley JP, Nigg M. 1996. The effect of an ankle orthosis on ankle range of motion and performance. J Orthop Sports Phys Ther 23:362-369.

Zuckerman JD, Gallagher MA, Lehman C, Kraushaar BS, Choueka J. 1999. Normal shoulder proprioception and the effect of lidocaine injection. J Shoulder Elbow Surg 8:11-16.

Part II

Primary Evaluation

The acute ankle sprain could be defined as the first event of ankle injury, or as a cause of primary damage. This damage may be exacerbated by further injuries. At this stage, accurate grading is important in order to specify the damage, decide on the appropriate treatment, and estimate the final outcome.

The most common mechanism of injury in acute ankle sprain is inversion injury, which leads to damage of the lateral ligaments and capsule. Medial ligamentous injuries, though rare, may cause chronic disability. Primary evaluation leads to accurate diagnosis of the extent of the injury, and scoring systems for evaluating the injured ankle allow quantifiable assessment of improvement of this injury.

The diagnostic modalities are discussed in the following chapters.

Chapter 6

Mechanics of Injury, Clinical Presentation, and Staging

Gideon Mann, MD; Meir Nyska, MD; Naama Constantini, MD; Y. Matan, MD;
Per Renström, MD, PhD; and Scott A. Lynch, MD

Ankle sprains usually occur when the foot is forcefully inverted when the ankle is plantarflexed; in this position the bony structure allows only minimal stability, the leverage is maximal, and the anterior talofibular ligament (ATFL), which is the weakest component of the lateral ligament of the ankle, is taut and exposed to injury. The degree of injury depends on the force exerted and on the range of abnormal motion that is enforced on the ankle. This force could be modified by timely muscle activation, external protection, and reasonable attention to the course or playing ground.

Grading systems of acute sprains are largely inaccurate and are often not practical for current clinical use. This chapter describes grading systems used by various authorities and in our local research and clinical work at The Meir Hospital, Kfar Saba, Israel; The Wingate Institute, Netanya, Israel; and Hadassah Hospital, Jerusalem, Israel.

■ Introduction

A certain lack of clarity surrounds the mechanics of ankle injury and staging. We often ask why such seemingly obvious and descriptive issues should involve so much vagueness. Further questions involve the practical implications of these issues, or what our knowledge of injury mechanism and clinical presentation, as well as a technical staging system, would add to decision making about and management of an injured athlete.

■ Mechanism of Injury

The load to failure of the lateral ligament of the ankle has been measured by various authorities. The ATFL has been shown to be the weakest component of the lateral ligament (Attarian et al. 1985; Siegler et al. 1998). The ATFL ligament has an approximate load to failure of 140 Newtons, the calcaneofibular ligament (CFL) of 350 Newtons, and the posterior talofibular ligament (PTFL) of 260 Newtons (Attarian et al. 1985). Others claim the PTFL is the strongest of the three (Anderson et al. 1954, 1962) and is rarely damaged (Broström 1966), though, when it is damaged, the talus dislocates out of the mortis (Anderson et al. 1954, 1962). A simple calculation will show that the combined force of the lateral ligament could not amount to more than 750-800 Newtons, which is far less than the force exerted by landing from a half-meter jump, and far inferior to the strength of the anterior cruciate ligament of the knee. This would probably at least partially explain the extremely high occurrence of this injury, which is reported in half the population (Coutts & Woodward 1965) and comprises 16-40% of sports-related injuries (Evans 1953; Garrick 1977; Mukerjee & Gangopadhyay 1983; Machlum & Daljord 1984; Liu & Jason 1994; Calliet 1997), ranging from 45% of injuries in basketball (Garrick 1977) to an incidence of 30-60% in military training (Balduini et al. 1987, Kahn et al. 1997, Kahn 1998), 25% in track & field (Mack 1982), and 20% in soccer (Sandelin et al. 1988, Ekstrand & Tropp 1990). The anatomy and biomechanics of the ankle joint are discussed in detail in other chapters of this text.

Sprains or ruptures of the lateral ligaments of the ankle most frequently occur when the foot is forcefully inverted while in the plantarflexed position (Garrick 1977; Knight 1978; Kristiansen 1981; Mukerjee & Gangopadhyay 1983; Mann et al. 1993; 1994, 1998; Calliet 1997), as illustrated by Renström and Lynch in chapter 20 of this book. This position brings the narrower part of the talus into the mortise and so places the ankle in an inherently precarious position (Calliet 1997) in which stability depends solely on ligament continuity. In this position, the ATFL is taut (Calliet 1997) and the leverage exerted by inversion of the outstretched foot outweighs the limited strength of the ATFL (Anderson et al. 1954, 1962). The mechanism of injury and the ligamentous and bony anatomy may also explain why the ATFL is so frequently torn in isolation in two-thirds of ankle sprains (Broström 1964). This ligament is also torn three times as often as the CFL (Niederm et al. 1981), while a combined CFL and ATFL tear is found in about a quarter of cases (Broström 1964, 1965), usually in the more severe injuries (Glasgow et al. 1980; Brand & Collins 1982). For the same reasons, isolated CFL, PTFL, or other injuries are rarely noted (Broström 1964, 1965), and the ATFL is probably ruptured in all cases of lateral ligament injuries (Broström 1966).

The extent of injury is directly related to the force exerted on the lateral ligament. The force would be reduced when injury occurs while walking on a level surface, and would be amplified by running, jumping, or when an opponent's weight and velocity is exerted on the medial side of the foot, as often occurs in basketball. Landing on a bump, a stone, or an opponent's foot would further enhance both the force and the amount of the ligament forced to elongate. The force would be reduced both by the peroneal muscle contracting and by preventive taping (Barret et al. 1991; Geyer et al. 1992; Karlsson & Andreasson 1992; Jerosch et al 1995; Guskiewicz & Perrin 1996; Kaminiski 1997; Trowe et al. 1997), bracing (Garrick & Requa 1988; Ryan et al. in US Army Report 1994; Amoroso et al 1998; Leaderson & Wredmark 1995; Fiolkowski et al. 1997), or a protective shoe (Shapiro et al. 1994; Barrett & Bilisko 1995; Ottaviani et al. 1995; Ricard et al. 1997). The effect of the brace or shoe would be most apparent as the injury commences and before extreme tilting occurs, as the torque has been shown to increase tenfold as foot inversion proceeds from 7 to 48 degrees (Ottaviani et al. 1995; Thonnard et al. 1996) (figure 6.1).

Certain factors may offer a mechanical disadvantage when an athlete is about to suffer an ankle sprain, namely joint laxity (Finsterbush & Pogrund 1982; van den Hoogenband et al. 1984; Anderson 1986; Baumhauer et al. 1995), weak plantarflexors (Baumhauer et al. 1995), a low "Tarsal Index" (Benink

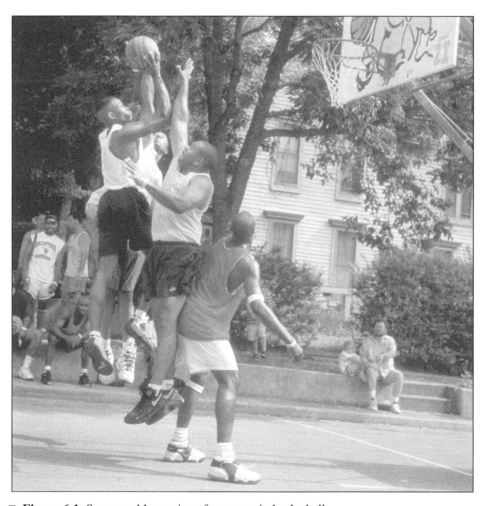

■ **Figure 6.1** Severe ankle sprains often occur in basketball.

1985), pes cavus (high arch), varus foot, or varus tibia (van Dijk 1994). The presence of these factors may call for enhanced protection and caution. Lavi in 1990 showed a certain tendency for soldiers with higher body mass index (BMI) to suffer ankle sprains. Our own work failed to disclose any relation between pes cavus, valgus heels, height, weight, BMI, or joint laxity and the occurrence of ankle sprains in 103 fighters of the Israel police force (Kahn et al. 1997; Kahn 1998) (figure 6.2).

■ Clinical Presentation and Staging

There is no standardized system for grading ankle injuries (see chapter 20 by Renström and Lynch). Grading is based on anatomical damage (Davis & Trevino 1995; Clanton 1999); clinical presentation (Jackson et al. 1974; Mann, Peri et al. 1993, Mann, Elishuv 1983; Mann et al. 1994, 1998), including pain, swelling, instability, and functional loss (Hamilton 1982; Kannus & Renstrom 1991; Kaikkonen et al. 1994, 1996); mechanism of trauma (Broström et al. 1965; Broström 1965; Dias 1979); stability (Davis & Trevino 1995; Clanton 1999); "severity" of the injury (Canale 1980, AMA standard nomenclature system) related to proposed treatment needed (Clanton 1999); or an undefined combination of any of the above. These are often far from objective or practical measures (Lindenfeld 1988), and grading by the "single" or "double" ligament damage method (Black et al. 1978; Cox 1985) would seem to be virtually impossible. Anatomical damage, pain, sensitivity, and functional impairment are

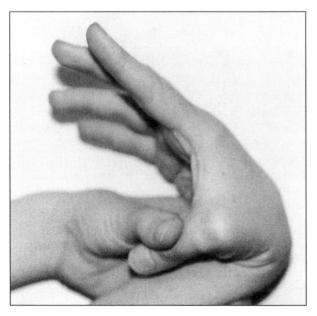

■ **Figure 6.2** Joint laxity may predispose a person to ankle sprains.

far from parallel, and measuring stability of an acutely injured ankle is obviously only theoretical. The following grading, or staging, systems for evaluating ankle sprains have been published and are currently in use.

Grading by Anatomic Damage or Severity of Injury

Determining which ligaments of the lateral ligament complex of the ankle have been damaged, and to what degree, seems an appealing method to grade the injury and has been used by various authorities.

The Anatomic System

This basic grading system is based on the number of ligaments of the lateral ligament complex that have been damaged (Clanton 1999):

- Grade I: ATFL sprain
- Grade II: ATFL and CFL sprains
- Grade III: ATFL, CFL, and PTFL sprains

AMA Standard Nomenclature System by Severity

The AMA (American Medical Association) has devised a simple classification system based on the severity of ligament injury (adapted from Clanton 1999):

- Grade 1: ligament stretched
- Grade 2: ligament partially torn
- Grade 3: ligament completely torn

Staging System Proposed by Davis & Trevino

In 1995, Davis & Trevino proposed a rather complicated system based on anatomical damage. The system attempts to combine the anatomical damage, severity of injury, additional injuries occurring to the ankle, and the grade of instability (table 6.1).

Grading by Clinical Presentation Symptoms

Jackson, Ashley, and Powell devised the following system in 1974:

- Mild sprain: minimal functional loss, no limp, minimal or no swelling, point tenderness, pain with reproduction of mechanism of injury
- Moderate sprain: moderate functional loss, unable to toe-rise or hop on injured ankle, limp when walking, localized swelling, point tenderness
- Severe sprain: diffuse tenderness and swelling, crutches preferred by patient for ambulation

Table 6.1 Davis & Trevino Staging System

Grade	Pathology	Instability
I	Stretch	None
II	Partial tear	Mild to moderate
IIIa	Complete tear of ATFL	Positive anterior drawer test
IIIb	Complete tear of ATFL and CFL	Positive anterior drawer and talar tilt tests
IIIc1	Complete tear of ATFL and CFL peroneal tendon tear	Positive anterior drawer and talar tilt tests Peroneal tendon stable in groove but tender to palpation
IIIc2	Complete tear of ATFL and CFL: peroneal tendon subluxation or dislocation	Positive anterior drawer and talar tilt tests Peroneal tendon subluxation or dislocation with resisted eversion and dorsiflexion
IVa	Complete tear of ATFL and CFL: avulsion fraction of fibula	Positive anterior drawer and talar tilt tests
IVb	Complete tear of ATFL and CFL: osteochondral fracture of talus	Positive anterior drawer and talar tilt tests
IVc	Complete tear of ATFL and CFL: lateral process fracture of talus	Positive anterior drawer and talar tilt tests

ATFL, anterior talofibular; CFL, calcaneofibular

Grading by Anatomic Damage and Clinical Presentation Symptoms

Hamilton and Kaikkonen proposed systems of grading that combined anatomic damage with patient symptoms.

Hamilton in 1982 graded acute ankle sprains as follows:

- Grade I: ligament stretch with no tear, little swelling or tenderness, minimal or no functional loss, and no mechanical joint instability

- Grade II: torn ATFL with intact CFL with partial tear, moderate pain, swelling, tenderness, some loss of joint motion, and mild joint instability

- Grade III: Tear of the entire lateral ligament complex with marked swelling, hemorrhage, and tenderness

Kaikkonen et al. 1994, whose research was based on other sources (Chapman 1975; Balduini & Tetziaff 1982; Dramond 1989; Lassiter et al. 1989; Kaikkonen et al. 1996), summarized the grading of ankle sprains as follows:

- Grade I (mild sprain): stretch of the ligaments without macroscopic tearing, little swelling or tenderness, slight or no functional loss, and no mechanical instability of the joint

- Grade II (moderate sprain): partial macroscopic tear of the ligaments with moderate pain, swelling, and tenderness, with some loss of motion and mild or moderate instability

- Grade III (severe sprain): complete rupture of the ligaments with severe swelling, hemorrhage, and tenderness, with loss of motion and considerable abnormal motion and instability

Grading for Outpatient Clinic Use

Following a developing need for a practical grading system to be used in the outpatient clinic for current research, we devised a grading system to be used both prospectively and retrospectively when a patient has been referred from the emergency room to the outpatient service (Mann et al. 1991, 1993, 1994, 1998; Peri 1992). Readers may photocopy this form "Scoring System for Acute Ankle Sprains" on page 58, for their own use.

The grading system is based on the separate grading of pain, swelling, and inability to walk, giving 0 to 3 points for each (0 = none, 1 = mild, 2 = moderate, 3 = severe) and calculating the total score: grade I, 1-3 points; grade II, 4-6 points; grade III, 7-9 points. The grading is done by the referring physician, the examining physician, nurse, physiotherapist, or by the patient.

We found the staging system practical, easy to use, and relatively accurate, as virtually all complications occurred in grade II and III sprains (see figure

6.3, a and b). Many people with sprains of grade I did not even return to the clinic for a second visit.

Grading System Related to Treatment Proposed by Clanton

In 1999, Clanton suggested a staging system related solely to treatment protocols requested. The system divided the injuries into only two classes, types I and II.

Type I

A type I injury is an ankle that is shown to be stable through clinical testing (see chapter 7). It may be necessary to use anesthesia to perform the testing. This type of ankle injury will require only symptomatic treatment. This would include nonsteroidal anti-inflammatory drugs, bandaging, and physical therapy aimed to regain motion, strength, and functional stability.

Type II

A type II injury will, upon clinical examination, yield positive results with both the anterior drawer and talar tilt tests, revealing that it is unstable. People with type II ankle injuries are divided into two groups:

■ **Group 1** patients will be nonathletes or older patients. They will require functional treatment, including 2 to 3 weeks of immobilization in a cast or walking boot, followed by a stirrup brace and ankle rehabilitation with Achilles stretching, peroneal strengthening, and proprioceptive reeducation.

■ **Group 2** will comprise young athletes. This group may be further divided into three types:

-**Type A** patients who, when tested, present with negative stress radiograph findings. These patients should be treated functionally, as described for Group 1.

-**Type B** patients will present with positive tibiotalar stress radiograph findings (talar tilt >15 degrees; anterior drawer >1 cm). They will require treatment by surgical repair.

-**Type C** patients will present with subtalar instability. They, too, should be treated functionally as described for Group 1.

■ References

Amoroso PJ, Ryan JB, Bickley B, Leitschuh P, Taylor DC, Jones BH. 1998. Braced for impact: Reducing military paratroopers' ankle sprains using outside-the-boot braces. J Trauma Sep 45(3):575-580.

Anderson KJ, Lecocq JF. 1954. Operative treatment of injury to the fibular collateral ligament of the ankle. J Bone Joint Surg Am 36:825-832.

Anderson KJ, Lecocq JF, Clayton ML. 1962. Athletic injury to the fibular collateral ligament of the ankle. Clin Orthop 23:126-160.

Anderson LJ. 1986. Ligamentous laxity and athletics. JAMA 256:527.

Attarian DE, McCrackin HK, DeVito DP. 1985. Biomechanical characteristics of human ankle ligaments. Foot Ankle Int 6:54-58.

Scoring System for Acute Ankle Sprains

Patient name: _____   Date: _____

Physician name: _____

Evaluator name: _____   Facility: _____

Instructions: Assign 0 to 3 points (0 = none; 1 = mild; 2 = moderate; 3 = severe) for each of the three subjects (pain, swelling, walking inability). Calculate total score to determine grade of sprain.

Subject/grading	0	1	2	3
Pain				
Swelling				
Walking inability				

Total Score:

Grade of Sprain:

(Grade I: 1-3 points; Grade II: 4-6 points; Grade III: 7-9 points)

From Meir Nyska and Gideon Mann, eds., 2002, *The Unstable Ankle* (Champaign, IL: Human Kinetics).

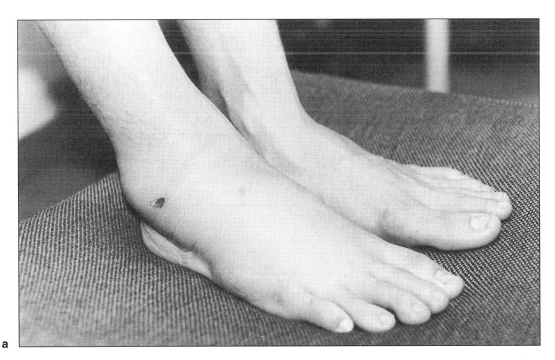

■ **Figure 6.3a** A grade III ankle sprain. Pain and swelling were severe, and the patient was unable to walk.

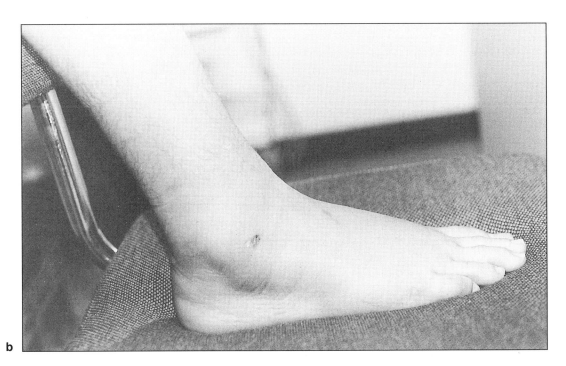

■ **Figure 6.3b** A grade III ankle sprain. Close-up of the injured ankle.

Attarian DE, McCrakin H J, Garrett WE. 1985. A biomechanical study of human lateral ankle ligaments and autogenous reconstructive grafts. Am J Sports Med 13:377-381.

Balduini FC, Tetziaff J. 1982. Historical perspective on injuries of the ligaments of the ankle. Clin Sports Med 1:3-12.

Balduini FC, Vegso JJ, Torg JS, Torg E. 1987. Management and rehabilitation of ligamentous injuries to the ankle. Am J Sports Med 4(5):364-380.

Barrett J, Bilisko T. 1995. The role of shoes in the prevention of ankle sprains. Sports Med 20(4):277-280.

Baumhauer JF, Alosa DM, Renstrom AF, Trevino S, Beynnon B. 1995. Test-retest reliability of ankle injury risk factors. Am J Sports Med 23(5):571-574.

Benink RJ. 1985. The constraint mechanism of the human tarsus: A roentgenological experimental study. Acta Orthop Scand Suppl 215:1-135.

Black HM, Brand R, Eichelberger MR. 1978. An improved technique for the evaluation of ligamentous injury in severe ankle sprains. Am J Sports Med 6(5):276-282.

Brand RL, Collins NMF. 1982. Operative management of ligamentous injuries to the ankle. Clin Sports Med 1:211.

Broström L. 1964. Sprained ankles I. Anatomic lesions in recent sprains. Acta Chir Scand 128:483-495.

Broström L. 1965. Sprained ankles III. Clinical observations in recent ligament ruptures. Acta Chir Scand 130:560-569.

Broström L. 1966. Sprained ankles VI. Surgical treatment of ligament ruptures. Acta Chir Scand 132:551-565.

Broström L, Liljedahl SO, Lindvald N. 1965. Sprained ankles II. Arthrographic diagnosis of recent ligament ruptures. Acta Chir Scand 129:485-499.

Calliet R. 1997. Foot and ankle pain. Philadelphia: FA Davis. p. 3-207.

Chapman MW. 1975. Part III. Sprains of the ankle. Instr Course Lect 24:294-306.

Clanton TO. 1999. Athletic injuries to the soft tissues of the foot and ankle. In Coughlin MJ, Mann RA, editors. Surgery of the Foot and Ankle, 7th ed. St Louis: Mosby. p. 1090-1209.

Coutts B, Woodward PE. 1965. Surgery and sprained ankles. Clin Orthop Related Res 42:81-90.

Cox JS. 1985. Surgical and nonsurgical treatment of acute ankle sprains. Clin Orthop (198):118-126.

Davis PF, Trevino SG. 1995. Ankle injuries. In Baxter DE, editor. The foot and ankle in sport. St. Louis: Mosby. p. 147-169.

Dias LS. 1979. The lateral ankle sprain: An experimental study. J Trauma 19(4):266-269.

Dramond JE. 1989. Rehabilitation of ankle sprains. Clin Sports Med 8:887-891.

Ekstrand J, Tropp H. 1990. The incidence of ankle sprains in soccer. Foot Ankle Int 11(1):41-44.

Evans DL. 1953. Recurrent instability of the ankle: A method of surgical treatment. Proc R Sco Med 46:343-344.

Finsterbush A, Pogrund H. 1982. The hypermobility syndrome. Musculoskeletal complaints in 100 consecutive cases of generalized joint hypermobility. Clin Orthop 168:124-127.

Fiolkowski P, Kaminski TW, Bauer JA. 1997. The effects of prophylactic ankle bracing on ankle biomechanics. J Athl Train 32(2):13.

Garrick JG. 1977. The frequency of injury, mechanism of injury and epidemiology of ankle sprains. Am J Sports Med 5:241-242.

Garrick JG, Requa RK. 1988. The epidemiology of foot and ankle injuries in sports. Clin Sports Med 7(1):29-36.

Geyer M, Bergmann C, Siebert E. Effect of taping in ballet dancers with overuse syndromes on stabilisation, proprioception and muscular activity by using electromyographic and 3-D motion analysis. Poster 76. ESSKA meeting: First World Congress of Sports Trauma, Fifth Congress of the European Society of Knee Surgery and Arthroscopy 25-29 May 1992, Palma de Mallorca, Spain.

Glasgow M, Jackson A, Jamieson AM. 1980. Instability of the ankle after injury to the lateral ligament. J Bone Joint Surg Br 62:196-200.

Guskiewicz KM, Perrin DH. 1996. Effect of orthotics on postural sway following inversion ankle sprain. J Orthop Sports Phys Ther 23(5):326-331.

Hamilton WG. 1982. Sprained ankles in ballet dancers. Foot Ankle Int 3(2):99-102.

Jackson DW, Ashley RL, Powell JW. 1974. Ankle sprains in young athletes: Relation of severity and disability. Clin Orthop 101:201-215.

Jerosch J, Hoffstetter I, Bork H, Bischof M. 1995. The influence of orthoses on the proprioception of the ankle joint. Knee Surg Sports Trauma Arth 3(1):39-46.

Kahn G. 1998. Ankle sprain prevention with an over-shoe brace in the military set-up [M.D. thesis]. Sackler Tel Aviv University Medical School, Tel Aviv, Israel. Directed by Mann G, Nyska M, Dvir Z.

Kahn G, Mann G, Nyska M, Zeev A, Lau J, Matan Y, Eliashuv O, Ben-Gal S, Constantini N, Siderer M. 1997. Ankle sprains. Prevention with an over-shoe brace in the military set up [M.D. thesis of G Kahn]. Tel Aviv: Tel Aviv University. Presented at the 14th International Jerusalem Symposium on Sports Injuries, February.

Kaikkonen A, Kannus P, Jarvinen M. 1994. A performance test protocol and scoring scale for the evaluation of ankle injuries. Am J Sports Med 22(4):462-469.

Kaikkonen A, Kannus P, Jarvinen M. 1996. Surgery versus functional treatment in ankle ligament tears. Clin Orthop 326:194-202.

Kaminiski TW. 1997. Modified Romberg balance test scores between uninjured and functionally unstable ankles. J Athl Train 32(2):25.

Kannus P, Renstrom P. 1991. Current concepts review: Treatment for acute tears of the lateral ligaments of the ankle. J Bone Joint Surg Am 73(2):305-312.

Karlsson J, Andreasson GO. 1992. The effect of external ankle support in chronic lateral ankle joint instability: An electromyographic study. Am J Sports Med 20:257-261.

Knight KL. 1978. Identification of ligament torn by forceful inversion of cadaver ankles in plantar and dorsiflexion. Med Sci Sports 10:38-42.

Kristiansen B. 1981. Evans' repair of lateral instability of the ankle joint. Acta Orthop Scand 52:679-682.

Lassiter TE Jr, Malone TR, Garret WE. 1989. Injury to the lateral ligaments of the ankle. Orthop Clin North Am 629-640.

Lavi O. 1990. A prospective study of risk factors for lateral ankle sprains, and the effect of training with 3/4 high shoe on the incidence of ankle sprains among recruits [M.D. thesis]. Jerusalem, Israel: Hebrew University, School of Medicine.

Leaderson J, Wredmark T. 1995. Treatment of acute ankle sprain: Comparison of semi-rigid ankle brace and compression bandage in 73 patients. Acta Orthop Scand 66:529-531.

Lindenfeld TN. 1988. The differentiation and treatment of ankle sprains. Orthop 11(1):203-206.

Liu SH, Jason WJ. 1994. Lateral ankle sprains and instability problems. Clin Sports Med 13:793-809.

Machlum S, Daljord OA. 1984. Acute sports injuries in Oslo: A one-year study. Br J Sports Med 18:181-185.

Mack RP. 1982. Ankle injuries in athletes. Clin Sports Med 1:71-84.

Mann G, Elishuv O, Perry C, Finsterbush A, Frankl U, Nyska M, Matan Y. 1994. Recurrent ankle sprain: Literature review. Israel J of Sports Med 104-113.

Mann G, Elishuv O, Lowe J. 1998. Repeated ankle sprain revisited: Pathology and pathogenesis. In Chan KM, Fu F, Maffulli N, Rolf C, Kurosaka M , Liu S, editors.

Controversies in orthopedic sports medicine. Baltimore: Williams & Wilkins. p. 445-459.

Mann G, Elishuv O, Nyska M, Chaimsky G, Finsterbush A, Perry C. 1993. Recurrent ankle sprain: Experience with modification of William Reefing technique. J Orthop Tech 8(3):361-376.

Mann G, Finsterbush A, Matan Y, Peri H, Frankl U. 1988. Capsular reefing with suture to the extensor digitorium muscle (by Williams) as treatment for recurrent ankle sprain. Paper presented at the Israel Orthopaedic Association Annual Meeting, December, Herziliya, Israel.

Mann G, Peri H, Nyska M, Matan Y, Frankl U, Finsterbush A. 1993. Ankle sprain: occurrence of chronic functional instability and its chronic relation to mechanical instability: A prospective study. Presented at the 9th International Jerusalem Symposium on Sports Injuries, January, Maale Hamisha, Israel.

Mukerjee K, Gangopadhyay P. 1983. Extensor digitorium brevis transfer in chronic unstable ankles. J Royal Col Surg Ed 28:250-255.

Niederm B, Anderson A, Vuust M. 1981. Rupture of the lateral ligament of the ankle: Operation of plaster cast. Acta Orthop Scand 52:579-587.

Ottaviani RA, Ashton-Miller JA, Kothari SU, Wojtys EM. 1995. Basketball shoe height and the maximal muscular resistance to applied ankle inversion and eversion moments. Am J Sports Med 23(4):418-423.

Peri H. 1992. Ankle sprains [M.D. thesis directed by G Mann, M Nyska, and A Finsterbush]. Hadassah-Hebrew University School of Medicine, Jerusalem, Israel.

Ricard MD, Saret JJ, Schulthies SS. 1997. Comparison of the amount and rate of inversion between high top and low top shoes. J Athl Train 32(2):13.

Sandelin J, Santavirta S, Lattila R, Vuolle P, Sarna S. 1988. Sports injuries in a large urban population: Occurrence and epidemiological aspects. Int J Sports Med 16(5):501-511.

Shapiro MS, Kabo JM, Mitchell PW, Loren G, Tsenter M. 1994. Ankle sprain prophylaxis: An analysis of the stabilizing effects of braces and tape. Am J Sports Med 22(1):78-82.

Siegler S, Block J, Schneck CD. 1998. The mechanical characteristics of the collateral ligaments of the human ankle joint. Foot Ankle Int 8:234-242.

Thonnard JL, Bragard D, Willems PA, Plaghki L. 1996. Stability of the braced ankle: A biomechanical investigation. Am J Sports Med 24:256-261.

Trowe B, Buxton BP, German TL, Joyner AB, McMillian JL, Tsang KKW. 1997. The effects of prophylactic taping on ankle joint motion and performance. J Athl Train 32(2):14.

U.S. Army Research Institute of Environmental Medicine. Impact of an outside-the-boot ankle brace on sprains associated with military airborne training. Natick MA. Report No. T95-1

van den Hoogenband CR, van Moppes FI, Stapert JW, Greep JM. 1984. Clinical diagnosis, arthroscopy, stress examination and surgical findings after inversion trauma of the ankle. Arch Orthop Trauma Surg 103(2):115-119.

van Dijk CN. 1994. On diagnostic strategies in patients with severe ankle sprain [Ph.D. thesis]. University of Amsterdam, Amsterdam.

Chapter 7

Scoring Systems Evaluating Ankle Function

Gideon Mann, MD; Meir Nyska, MD; and Y. Matan, MD

In 1975, Good et al. published a grading system based on four categories for evaluating the outcome of ankle injuries: excellent, good, fair, and poor. Since then, another five scoring scales have been suggested for evaluating the outcome of ankle sprains, evaluating the success of conservative treatment protocols, assessing the success of surgical procedures, or evaluating the severity and prognosis of an ankle sprain at the acute stage of injury. The various scoring systems are discussed in this chapter.

■ Function and Desirable Characteristics

Development of ankle scoring systems would be expected as part of the growing accuracy required for evaluation of acute ankle injury treatment protocols and evaluation of various surgical techniques for ankle reconstruction. Realizing their obvious importance in obtaining objective knowledge on the well-being of the previously injured athlete, and understanding the complexity of success and failure, it seems both unusual and surprising that scoring systems were not developed earlier and are still rarely seen in current use.

Scoring systems are devised to combine the various functional, clinical, objective measurement, and possibly radiological findings that are used to assess the "good," "fair," or "poor" result of an injury or mode of treatment. A scoring system should include the major findings that determine the "result" and should include enough factors to make the scoring system accurate, reliable, and reproducible, but not include so many factors as to make its use impractical. The factors included should be practical enough to be available for each patient (the system should not include, for example, an MRI or a 10K run) and should preferably be completed by a physician or physiotherapist not involved in the conservative or surgical treatment protocol being tested. The maximum number of points should be easily and readily calculated (a maximal of 10, 20, 50, or 100 points).

■ Various Scoring Systems

Scoring systems for hip (Anderson 1972; d'Aubigne & Postel 1954; Harris 1969; Larsson 1974) or knee (Larsson 1974; Lysholm & Gillqvist 1982; Oretorp et al. 1979) evaluation have been in use for the last three decades. An evaluation system for ankle fractures was suggested in the early 1980s (Olerod & Molander 1984). In 1979, Sefton et al. used a simple system to evaluate surgically treated unstable ankles based on Good, Jones, and Livingstone (1975). He categorized the results into "excellent," "good," "fair," and "poor" (table 7.1).

The first scoring system for surgically repaired ankle sprains was devised by St. Pierre et al. in 1982, but it failed to gain popularity (table 7.2). St. Pierre's system is based on separate evaluation of activity level, pain, swelling, and functional instability. Each was evaluated as excellent (0), good (1), fair (2), or failure (3), and the results were summarized as follows: 0 = excellent; 1 = good; 2-6 = fair; greater than 6 = failure.

Scoring System of Karlsson and Peterson

Karlsson and Peterson (1991) published a scoring system based on eight functional observations (table 7.3): pain, swelling, subjective instability, stiffness, stair climbing, running, work activities, and use of external support. Each item was allowed a certain number of points, amounting to a total maximum of 100 points. The scoring scale showed a good correlation to a visual analog estimation of ankle function as compiled by the patient, and a good correlation to the

Table 7.1 Sefton Scoring Scale

Grade 1	Full activity, including strenuous sport No pain, swelling, or giving way
Grade 2	Occasional aching only after strenuous exercise No giving way or feeling of apprehension
Grade 3	No giving way but some remaining apprehension, especially on rough ground
Grade 4	Recurrent instability and giving way in normal activities, with episodes of pain and swelling

Reprinted from Sefton et al. 1979.

Table 7.2 St. Pierre Functional Scale for Evaluation of Ankle Function After Reconstruction

Excellent	Good	Fair	Failure
Level of activity after treatment			
0 - Full return to activity and athletics	1- Return to full activity with support	2 - Unable to return to athletics	3 - Decreased activity
Intensity of pain			
0 - No pain	1 - Mild pain	2 - Moderate pain	3 - Severe pain
Swelling			
0 - No swelling	1 - Swells after exercise	2 - Swells after routine activity	3 - Swells all of the time
Functional instability			
0 - No evidence of instability (no sprains)	1 - Mild instability (1 sprain/year)	2 - Moderate instability (2-3 sprains/year)	3 - Severe instability (greater than 3 sprains/year)

Reprinted from St. Pierre et al. 1982.

Scale:

Grade of operative repair	Functional result
0	Excellent
1	Good
2-6	Fair
> 6	Failure

functional score of St. Pierre, to the talar anterior translation, and to the talar tilt.

Scoring System of Mann et al.

In 1991 we found a need to develop a scoring system to be used in following up acute ankle sprains as well as surgically treated patients. The system was first used in the MD thesis of H. Peri (1992) and first presented at the International Jerusalem Symposium on Sports Injuries (Mann, Matan et al. 1993). The system was later published in various publications (Mann, Elishuv et al. 1993, 1994, 1998) and presented on a number of occasions.

The scoring system was based on two tables: an objective score (table 7.4a) (36 points) and a functional score (table 7.4b) (64 points) amounting to a total maximum score of 100 points. The system emphasized the functional ability of the athlete while allowing less points to purely nonfunctional measurements such as radiological findings (tilt and drawer) or range of motion.

The objective measurement table (table 7.4a, 36 points) included the modified Romberg Test, jump from height, figure-eight run, cutting ability, swelling, sensitivity to pressure, drawer test (in millimeters), tilt test (in degrees), dorsiflexion, plantarflexion, varus heel, and crepitation, with a

Table 7.3 Karlsson and Peterson Scoring System for Ankle Function

	Degree	Score
Pain	None During exercise (training, etc.) Walking on uneven surface Walking on even surface Constant (severe)	20 15 10 5 0
Swelling	None After exercise Constant	10 5 0
Instability (subjective)	None 1-2/year (during exercise) 1-2/month (during exercise) Walking on uneven ground Walking on even ground Constant (severe) using ankle support	25 20 15 10 5 0
Stiffness	None Moderate (morning, after exercise) Marked (constant, severe)	5 2 0
Stair climbing	No problems Impaired (instability) Impossible	10 5 0
Running	No problems Impaired Impossible	10 5 0
Work activities	Same as pre-injury Same work, less sports, normal leisure activities Lighter work, no sports, normal leisure activities Severely impaired work capacity, decreased leisure activities	15 10 5 0
Support	None Ankle support during exercise Ankle support during daily activities	5 2 0

Adapted from Karlsson and Peterson 1981.

Table 7.4a Objective Scoring System

		Score	1 wk	6 wks	12 wks	6 mos	1 yr
Romberg Test modifications (30 sec.)	No side-to-side difference (up to 5 sec) Slight difficulty (5 to 15 sec) Difficult (over 15 sec difference)	9 4 0					
Jump 30 cm	Symmetrical landing Careful at landing Lands on one leg	3 2 0					
Figure-eight run	Free Limited Impossible	3 2 0					
Cutting	Free Limited Impossible	3 2 0					
Swelling	None Mild Obvious	3 2 0					
Sensitivity	None Mild Obvious	3 2 0					

		Score	1 wk	6 wks	12 wks	6 mos	1 yr
Drawer	Like other side Mild up to 4 mm Severe over 4 mm	2 1 0					
Tilt	Like other side Mild up to 5° Severe over 5°	2 1 0					
Dorsiflexion	Like other side Loss up to 10° Loss over 10°	2 1 0					
Plantarflexion	Like other side Loss up to 10° Loss over 10°	2 1 0					
Varus of heel	Like other side Loss up to 10° Loss over 10°	2 1 0					
Crepitation	None Mild Obvious	2 1 0					

Part I of the system devised by Mann, Peri, and Finsterbush 1991. The total possible score for the objective scoring system is 36 points.

Table 7.4b Functional Scoring System

		Score	First visit	6 wks	12 wks	6 mos	1 yr
Recurrent sprain	None Once in 3 months Once in 1 or 2 months Once a week/any activity	28 20 10 0					
Sports	Full return as before Return at lower level Return to noncompetitive sport Did not return to sport	10 7 4 0					
Daily activity	Can run on any surface Can run only on flat surface Can walk but not run on any surface Can walk only on flat surface Difficulty walking and daily activity	12 9 6 3 0					
Walking slant 45°	No limitations Difficult Impossible	5 3 0					
Pain	None After stressful sports After nonstressful sports Without physical activity Severe and frequent	5 4 3 2 0					
Orthopedic instrumental use	Not using Elastic support only Firm (hard) support	4 2 0					

Part II of the system devised by Mann, Peri, and Finsterbush 1991. The total possible score for the functional scoring system is 64 points.

total of 12 measurements. The functional table (table 7.4b, 64 points) included frequency of recurrent sprain, sports activity, daily activities, walking on a slant, pain, and use of orthopedic supports, with a total of 36 functions.

The combined scoring system showed a significant correlation with the late occurrence or nonoccurrence of chronic functional instability (p = .005). We have found this scoring system to be both accurate and practical for use in the clinical or research setting for evaluating the outcome of athletes who have been either conservatively or surgically treated for ankle sprains.

The objective and functional scoring systems have a maximum combined score of 100 points.

Scoring System of Kaikkonen et al.

In 1994, Kaikkonen et al. published a scoring system for evaluating ankle injuries (table 7.5). The system was based on three questions chosen after assessment of 11 functional inquiries, two clinical measurements, two strength tests, one functional test, and one balance test. The total number of factors assessed would thus amount to nine, with a maximum score of 100 points.

The authors found a significant correlation of the system to isokinetic ankle strength, patients' subjective evaluations of their own recovery, and patients' subjective functional assessments (Kaikkonen 1994).

Table 7.5 Scoring Scale[a] for Subjective and Functional Follow-Up Evaluation

Questions	Subjective assessment of the injured ankle	
	no symptoms of any kind[b]	15
	mild symptoms	10
	moderate symptoms	5
	severe symptoms	0
	Can you walk normally?	
	yes	15
	no	0
	Can you run normally?	
	yes	10
	no	0
Functional test	Climbing down stairs[c]	
	< 18 seconds	10
	18 to 20 seconds	5
	> 20 seconds	0
Strength tests	Rising on heels with injured leg	
	> 40 times	10
	30 to 39 times	5
	< 30 times	0
	Rising on toes with injured leg	
	> 40 times	10
	30 to 39 times	5
	< 30 times	0
Balance test	Single-limb stance with injured leg	
	> 55 seconds	10
	50 to 55 seconds	5
	< 50 seconds	0
Clinical measurements	Laxity of the ankle joint (ADS)	
	stable (≤ 5 mm)	10
	moderate instability (6-10 mm)	5
	severe instability (> 10 mm)	0
	Dorsiflexion range of motion, injured leg	
	≥ 10°	10
	5°-9°	5
	< 5°	0

[a] Total: Excellent = 85-100; Good = 70-80; Fair = 55-65; Poor ≤ 50.

[b] Pain, swelling, stiffness, tenderness, or giving way during activity (mild, only one of these symptoms is present; severe, four or more of these symptoms are present).

[c] Two levels of staircase (length, 12 m) with 44 steps (height, 18 cm; depth, 22 cm).

Adapted from Kaikkonen, Kannus, and Jarvinen 1994.

Scoring System of de Bie et al.

In 1997, de Bie et al. published a scoring system to be used in acute ankle sprains not subjected to surgery (table 7.6). The system is based on functional evaluation of pain, stability, weight bearing, swelling, and the walking pattern, with a maximum obtainable score of 100 points. The system was used to enable prognosis in acute injuries and gave a good correlation with the four-week outcome in 81% of patients, and with the two-week outcome in 97% of patients (de Bie et al. 1997).

The diversity of approaches and opinions has brought together a working group that is attempting to assess and formulate an ankle scoring system protocol that can be both widely accepted and practical. This group was initiated by Smith and Nephew Co. and met in Orlando, Florida, during the International Federation of Sports Medicine/American College of Sports Medicine (FIMS/ACSM) joint meeting in May 1998. The work of this group is in process and has not yet been completed. (Working team 1998).

■ References

Anderson G. 1972. Hip assessment: A comparison of nine different methods. J Bone Joint Surg Am 54:621-625.

d'Aubigne MD, Postel M. 1954. Functional results of hip arthroplasty with acrylic prosthesis. J Bone Joint Surg Am 36:451-475.

de Bie RA, de Vet HC, van den Wildenberg FA, Lenssen T, Knipschild PG. 1997. The prognosis of ankle sprains. Int J Sports Med 18(4):285-289.

Good CJ, Jones MA, Livingstone BN. 1975. Reconstruction of the lateral ligament of the ankle. Injury 7:63-65.

Harris WH. 1969. Traumatic arthritis of the hip after dislocation and acetabular fractures: Treatment by mold arthroplasty. J Bone Joint Surg Am 51:737-754.

Kaikkonen A, Kannus P, Jarvinen M. 1994. A performance test protocol and scoring scale for the evaluation of ankle injuries. Am J Sports Med 22(4):462-469.

Karlsson J, Peterson L. 1991. Evaluation of ankle joint function: the use of a scoring scale. Foot Ankle Int 1:15-19.

Larsson R. 1974. Rating sheet for knee function. In Smillie I, editor. Diseases of the knee joint. Philadelphia: Churchill Livingstone. p. 29-30.

Lysholm J, Gillqvist J. 1982. Evaluation of knee ligament surgery results with special emphasis on the use of a scoring scale. Am J Sports Med 10:150-154.

Table 7.6 Functional Score for Assessment of Acute Lateral Ankle Sprains (Not Subjected to Surgery) in Aim of Anticipating Their Prognosis

Category	Item	Score
Pain	None	35
	During sports	30
	During running on nonlevel surface	25
	During running on level surface	20
	During walking on nonlevel surface	15
	While carrying load	10
	Constant pain	5
Instability	None	25
	Sometimes during sports (less than once a day)	20
	Frequently during sports (daily)	15
	Sometimes during ADL* (less than once a day)	10
	Frequently during ADL (daily)	5
	Every step	0
Weight bearing	Jumping	20
	Standing on toes of injured leg	15
	Standing on injured leg	10
	Standing on two legs	5
	None	0
Swelling	None	10
	Light	6
	Mild	3
	Severe	0
Gait pattern	Running	10
	Normal gait	6
	Mild limp	3
	Severe limp	0

*ADL: activities of daily living

Adapted from de Bie et al. 1997.

Mann G, Elishuv O, Lowe J, Finsterbush A, Frank U, Nyska M, Matan Y. 1994. Recurrent ankle sprain: Literature review. Israel J Sports Med January:104-108.

Mann G, Elishuv O, Nyska M, Chaimsky G, Finsterbush A, Perry C. 1993. Recurrent ankle sprain: Experience with modification of William Reefing technique. J Orthop Tech 8(3):361-376.

Mann G, Elishuv O, Lowe J, Finsterbush A, Constantini N, Matan Y, Nyska M. 1998. Repeated ankle sprain revisited: Pathology and pathogenesis. In Chan KM, Fu F, Maffulli N, Rolf C, Kurosaka M, Liu S, editors. Controversies in orthopedic sports medicine. Baltimore: Williams & Wilkins. p. 445-449.

Mann G, Matan Y, Frankel U, Nyska M, Peri H, Soran A, Milgrom M, Finsterbush A. 1993. Ankle sprain: occurrence of chronic functional instability and its chronic relation to mechanical instability: a prospective study. Presented at the Ninth International Jerusalem Symposium on Sports Injuries, Jerusalem, Israel, January.

Olerod C, Molander H. 1984. A scoring scale for symptom evaluation after ankle fractures. Arch Orthop Trauma Surg 103:190-194.

Oretorp N, Gillqvist J, Liljedahl SO. 1979. Long term results of surgery for non-acute antero-medial rotatory instability of the knee. Acta Orthop Scand 50:329-336.

Peri H. 1992. Ankle sprains [MD thesis directed by G Mann, M Nyska, and A Finsterbush]. Hadassah-Hebrew University School of Medicine.

Sefton GK, George J, Filton JM, McMullen H. 1979. Reconstruction of the anterior talo-fibular ligament for the treatment of the unstable ankle. J Bone Joint Surg Br 61:352-54.

St. Pierre R, Allman F, Bassett FH III, Goldner JL, Fleming LL. 1982. A review of lateral ankle ligamentous reconstruction. Foot Ankle Int 3:114-123.

Working team for composing an accepted international ankle evaluation scoring system. Meeting was held during the ACSM annual meeting in Orlando, Florida, May 1998 and was initiated by Smith and Nephew Corporation. The group included A. Renström, J. Karlsson, P. Vaes, G. Mann, and C.N. van Dijk.

Chapter 8

Diagnostic Aspects of Chronic Ankle Instability

Beat Hintermann, MD

Inversion ankle injuries are the most common musculoskeletal complaint in the emergency room. Ankle sprains result from a sudden, violent inversion and flexion stress to the hindfoot. The lateral ligament complex is overwhelmed as the weightbearing force passes lateral to the body of the talus and is partially absorbed by the lateral ligaments. The degree of damage determines the severity of the sprain—mild, moderate, or severe. Because ankle sprains are so common, they are often regarded lightly by both the patient and the examining physician. This can lead to inadequate assessment and treatment, which can significantly prolong recovery. Such a negligent attitude can have consequences other than a prolonged recovery. The anatomy of the hindfoot is complex, and many other structures may be injured by mechanisms similar to those that produce the common ankle sprain. When these injuries are missed, the opportunity for early diagnosis and treatment is lost. The purpose of the present chapter is to outline a method of approaching the patient with chronic ankle instability.

■ The Problem

Most patients recover from their sprain in a matter of weeks, depending on the severity of the injury. Although the accepted time for recovery is arbitrary, 3 months would seem sufficient time for the patient with a routine ankle sprain to recover and return to full activities. There is, however, no estimate available for the number of injuries that are misdiagnosed as ankle sprains. The incidence of chronic ankle instability after acute lateral ankle sprains has been estimated as being from 10% to 30% (Peters et al. 1991).

■ Examination

A thorough examination is crucial, and it must include a history and physical examination. It may also involve radiological examination, other imaging methods, or arthroscopy.

■ **History.** The most important diagnostic tool for assessing the patient with chronic ankle instability is taking the time to obtain an adequate history of the events leading up to the current problem. It is tremendously important to determine as accurately as possible the mechanism of injury and the site of the initial pain and swelling. Medial ankle sprains are rare, and pain and swelling in this area is often a result of a posterior tibial tendon injury. A lateral ankle injury sustained in a ski boot suggests a peroneal tendon injury. Recurrent lateral ankle injuries with a familial history of cavus feet may lead to a diagnosis of neuromuscular imbalance. Most important in diagnosis of chronic ankle instability is a history of ankle insecurity, instability, and giving way (Mann et al. 1994).

■ **Physical examination.** The examination includes the observation of the patient's gait for altered stance on the affected site. Chronic ankle instability can make toe walking difficult. Limited hindfoot inversion and eversion combined with a history of repeated sprains suggest the diagnosis of tarsal coalition. The anterior drawer and clinical talar tilt test should be performed and the results compared to the results of the opposite site.

■ **Radiological examination.** Plain radiographs of the ankle and hindfoot should include anterior-posterior (AP) and lateral views. If ankle or subtalar instability is suspected, inversion stress tests and anterior drawer tests can be useful. Because wide variations of physiological laxity are present in 4% to 5% of the population, radiological diagnosis of lateral ankle instability may be highly unreliable (Anderson et al. 1962).

■ **Further imaging methods.** A 99Tc bone scan can be used as a screen to locate abnormalities. It can be particularly useful in differentiating between bony and soft tissue problems, and thus it should be used before choosing between a CT scan or MRI for further information. Today, in general, there is a very limited role for arthrograms, tomograms, or tenograms.

■ **Arthroscopy.** Ankle arthroscopy has become a firmly established diagnostic and therapeutic tool in the management of disorders involving the ankle. When chronic lateral ligamentous instability remains despite conservative treatment, surgery may by necessary for stabilizing the ankle joint. In 1990 we started to routinely assess the ankle joint by arthroscopy before the surgical restoration of the ligaments (Schäfer & Hintermann 1996). The 110 arthroscopies we performed have demonstrated that abnormalities of different structures are involved in chronic ankle instability, and there is no single entity causing it. This is especially true for the lateral and medial ligaments. Although 12 of the 110 ankle joints that were arthroscopically investigated did not demonstrate instability clinically and radiologically, the patients complained nonetheless about insecurity, instability, and giving way. Arthroscopic assessment revealed a rotational instability in all these patients (figure 8.1).

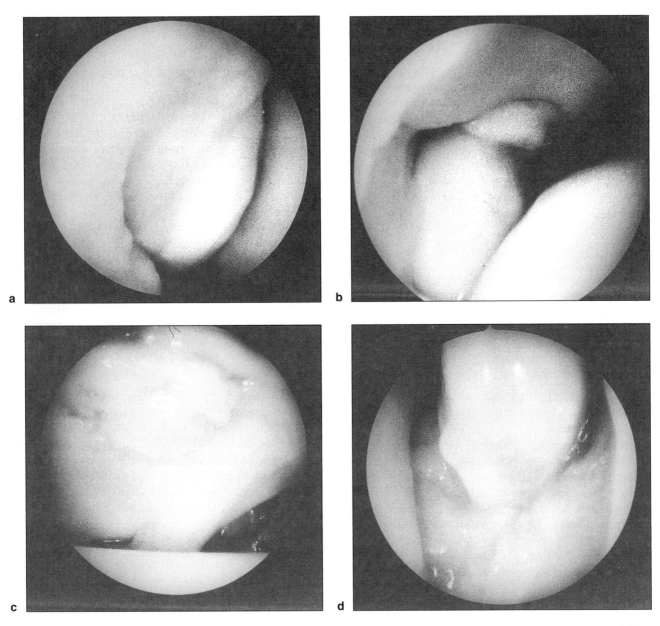

■ **Figure 8.1** Arthroscopy of a 36-year-old male patient suffering from recurrent ankle sprains, insecurity, and instability: *(a)* anterior view of the fibula showing the distal insertion of the anterior syndesmosis, while the ATFL and CFL ligaments were absent; *(b)* anterior view of the lateral ankle mortise demonstrating a moderate instability; *(c)* the complex ankle instability allowed direct view of the medial aspect of the fibula and the posterior syndesmosis; *(d)* anterior view of the medial malleolus showing no deltoid ligament.

A 36-Year-Old Male Patient Suffering From Recurrent Ankle Sprains, Insecurity, and Instability

During the 18 months after a severe ankle sprain, conservative treatment of the patient whose ankle is pictured in figures 8.1 and 8.2 had failed. The patient was referred to our clinic by the insurance company for final expertise. Clinical and radiological examination did not evidence instability of the ankle joint. Arthroscopy under regional anesthesia revealed a significant rotational instability in the presence of a relevant lesion of the lateral and medial ligaments (5-mm 30° optic, no traction device, insufflation with carbon dioxide gas) (see figure 8.1a-d for arthroscopic images). Immediately after the arthroscopic examination, the patient was brought to the radiology department to document the significant combined lateral and medial instability, where stress radiographs were performed still under full regional anesthesia. For the radiograph images, see figure 8.2, a-c. Surgical exploration during open surgical reconstruction performed 6 weeks later revealed a huge scar tissue complex, and the fact that the lateral ligaments (CFL and ATFL) were completely detached from the fibula. The fibula could thus easily translate anteriorly and posteriorly, whereas the remaining lateral ligament complex still stabilized talus and calcaneus. The lateral ligament complex was reattached to the fibula (figure 8.3), and the medial ligament was also reconstructed (not shown in figure 8.3).

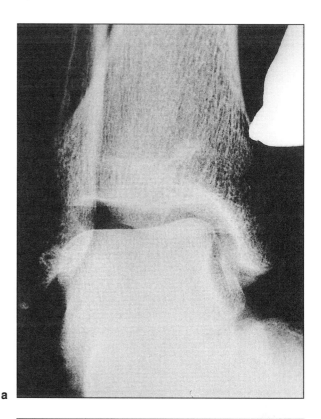

a

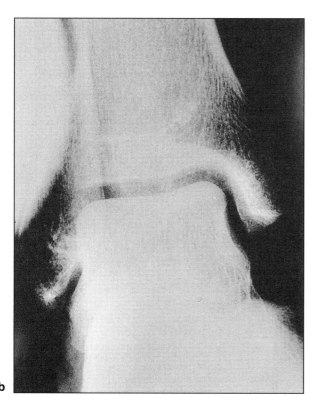

b

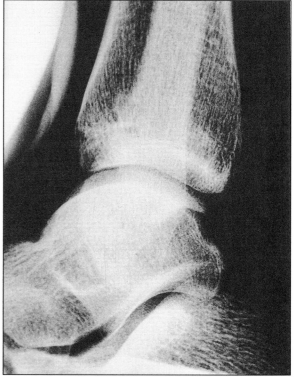

c

■ **Figure 8.2** Radiographs of ankle shown in figure 8.1: *(a)* lateral stress ("talar tilt") demonstrating mild lateral instability; *(b)* medial stress ("reversed talar tilt") demonstrating no medial instability; *(c)* anterior translation stress ("drawer test") demonstrating no anterior instability.

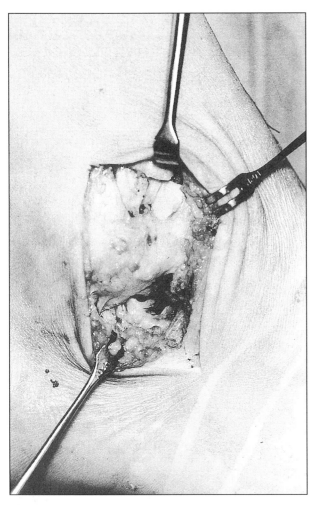

■ **Figure 8.3** Photo showing the intraoperative situs of the ankle shown in figures 8.1 and 8.2.

■ Conclusions

There is no doubt that chronic symptoms after ankle sprains require very careful evaluation. A history of ankle insecurity, instability, and giving way is far more important in diagnosis than the physical and radiological examination. When chronic ankle instability remains despite conservative treatment and surgery is advised, arthroscopy is a very effective diagnostic tool to preoperatively assess the ankle joint and the different structures that might be involved. This is especially relevant because there are always many possible causes of any case of chronic ankle instability.

■ References

Anderson KJ, Lecocq JK, Clayton ML. 1962. Athletic injury to the fibular collateral ligament of the ankle. Clin Orthop Rel Res 23:146-160.

Mann G, Eliashuv O, Perry C, Finsterbush A, Frankl U, Nyska M, Mattan Y. 1994. Recurrent ankle sprain: literature review. Israel J Sports Med: 104-113.

Peters JW, Trevino SG, Renström PA. 1991. Chronic lateral ankle instability: a review. Foot Ankle 12:182-191.

Schäfer D, Hintermann B. 1996. Arthroscopic assessment of the chronic unstable ankle joint. Knee Surg Sports Traumat Arthroscopy 4:48-452.

Part III

Diagnostic Approaches to Ankle Sprain

Plain radiography is the mainstay in evaluation of the injured ankle. There is still controversy regarding the usefulness of taking plain radiographs in the emergency facility. However, the combination of physical examination and meticulous evaluation of standard radiographic views of the ankle during the acute sprain may lower the high rate of missed diagnosis. Familiarity with the common fractures that may occur in acute ankle sprain and the different modalities of imaging will lead to correct diagnosis and optimized treatment. The imaging of the injured ankle includes three main categories:

1. Noninvasive techniques such as plain radiography, bone scan, computed tomography, and magnetic resonance imaging may demonstrate mainly anatomical injuries to the bony and soft tissue.

2. Semi-invasive techniques, such as stress radiographs and arthrography, contribute to the dynamic understanding of the injury.

3. Invasive techniques, such as arthroscopy, evaluate the anatomical defect and enable immediate treatment of the lesion.

Chapter 9

Radiographic Assessment of Acute Ankle and Hindfoot Injuries

Ehud Rath, MD, and Ilan Shelef, MD

Radiographs of the acutely injured ankle and foot add valuable information for the diagnosis in the emergency setting. These radiographs account for more than 10% of emergency department radiographs (Svenson 1988) and are second only to chest and C-spine radiographs in the frequency of ordering (Brunswick, Ilkhanipour, Seaberg, & McGill 1996; Brunswick, Ilkhanipour, Fuchs, & Seaberg 1996). Foot radiographs are among the most frequently misinterpreted (Brunswick, Ilkhanipour, Fuchs, & Seaberg 1996), mainly because of congestion of relatively small bones in the foot, their unique relationships, and overlapping of these bones on many of the radiographs (Heckman et al. 1996).

Several factors should be considered before ordering specific views. Each injury is associated with a certain mechanism, hence taking a careful history is crucial. The injury pattern, point of maximal tenderness, and plain radiographs usually make it possible to identify most problems. If the diagnosis remains unclear, special views and other modalities may be useful. A careful examination is crucial for ordering the right views.

This chapter discusses indications for foot and ankle radiographs in the emergency setting, and gives guidelines for interpreting them. Table 9.1 lists the differential diagnoses of the post-traumatic painful ankle and hindfoot. Table 9.2 sums up the trauma series radiographs and additional relevant radiographs.

Table 9.1 Differential Diagnoses of Ankle and Hindfoot Pain of Traumatic Origin

Area of maximal tenderness	Bone injury	Soft tissue injury
Anterolateral	Lateral malleolus Talar dome	Anterior talofibular ligament
Posterolateral	Lateral malleolus Trigonoid process	Posterior talofibular ligament
Inferolateral	Lateral malleolus Lateral process of talus Calcaneus Cuboid Base of 5th metatarsal	Calcaneofibular ligament
Medial	Medial malleolus Talar dome Sustentaculum tali Medial tubercle of talus	Deltoid ligament Posterior tibial tendon Spring ligament
Anterior	Tibial plafond Talar neck Talar dome	Tibiofibular sindesmosis
Posterior	Calcaneus Body of talus	Achilles tendon Flexor hallucis longus

Table 9.2 Trauma Series Radiographs and Special Views for Ankle and Hindfoot

Region	Trauma series*	Special radiographs	Additional imaging recommended
Ankle	AP, lateral, mortise		Stress views Stress tenography
Talus	Dome–mortise Neck–lateral	Canale view	CT scan
Calcaneus	AP, lateral, oblique	Broden's view Harris axial view	CT scan
Lesser tarsals, Lisfranc joint	AP, lateral, oblique	Weightbearing radiographs	

*Radiographic assessment of ankle and foot trauma begins with ankle or foot trauma series according to clinical judgment of the examiner. The approach should be based upon guidelines for radiographs suggested.

■ Ankle Injuries—Indications and Radiograph Interpretation

The majority of ankle injuries are sprains and strains with no skeletal involvement (Vargish et al. 1983; Sujitkumar et al. 1986). The question of whether to perform radiographs in every acutely injured ankle has been raised many times (Svenson 1988; Vargish et al. 1983; David 1989; DeLacy & Bradbrooke 1979; Tandeter & Shvartzman 1997). The Ottawa ankle rules are a set of decision rules for the use of radiography in ankle injury, developed by Stiell in the early 1990s to reduce radiographic procedures and cost. They suggest clinical guidelines for ordering ankle radiographs after injury (Stiell, Greenberg et al. 1992; Stiell, McKnight et al. 1992). Pain near the malleoli, inability to bear weight, or bone tenderness at the posterior edge of either malleoli dictates the need for ankle radiographs (Stiell, Greenberg et al. 1992; Dunlop et al. 1986). Foot radiographs should be ordered if there is pain in the midfoot zone and either tenderness at the base of the fifth metatarsal or navicular, or inability to bear weight for four steps. Adhering to these rules, 100% sensitivity and 40.1% specificity were reported with a reduction of 36.0% of ankle radiographic series ordered. The Ottawa ankle rules led to a decrease in use of foot and ankle radiography, waiting times, and costs, without patient dissatisfaction or missed fractures (Stiell et al. 1994; Anis et al. 1995). Other authors were unable to validate the Ottawa rules with 100% sensitivity (Lucchesi et al. 1995; Verma et al. 1997) but agree that they were more sensitive than clinical suspicion alone. No combination of physical findings can distinguish with 100% certainty between fractured and nonfractured ankles, and some authors conclude that radiographs should be performed for every acutely injured ankle (Svenson 1988).

Plain radiographic evaluation of the ankle should include anteroposterior, lateral, and mortise views (Geissler et al. 1996). A radiograph of the opposite side is sometimes necessary to determine normal measurements for the individual patient.

■ Technical Notes

The orthopedist should be familiar with the technical aspects of taking the radiograph. Diagnosis is based on at least two-plane radiographic evaluation. Specific oblique views may help for further investigation.

■ **The anteroposterior view** (figure 9.1) is taken in the supine position with a small sandbag under the knee to relieve strain. The position of the ankle is adjusted by flexing and pronating the foot so that the long axis is vertical. Slight inversion is used to open the talofibular articulation. The central ray is directed vertically to the midpoint of the malleoli. This view demonstrates the lower end of the tibia and fibula and the tallar dome. The tibiofibular articulation is not clearly visualized because the two bones overlap in this view.

■ **The lateral view** (figure 9.2) should be performed with the medial side of the ankle in contact with the film holder. The midline of the film should be parallel with the long axis of the leg, and the patella will be perpendicular with the horizontal plain. The central ray is directed vertically through the ankle joint. The lateral view demonstrates well the relationships between the body of the talus and the articulation surface of the distal tibia. These structures should be congruent: The joint space should

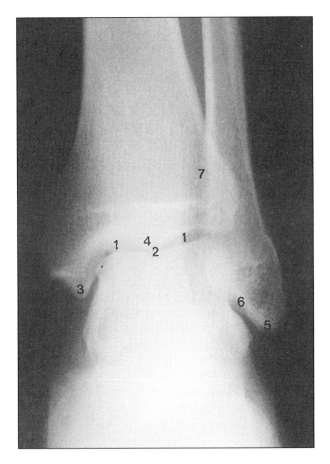

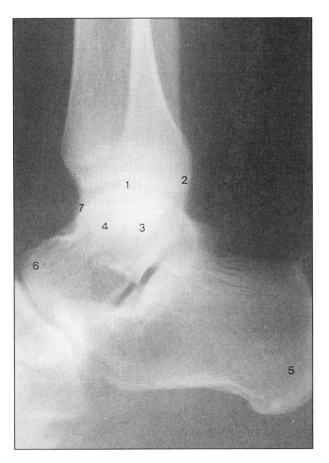

■ **Figure 9.1** Ankle anteroposterior projection, normal anatomy: *(1)* ankle joint; *(2)* trochlear surface of the talus; *(3)* medial malleolus; *(4)* promontory of tibia; *(5)* lateral malleolus; *(6)* malleolus fossa; *(7)* distal tibiofibular joint.

■ **Figure 9.2** Ankle lateral projection, normal anatomy: *(1)* ankle joint; *(2)* promontory of tibia; *(3)* lateral malleolus; *(4)* medial malleolus; *(5)* calcaneus; *(6)* talus; *(7)* trochlear surface of the talus.

measure the same at both the anterior and posterior regions.

■ **The mortise view (medial oblique)** (figure 9.3) is the best one for seeing the malleoli and their articular surfaces (Daffner 1990). The joint space is uniform from the lateral to the medial aspect and should not exceed 4 mm in width (Griffiths 1986). Malleolar fractures are easily noticed in these views. Fractures of the posterior tibial malleolus are harder to interpret from the plain radiograph (Ferries et al. 1994). Compared with a CT scan, these radiographs do not give consistent, reproducible, or reliable measurements of the fragment. Because operative stabilization of the posterior fragment has been recommended for fragments that occupy more than 25-33% of the articular surface, it is important to measure them accurately.

Soft tissue injuries make up the majority of ankle injuries and are not demonstrated directly on plain radiographs. Knowing the normal bony relationships is fundamental to understanding when to suspect

instability and proceed to evaluation with stress radiographs.

■ Radiographs of Specific Injuries

Crowding of bones around the foot and ankle makes some injuries difficult to diagnose with routine plain radiographs. Special views may be necessary to reveal the fracture or ligamentous insufficiency. Using indirect measurements helps to disclose syndesmotic and ligamentous injuries.

Tibiofibular Syndesmotic Diastasis

The syndesmosis ligament complex includes the tibiofibular ligaments and the interosseous membrane. Isolated complete syndesmosis injury without fracture is rare and usually occurs in conjunction with rupture of the deltoid ligament (Renström 1994). The tibiofibular clear space and the tibiofibular overlap are used to evaluate the integrity of the syndesmosis on AP and mortise views (Harper & Keller 1989)

In another cadaveric study done by Ebraheim et al. (1997), a CT scan proved to be more sensitive than static radiographs for detecting minor degrees of syndesmotic injury in cases of up to 3-mm syndesmotic diastases.

Stress views may be used to evaluate the presence of syndesmotic disruption. External rotation force is applied to the ankle while the upper portion of the leg is stabilized. Measurements of anatomical diastasis on the stress lateral radiographs are more sensitive than measurements on the mortise radiographs (Xeno et al. 1995).

Ankle Ligamentous Instability— Radiographic Evaluation

Stress radiographs assess indirectly the integrity of the stabilizing ligaments of the ankle. Anteroposterior and mortise views are taken while stress is applied to the ankle in various positions of neutral, flexion, internal rotation, or external rotation.

Stress views of the contralateral ankle are mandatory for comparison. The anterior talofibular and calcaneofibular ligaments function together at all positions of ankle flexion to provide lateral stability (Colville et al. 1990). Strain in the anterior tibiofibular ligament increases with plantarflexion, internal rotation, and inversion (Colville et al. 1990; Larsen 1985). A talar tilt double that of the tilt at the uninjured ankle, or a talar tilt of more than 10° to 15° indicates a tear of the anterior talofibular and calcaneofibular ligaments (Geissler et al. 1996)*. Grace (1984) used autopsy specimens to evaluate the degree of ligamentous injury with appearance of radiographic abnormality. Ankle ligaments were surgically divided to produce various single and combined lesions. A significant talar tilt occurred only when more than one component of the lateral ligaments had been divided. Anterior displacement of the talus as measured from the posterior lip of the tibia to the nearest part of the talar dome was greatest with the foot plantigrade. Medial ankle instability is not common. The deltoid ligamentous complex is assessed on eversion stress.

Stress tenography under local anesthesia may identify the severity of ligamentous injury (Evans & Frenyo 1979). The extent of talar tilt of the injured ankle as compared with that of the uninjured ankle is assessed on standard inversion radiographs. With the aid of the tenograms, it is possible to identify whether the instability is the result of a rupture of the anterior talofibular ligament alone or the result of a combination of a rupture of both this ligament and the calcaneofibular ligament (Evans et al. 1984).

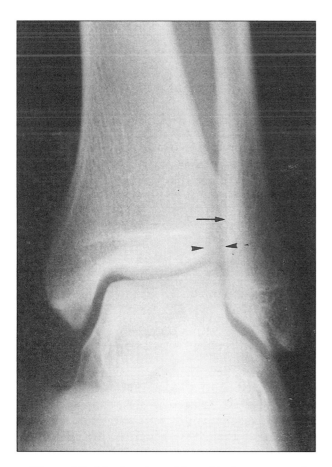

■ **Figure 9.3** Mortise view of the ankle demonstrates the clear space (arrowheads) and the tibiofibular overlap (arrow).

(figures 9.1-9.3). The clear space is measured 1 cm above the distal tibial articular surface. It is defined by measuring the distance between the lateral border of the posterior tibia and the medial border of the fibula. A normal clear space is less than 6 mm. The tibiofibular overlap should measure more than 1 mm on the mortise view and more than 6 mm on the AP view. In a cadaveric study done by Harper and Keller (1989), a clear space greater than 6 mm on both views was the most reliable predictor of early syndesmotic widening.

To determine the degree of variability among individuals, as well as gender differences, in measurements of the tibiofibular clear space and the tibiofibular overlap, Ostrum et al. (1995) investigated the anatomy of the syndesmosis as ratios of the potentially variable values to fixed landmarks. The ratio of the tibiofibular overlap to the fibular width averaged 54%, and the ratio of the tibiofibular clear space to the fibular width averaged 30%, with no statistically significant difference due to gender.

---

*Editors' remark: This is not a consensus agreement. Others use a side-to-side difference of 5° or more to diagnose mechanical instability.

Osteochondral Lesions of the Talar Dome

Osteochondral lesions of the talar dome are a relatively common cause of ankle pain and disability. These fractures are often overlooked in the initial evaluation. Stage I osteochondral fractures show no diagnostic changes on plain radiographs, and stage II lesions are usually subtle and, therefore, are often overlooked by both radiologists and clinicians (Anderson et al. 1989). The two most common sites for these lesions are the anterolateral and posteromedial corners of the talar dome (Prokuski & Saltzman 1997). The lateral lesion is usually associated with trauma (Canale & Belding 1980). Medial lesions are often bilateral and not necessarily traumatic. A mortise view in plantarflexion may better delineate a posteromedial lesion. Ankle dorsiflexion may show an anterolateral lesion (Stone 1996).

Because osteochondral lesions of the talar dome may coexist with lateral ligament laxity, stress radiographs should be obtained if ligament laxity is identified on clinical examination.

If there is a clinical suspicion of an osteochondral fracture but the plain radiographs appear to be negative, cintigraphy should be used. A CT scan accurately assesses the location, size, and intactness of the lesion (figure 9.4).

Fractures of the Lateral Process of the Talus

This rare type of fracture should be suspected in a patient with an inversion type ankle injury. Fractures of the lateral process of the talus are common after snowboard injuries and have been reported to represent 34% of ankle fractures in those patients (Kirkpatrick et al. 1998). Since plain radiographs often miss it, a CT scan should be considered for a patient with severe ankle sprain who cannot bear weight on the injured side. An AP radiograph of the ankle with the foot in 45° of internal rotation and the ankle in 30° of plantarflexion exposes the lateral process better than the AP at neutral position (Prokuski & Saltzman 1997).

Because routine radiographs failed to determine either the size or comminution of the fractured process, CT imaging should be routinely performed (Ebraheim et al. 1994).

Talar Neck Fractures

Talar neck fractures should be diagnosed as early as possible since displaced talar neck fractures are associated with avascular necrosis of the body of the talus. This complication is a major cause for poor results (Faciszewski et al. 1990; Hawkins 1998). The talar neck is well demonstrated on the lateral view (figure

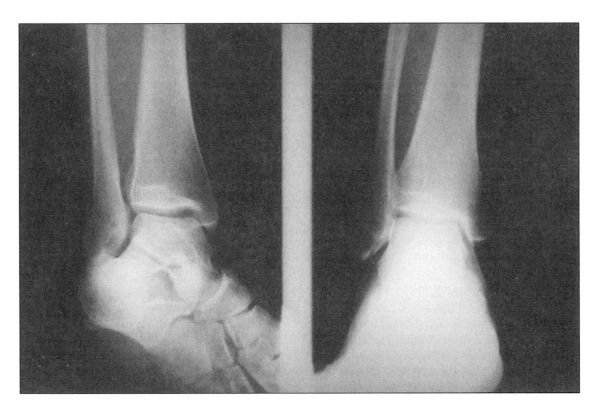

■ **Figure 9.4** Medial osteochondral lesion almost unremarkable on AP radiograph. Improved visualization may occasionally be obtained with foot in plantar flexion.

9.5). However, maximum equinus with pronation is reported to be the best position to demonstrate the talar neck on the AP. The radiograph tube should be directed cephalad at a 75° angle from the horizontal plane (Canale & Kelly 1978). This view, described by Canale, enables one to detect any offset or varus deformity of the head and neck of the talus.

Fractures of the Posterior Process of the Talus

The posterior process of the talus has two tubercles—medial and lateral. Between these tubercles passes the flexor hallucis longus. The lateral tubercle is longer than the medial, hence fractures of it are much more commonly seen. This tubercle is seen in profile on the lateral radiograph. It is hard to demonstrate these fractures on plain radiograph, therefore a CT scan should be done once this type of fracture is suspected.

Calcaneus

Radiographic assessment of the largest tarsal bone includes dorsoplantar (anteroposterior), lateral, oblique, Broden's view, and Harris axial calcaneal projections (Prokuski & Saltzman 1997; Koval & Sanders 1993; Sanders & Gregory 1995).

For dorsoplantar view (figure 9.6), the patient is in the supine position with a fully extended leg. The film is placed under the ankle, and a long strip of bandage or a sandbag holds the ankle in dorsiflexion. The central ray is directed at the cranial angle of 40° to the long axis of the foot. The anteroposterior view demonstrates extension of a fracture line into the calcaneocuboid joint, lateral displacement of the calcaneus, and subluxation of the talonavicular joint.

The lateral view of the heel (figure 9.7) is included in the lateral ankle view. It accentuates the

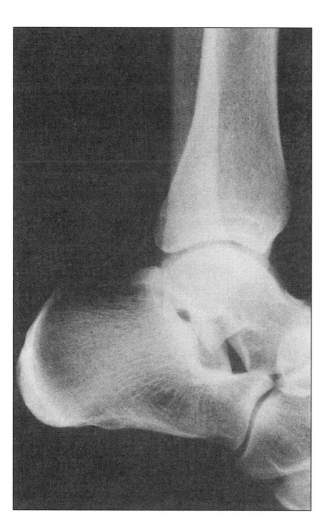

■ **Figure 9.5** Talar neck fracture.

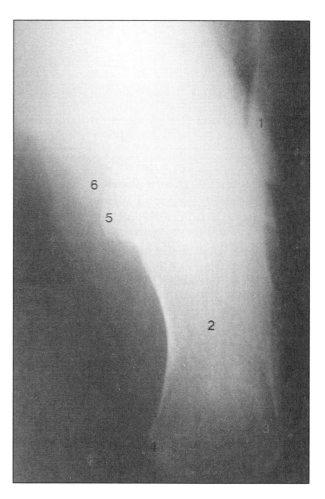

■ **Figure 9.6** Calcaneus axial projection (Harris view), normal anatomy: *(1)* lateral malleolus of fibula; *(2)* calcaneus; *(3)* lateral process of calcaneus; *(4)* medial process of calcaneus; *(5)* sustentaculum tali of calcaneus; *(6)* medial malleolus of tibia.

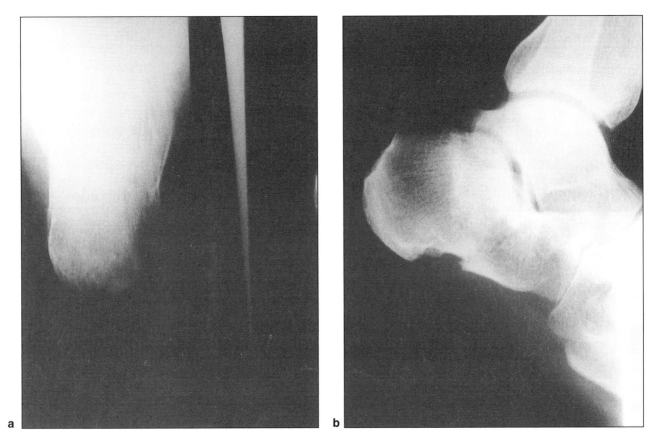

■ **Figure 9.7** Fracture of calcaneus. *(a)* An axial view demonstrates varus-valgus alignment; and *(b)* a lateral view demonstrates loss of valcaneal height and extension into the calcaneocoboid joint.

fracture. Most intra-articular calcaneal fractures will be demonstrated by this view. Boehler's angle will be reduced as a result of height loss of the posterior facet. Gissane's angle will usually increase. When only the lateral half of the posterior facet is displaced, calcaneal height may be normal, along with normal Boehler's angle. A double density at the level of the posterior facet will result as the fractured part of the facet is rotated. Fracture of the tuberosity, calcaneocuboid joint involvement, and subtalar subluxation should also be noticed on the lateral view.

Oblique projections delineate the subtalar joint and show articular involvement of the fracture. Broden's view (Broden 1949) is obtained with the patient supine, the foot in neutral flexion, and the leg internally rotated 30° to 40°. The posterior calcaneal articular facet is shown as the beam is centered on the lateral malleolus and the tube moves from 10° to 40° toward the head. Broden's views are also taken intraoperatively by fluoroscopy to control reduction of the posterior facet.

Harris axial heel view shows varus and valgus displacement of the heel, sustentaculum tali fragment, body, and posterior facet. Because most calca-

neal fractures result from falls from height, associated fractures are frequent. Views of the ipsilateral ankle and the dorsolumbar spine should be obtained in all patients who have sustained a calcaneal fracture.

Tarsometatarsal Injuries

The articulations of the midfoot and forefoot are named after the French physician Jacques Lisfranc, 1790-1847, who first described amputation through that joint. Lisfranc joint injuries are not common and are often misdiagnosed (Burroughs et al. 1998). It has been estimated that up to 20% of cases of significant Lisfranc joint injury are overlooked on the initial radiographs (Heckman & Rockwood 1996). Since prognosis of the undertreated Lisfranc injury is poor, careful physical examination with a high index of suspicion is crucial. Swelling over the midfoot and pain on palpation along the tarsometatarsal articulations should raise suspicion for Lisfranc injury. Plantar hematoma at the midfoot was reported to be associated with this injury (Ross et al. 1996).

Routine radiographic evaluation of the Lisfranc joint includes anteroposterior, lateral, and 30° oblique views. The anteroposterior projection should include the uninjured foot for comparison. The articulations and its complex bony configuration form the transverse arch of the midfoot. The second metatarsal is the keystone to that arch (Vuori & Aro 1993). Certain alignments should be noted systematically on this view:

1. The lateral aspect of the first metatarsal base aligns with the lateral border of the medial cuneiform.

2. Continuity should exist between the medial border of the second metatarsal and the medial border of the middle cuneiform.

3. The medial surface of the cuboid and the medial side of the base of the fourth metatarsal form an unbroken line.

The oblique view gives more details on the bases of the lateral metatarsals:

1. The lateral border of the third metatarsal is continuous with the lateral border of the lateral cuneiform.

2. The medial border of the fourth metatarsal is in a straight line with the medial border of the cuboid. The articulation of the cuboid and base of the fifth metatarsal is best appreciated on this view. Only the medial part of the fifth metatarsal articulates with the cuboid. The lateral part extends laterally and proximally.

The lateral view may demonstrate dorsal or plantar displacement of the metatarsal bases. In this view, the metatarsals should align with the tarsal bones.

Not all injuries to the Lisfranc joint are detected on routine radiographs. Spontaneous reduction may obscure instability that results from a ligamentous tear. Stress radiographs should be obtained when the mechanism of injury was axial loading on a plantarflexed foot, and palpation of the tarsometatarsal joints elicits local tenderness (Prokuski & Saltzman 1997). Stress radiographs are taken while abduction and adduction force is applied to the foot. The foot should be anesthetized locally.

Weightbearing AP views add important information regarding the stability of the medial joints (Faciszewski et al. 1990). Radiographs that reveal flattening of the longitudinal arch on weight bearing are associated with a poor prognosis. An ankle block may be necessary if the patient is in great pain and cannot tolerate weight bearing (Trevino & Kodros 1995). To achieve a reliable result, weightbearing radiographs should be taken 1 to 2 weeks after injury and pain relief. Radiographs of the uninjured side should be compared. Flattening of the longitudinal

arch after an injury of the Lisfranc joint is an indication for surgery (Faciszewski et al. 1990).

■ Summary

In this chapter we have outlined the indications and technique to obtain radiographic views of the foot and ankle after injury. It should be kept in mind that most injuries to the foot and ankle include soft tissues only, and recalling the Ottawa rules would allow logical decisions concerning the necessity and choice of imaging. Meticulous anamnesis concerning the mechanism of trauma and a detailed physical examination would best define the radiographic view to be applied in the specific injury in order to disclose a fracture or dislocation as demonstrated in the second part of this chapter.

■ References

Anderson IF, Crichton KJ, Grattan ST, Cooper RA, Brazier D. Osteochondral fractures of the dome of the talus. J Bone Joint Surg Am 1989;71(8):1143-1152.

Anis AH, Stiell IG, Stewart DG, Laupacis A. Cost-effectiveness analysis of the Ottawa Ankle Rules. Ann Emerg Med 1995;26(4):422-428.

Broden B. Roentgen examination of the subtaloid joint in fractures of the calcaneus. Acta Radiol 1949;3:85-91.

Brunswick JE, Ilkhanipour K, Fuchs S, Seaberg D. Emergency medicine resident interpretation of pediatric radiographs. Acad Emerg Med 1996;3(8):790-793.

Brunswick JE, Ilkhanipour K, Seaberg DC, McGill L. Radiographic interpretation in the emergency department. Am J Emerg Med 1996;14(4):346-348.

Burroughs KE, Reimer CD, Fields KB. Lisfranc injury of the foot: a commonly missed diagnosis. Am Fam Physician 1998;58(1):118-124.

Canale ST, Belding RH. Osteochondral lesions of the talus. J Bone Joint Surg Am 1980;62(1):97-102.

Canale ST, Kelly FBJ. Fractures of the neck of the talus: Long-term evaluation of seventy-one cases. J Bone Joint Surg Am 1978;60:143-156.

Colville MR, Marder RA, Boyle JJ, Zarins B. Strain measurement in lateral ankle ligaments. Am J Sports Med 1990;18(2):196-200.

Daffner RH. Ankle trauma. Radiol Clin North Am 1990;28(2):395-421.

David HG. Value of radiographs in managing common foot injuries. Br Med J 1989;298(6686):1492-1493.

DeLacy GJ, Bradbrooke S. Rationalizing requests for X-ray examination of acute ankle injuries. Br Med J 1979;1597-1598.

Dunlop MG, Beattie TF, White GK, Raab GM, Doull RI. Guidelines for selective radiological assessment of inversion ankle injuries. Br Med J 1986;293(6547):603-605.

Ebraheim NA, Lu J, Yang H, Mekhail AO, Yeasting RA. Radiographic and CT evaluation of tibiofibular syndesmotic diastasis: a cadaver study. Foot Ankle Int 1997;18(11):693-698.

Ebraheim NA, Skie MC, Podeszwa DA, Jackson WT. Evaluation of process fractures of the talus using computed tomography. J Orthop Trauma 1994;8(4):332-337.

Evans GA, Frenyo SD. The stress-tenogram in the diagnosis of ruptures of the lateral ligament of the ankle. J Bone Joint Surg Br 1979;61:347-351.

Evans GA, Hardcastle P, Frenyo AD. Acute rupture of the lateral ligament of the ankle. To suture or not to suture? J Bone Joint Surg Br 1984;66(2):209-212.

Faciszewski T, Burks RT, Manaster BJ. Subtle injuries of the Lisfranc joint. J Bone Joint Surg Am 1990;72:1519-1522.

Ferries JS, DeCoster TA, Firoozbakhsh KK, Garcia JF, Miller RA. Plain radiographic interpretation in trimalleolar ankle fractures poorly assesses the posterior fragment size. J Orthop Trauma 1994;8(4):328-331.

Geissler WB, Tsao AK, Hughes JL. Rockwood CA, Green DP, Bucholz RW, Heckman JD, editors. Fractures in adults. 4th ed. Philadelphia: Lippincott-Raven; 1996; 31, Fractures and injuries of the ankle. p. 2201-2266.

Grace DL. Lateral ankle ligament injuries. Inversion and anterior stress radiography. Clin Orthop 1984;183:153-159.

Griffiths HJ. Trauma to the ankle and foot. Crit Rev Diagn Imaging 1986;26:45-105.

Harper MC, Keller TS. A radiographic evaluation of the tibiofibular syndesmosis. Foot Ankle 1989;10:156-160.

Hawkins LG. Fractures of the neck of the talus. J Bone Joint Surg Am 1998;52:991-1002.

Heckman JD. Rockwood CA, Green DP, Bucholz RW, Heckman JD, editors. Fractures in adults. 4th ed. Philadelphia: Lippincott-Raven; 1996; 32, Fractures and dislocations of the foot. p. 2267-2405.

Kirkpatrick DP, Hunter RE, Janes PC, Mastrangelo J, Nicholas RA. The snowboarder's foot and ankle. Am J Sports Med 1998;26(2):271-277.

Koval KJ, Sanders R. The radiologic evaluation of calcaneal fractures. Clin Orthop 1993;290:41-46.

Larsen E. Experimental instability of the ankle: A radiographic investigation. Clin Orthop 1985;204:193-200.

Lucchesi GM, Jackson RE, Peacock WF, Cerasani C, Swor RA. Sensitivity of the Ottawa rules. Ann Emerg Med 1995;26(1):1-5.

Ostrum RF, De Meo P, Subramanian R. A critical analysis of the anterior-posterior radiographic anatomy of the ankle syndesmosis. Foot Ankle Int 1995;16(3):128-131.

Prokuski LJ, Saltzman CL. Challenging fractures of the foot and ankle. Radiol Clin North Am 1997;35(3):655-670.

Renström PAFH. Persistently painful sprained ankle. Am Acad Orthop Surg 1994;2(5):270-280.

Ross G, Cronin R, Hauzenblas J, Juliano P. Plantar ecchymosis sign: a clinical aid to diagnosis of occult Lisfranc tarsometatarsal injuries. J Orthop Trauma 1996;10(2):119-122.

Sanders R, Gregory P. Operative treatment of intraarticular fractures of the calcaneus. Orthop Clin North Am 1995;26(2):203-214.

Stiell IG, Greenberg GH, McKnight RD, Nair RC, McDowell I, Worthington JR. A study to develop clinical decision rules for the use of radiography in acute ankle injuries. Ann Emerg Med 1992;21:384-390.

Stiell IG, McKnight RD, Greenberg GH, McDowell I, Nair RC, Wells GA, Johns C, Worthington JR. Implementation of the Ottawa ankle rules. JAMA 1994;271(11):827-832.

Stiell IG, McKnight RD, Greenberg GH, Nair RC, McDowell I, Wallace GJ. Interobserver agreement in the examination of acute ankle injury patients. Am J Emerg Med 1992;10(1):14-17.

Stone JW. Osteochondral lesions of the talar dome. Am Acad Orthop Surg 1996;4(2): 63-73.

Sujitkumar P, Hadfield JM, Yates DW. Sprain or fracture? An analysis of 2000 ankle injuries. Arch Emerg Med 1986;3(101):106

Svenson J. Need for radiographs in the acutely injured ankle (letter). Lancet 1988;1(8579):244-245.

Tandeter HB, Shvartzman P. Acute ankle injuries: clinical decision rules for radiographs. Am Fam Physician 1997;55(8):2721-2728.

Trevino SG, Kodros S. Controversies in tarsometatarsal injuries. Orthop Clin North Am 1995;26(2):229.

Vargish T, Clarke WR, Young RA, Jensen A. The ankle injury—indications for the selective use of x-rays. Injury 1983;14(6):507-512.

Verma S, Hamilton K, Hawkins HH, Kothari R, Singal B, Buncher R, Nguyen P, O'Neill M. Clinical application of the Ottawa ankle rules for the use of radiography in acute ankle injuries: an independent site assessment. Am J Roentgenol 1997;169(3):825-827.

Vuori JP, Aro HT. Lisfranc joint injuries: trauma mechanisms and associated injuries. J Orthop Trauma 1993;35(1):40-45.

Xeno JS, Hopkinson WJ, Mulligan ME, Olson EJ, Popovic NA. The tibiofibular syndesmosis. Evaluation of the ligamentous structures, methods of fixation, and radiographic assessment. J Bone Joint Surg Am 1995;77(6):847-856.

Chapter 10

Imaging of Ankle Injuries

Yaakov H. Applbaum, MD

This last decade has witnessed an increase in the application of imaging techniques to the diagnosis and management of ankle disorders. In the past, plain radiographs, including stress films and contrast studies, allowed only an indirect view of the soft tissues and bone marrow. Ultrasonography, computed tomography (CT), nuclear medicine, and magnetic resonance imaging (MRI) have brought an explosion of new information. The clinical impact of this information and the most useful way to capitalize on it have yet to be determined. In this chapter we will demonstrate the current uses of these modalities in ankle injuries.

■ Techniques

Radiographic evaluation of the ankle accounts for 10% of all radiographic examinations requested from the emergency department. The use of radiographs in the emergency room is discussed in chapter 9. Radiographs have an important role in diagnosing fractures and other gross osseous abnormalities. However, plain radiographs rely on indirect signs in the assessment of the soft tissues, joints, and bone marrow, and are therefore limited. Special techniques discussed in this chapter, such as arthrography and tenography, in which radio-opaque contrast agents are introduced into the joint or tendon sheath, allow an indirect view of joints, tendons, and ligaments. Stress radiographs add a functional dimension to the assessment of ankle ligaments. Although these techniques are effective, they focus on a narrow clinical problem and are time-consuming.

Ultrasonography has been gaining wide acceptance as a diagnostic tool in musculoskeletal medicine in certain clinical settings. Ultrasonography utilizes the echoes from high frequency sound waves that reflect from tissues to create an image. Ultrasonic waves cannot penetrate cortical bone well and are useful in the study of superficial structures. In the ankle region, ultrasound imaging can demonstrate abnormalities of tendons and ligaments, as well as joint effusions (Fessell et al. 1998). Although ultrasonography has the advantage of being rapid, inexpensive, and widely available, it must be performed by an experienced operator with advanced equipment.

Nuclear medicine bone scanning is a highly sensitive but often nonspecific technique for focal and diffuse bone lesions. MRI has superseded it in many applications, but nuclear medicine has the advantage of allowing easy imaging of large areas and is usually less expensive than MRI.

Computed tomography (CT) is a technique that utilizes computers to construct cross-sectional images from x-rays projected on electronic detectors. It is more sensitive to differences in tissue density than film radiography, and the cross-sectional images add important information in areas with complex anatomy such as joints. In the ankle region, CT is invaluable in assessing fractures and other bony abnormalities. In soft tissues, CT has a more limited role and has been surmounted primarily by MRI and ultrasonography.

In MRI, powerful magnets and radiofrequency transmitter-receivers are used to create images of the body. MRI is sensitive to differences in tissues not dependant on density, adding information essential for diagnosis. In addition, MRI allows cross-sectional images in planes not easily attainable by CT. MRI has definite advantages in the imaging of cartilage and bone marrow. No other imaging technique is as versatile. The disadvantages of MRI include its high price and limited availability. Furthermore, claustrophobic patients and patients with biomedical implants (such as pacemakers, cochlear implants, and intracranial vascular clips) may be unable to undergo the examination.

■ Ligament Injuries

Stress radiographs, in which lateral, medial, or anterior stress are applied to the ankle joint, have been widely accepted as a tool for assessment of ankle ligament injury (figure 10.1). The standardization of

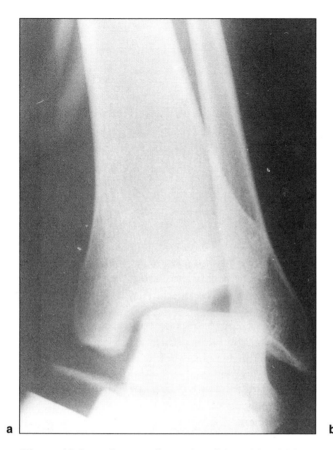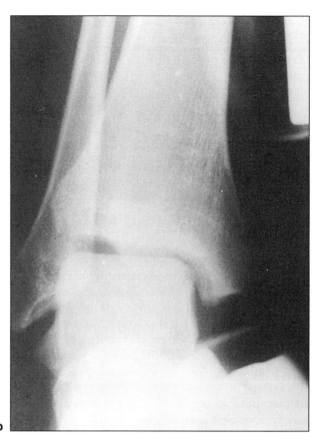

■ **Figure 10.1** *(a)* Stress radiography of the ankle with inversion stress, anteroposterior view. Increased angle due to lateral ligament injury. *(b)* Normal comparison view.

the stress applied to the ankle has added a measure of reproducibility. However, there is a lack of agreement on the threshold for pathology. Studies comparing stress radiography with direct images of the ankle obtained with MRI have demonstrated a low sensitivity for ligament tears (Breitenseher, Trattnig et al. 1997). Furthermore, the criteria for distinguishing a tear of a single ligament from multiple ligament tears are not well established.

The components of the lateral and medial ligament complexes can be imaged by ultrasound, CT, or MRI. Acute injury to the ligaments can be assessed by ankle arthrography and peroneal tenography. However, the utility of imaging ligaments depends on its impact on diagnosis and on the treatment plan. Because functional treatment is the standard of care in lateral ankle sprains, the role of imaging is limited to specific clinical subsets (Anzilloti et al. 1996; Zanetti et al. 1997).

Lateral Ligaments

The lateral ligament complex of the ankle consists of the anterior talofibular, calcaneofibular, and posterior talofibular ligaments. The lateral ligaments are the most commonly injured ligaments. Of the lateral ligaments, the anterior talofibular ligament is injured most often. Calcaneofibular ligament injury is usually seen accompanying anterior talofibular ligament injury. The posterior talofibular ligament is least commonly injured and then only in conjunction with the injury of the other two lateral ligaments.

Ligament injury is graded from grade I, with failure of only some fibers, to grade III, with complete ankle ligament tear and instability.

Ankle arthrography can be used to demonstrate ligament tears with a reported accuracy of 75%-90% (Fordyce & Horn 1972). With anterior talofibular ligament tears, contrast is seen inferior and lateral to the lateral malleolus. In tears of the calcaneofibular ligament, there is filling of the peroneal tendon sheath. However, in recurrent ankle ligament injury, these findings may be due to prior injury or may be absent due to scarring.

The ligaments can be imaged with ultrasonography using high resolution, high frequency transducers. When injured, the ligaments may appear discontinuous, bulbous, or wavy with low echogenicity in and around the ligament (figure 10.2).

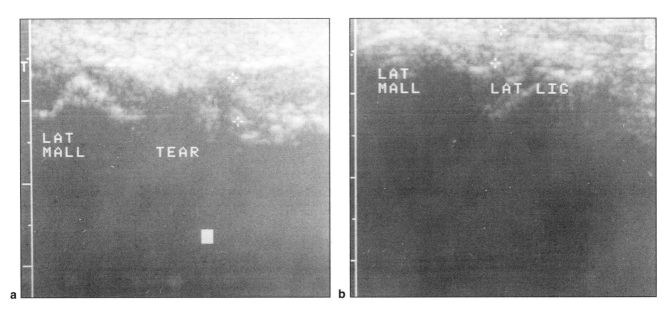

■ **Figure 10.2** Ultrasound of lateral ligaments of the ankle. *(a)* Tear of anterior talofibular ligament with hypoechoic gap. *(b)* Normal comparison.

On MRI, the lateral ligaments are best imaged with coronal and axial images with 10° to 20° dorsiflexion for the anterior and posterior talofibular ligaments. The calcaneofibular ligament is best imaged in axial images with 40° to 50° of plantarflexion (Schneck et al. 1992). The MRI findings associated with ligament tears include waviness, thickening or thinning of a portion of the ligament, or even complete disruption. Surrounding hemorrhage or edema with increased joint or peroneal sheath fluid are secondary signs of lateral ligament injury.

There are problems involved with using MRI for diagnosing lateral ligament injury. The lateral ligaments are not always visualized, and increased signals may be normal in the posterior talofibular ligament (Link et al. 1993; Noto et al. 1989).

MRI arthrography in which contrast medium is injected into the ankle joint before MRI has been shown to overcome some of these problems, and it is a sensitive tool even in chronic ankle ligament injuries. The contrast delineates the ligaments and allows more accurate diagnosis and staging of lateral ankle injuries than are possible with other imaging techniques (Chandnani et al. 1994).

Medial Ligaments

The tibial collateral, or deltoid, ligament and the inferior calcaneonavicular, or spring, ligament make up the medial ligament complex. The deltoid ligament is divided into superficial and deep portions. The superficial portion arises from the anterior medial malleolus and inserts anteriorly into the navicular bone, medially into the calcaneus, and posteriorly to the talus. The deep portion of the deltoid ligament runs from the medial malleolus to the talus.

The spring ligament is supported in part by the superficial anterior deltoid ligament. Injuries to the medial ligament most commonly include avulsion fractures of the medial malleolus. Tears of the deltoid ligament are associated with more severe injury and are often accompanied by injury to the lateral ligaments. Widening of the ankle mortise is seen on radiography. These tears are usually complete.

The deltoid ligament is usually visualized on MRI in the coronal plane, especially with 20° to 40° plantarflexion. Axial images can also be helpful. The MRI signs of ligament tear are similar to those of other ligaments (figure 10.3).

Inferior Tibiofibular Ligaments

The inferior tibiofibular joint, or syndesmosis, is stabilized by the anterior tibiofibular ligament, the superficial and deep posterior tibiofibular ligaments, and the interosseous ligament. The inferior tibiofibular syndesmosis is involved in 10% of all ankle injuries. Conventional and stress radiography may demonstrate diastasis of the tibiofibular joint, but consensus is lacking on the criteria for diagnosis. This is due to variations in anatomy and difficulty in standardizing technique.

The syndesmotic ligaments can be imaged on MRI. However, nonvisualization of the ligaments

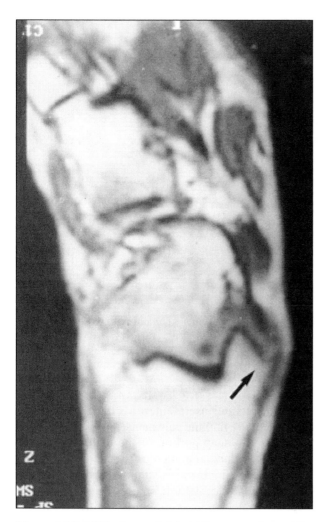

Figure 10.3 MRI of tear of deltoid ligament. Coronal T1 weighted spin echo image demonstrates lack of continuity between the medial malleolus and the posterior deltoid ligament.

without other signs is an unreliable predictor of ligament tear. Increased signal intensity on T2 weighted images, abnormal course, and wavy contour are other signs of ligament tear. The anterior tibiofibular ligament is most commonly injured (Vogl et al. 1997).

Injury to the Sinus Tarsi and Its Ligaments

The sinus tarsi is an anatomic space between the talus, calcaneus, and navicular bone. It is located anterior to the posterior talocalcaneal joint. It contains the talocalcaneal interosseous ligament, cervical ligament, fatty tissues, and blood vessels. The sinus tarsi syndrome, characterized by lateral foot pain, hindfoot instability, and tenderness over the sinus tarsi, is associated with ankle inversion trauma in 70% of patients (Klein & Spreiter 1993). In 43% of patients with acute ankle sprain, tarsal sinus abnormalities are seen on MRI. The most common finding is replacement of the normal fat in the sinus tarsi by decreased

signal intensity on T1 weighted images and increased signal intensity on STIR images (Breitenseher, Haller et al. 1997) (figure 10.4).

■ Tendon Injuries

Radiographs may demonstrate soft tissue swelling or other changes in tissue contour, tendon calcification, or proliferation of bone. However, radiographs are insensitive and usually not specific for tendon disorders. Soft tissue changes are best appreciated where the tendon is close to the skin or surrounded by fat.

High resolution ultrasonography is a useful tool in the evaluation of tendon abnormalities. It is limited by the experience of the operator, the quality of the equipment, and the location of the tendon.

CT can be used to image the tendons around the ankle. Although it is inferior to MRI in differentiating edema and fluid from scar tissue and in demonstrating small amounts of fluid, it is superior in depicting calcifications and avulsion fractures (Cheung et al. 1992).

Achilles Tendon

The Achilles tendon is formed from the gastrocnemius and soleus tendons. In axial cross-section, the Achilles tendon has a crescentic appearance with a rounded posterior aspect and a flat or slightly concave anterior aspect. Immediately above its insertion into the calcaneus, the tendon appears more ovoid. The Achilles tendon does not have a tendon sheath—only a peritenon. The Achilles tendon, although the strongest tendon in the lower leg, is the most commonly injured tendon in the ankle. Most injuries to the Achilles tendon occur approximately 2 to 6 cm proximal to its insertion, possibly because of a decreased blood supply to that area.

Injury to the Achilles tendon occurs most commonly through indirect forces, forced dorsiflexion, or overpronation, and is due to an acute event superimposed on a degenerated tendon. The typical patient is a poorly conditioned male between the ages of 30 and 50 who is involved in strenuous activity. Complete tears are seen as a discontinuity of the tendon. The gap is filled with blood or edema that in MRI images appears as increased signal (figure 10.5). This gap is seen as a hypoechoic region with ultrasonography. Partial tears are more difficult to diagnose and may demonstrate discontinuity of tendon fibers or thickening of the tendon (figure 10.6). MRI is considered the most accurate imaging modality. In MRI, increased signal is often noted in the tendon. MRI and ultrasound play a role in the selection of patients for surgical repair of tears. The site of the tear, the extent of the tear, and the size of the gap are all important parameters.

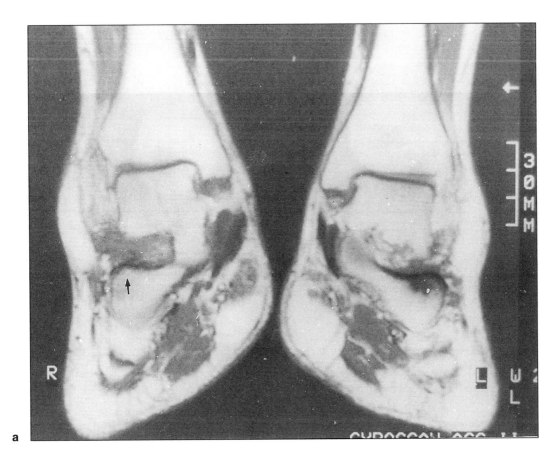

a

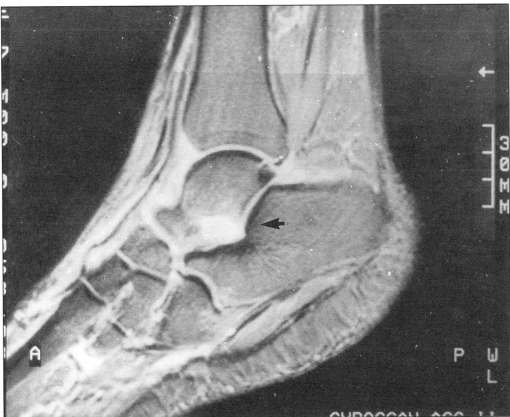

b

■ **Figure 10.4** MRI of sinus tarsi. *(a)* Coronal T1 weighted spin echo image demonstrates decreased signal intensity in sinus tarsi compared to the normal left ankle. *(b)* Sagittal STIR image demonstrates increased signal intensity in tarsal sinus.

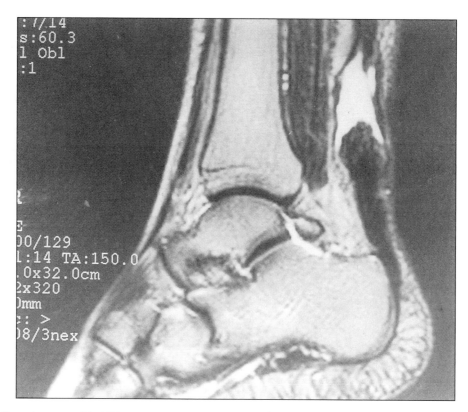

■ **Figure 10.5** Complete tear of Achilles tendon. Lateral T2 weighted fast spin echo MR image demonstrates tendon gap with thickened tendon edges and fluid in gap.

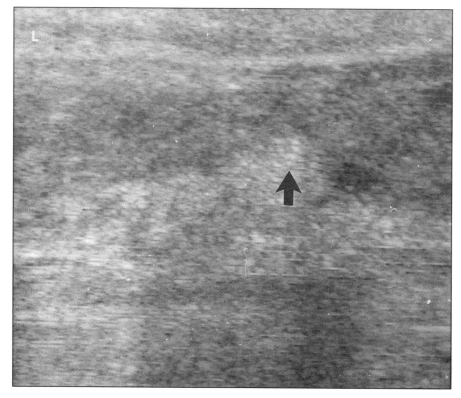

■ **Figure 10.6** Partial tear of the Achilles tendon. Sagittal ultrasound image demonstrates thinning of the tendon with thickened edges.

Inflammation in and around the Achilles tendon may be acute or chronic and is usually due to overuse of the ankle and foot, although systemic rheumatic disorders may be implicated. There is often surrounding inflammation. Tendon enlargement (manifested as rounding of the anterior border on axial images) and increased signal in the tendon on MRI are signs of tendinitis. Increased signal in the surrounding soft tissues on T2 weighted or STIR images are signs of peri- or paratendinitis.

Achilles tendon injury and inflammation may be associated with retrocalcaneal bursitis, and this structure must be evaluated.

Tibialis Posterior Tendon

The tibialis posterior tendon is the second most commonly injured tendon of the ankle. It is the most anterior of the flexor tendons. After curving under the medial malleolus, it inserts on the navicular, the cuneiforms, and the bases of the second to fourth metatarsal bones. Tendon tears and dysfunctions are most common in middle-aged patients, often with an underlying systemic articular disease, but have also been described in young athletes. An accessory navicular bone may also predispose individuals to tendon injury (Miller et al. 1995) (figure 10.7).

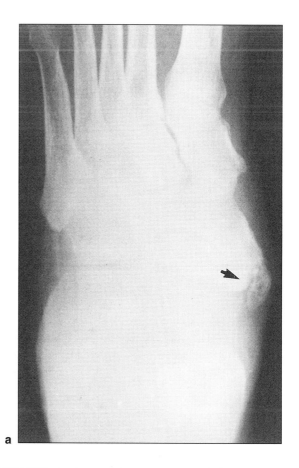

a

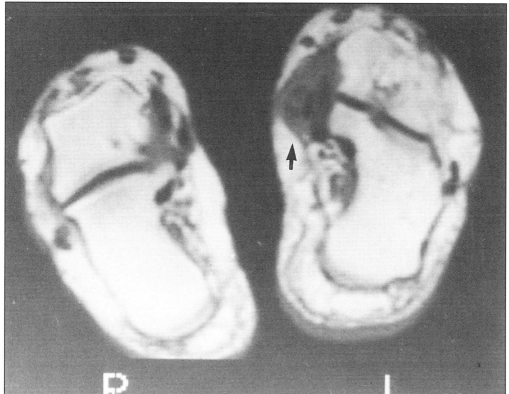

b

■ **Figure 10.7** Partial tear of the posterior tibialis tendon associated with os navicularis. *(a)* Radiograph of the foot demonstrates os navicularis. *(b)* T1 weighted spin echo axial MR image. Partial tear of the posterior tibialis tendon is seen with irregularity of the tendon and dilation of the tendon sheath.

Routine and weightbearing radiographs present a number of findings: increased talocalcaneal angle, lateral navicular subluxation, and pes planus. These are due to weakness of inversion of the foot, may appear later in the clinical course, and are less useful in early diagnosis. A diagnosis of tendon tear can be made with ultrasonography (figure 10.8). CT and MRI are accurate in the evaluation of degenerative changes as well as in evaluation of inflammation and tears. MRI is more accurate than CT and is superior in demonstrating vertical splits, edema, synovial fluid, and degeneration. CT is superior to MRI in showing associated bone changes such as periostitis, dislocations, and osteoarthritis (Rosenberg et al. 1988).

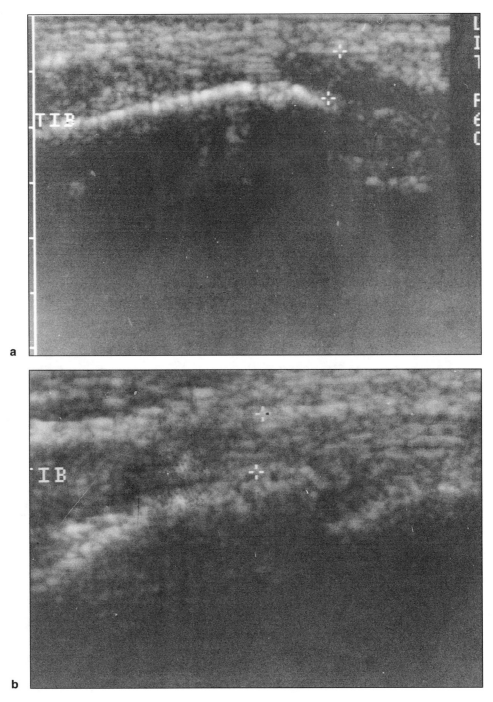

■ **Figure 10.8** Ultrasound of posterior tibialis tendon tear—oblique coronal view. (a) Tear of the tendon with thickened edges. (b) Normal comparison.

Peroneal Tendons

The peroneus longus and peroneus brevis tendons are closely related in their course behind and under the lateral malleolus, with the peroneus brevis tendon located anteriorly to the peroneus longus tendon. In this area, the tendons share a common tendon sheath and are held in place by the superior peroneal retinaculum.

The peroneal tendons may subluxate or dislocate, tear or become inflamed, or be entrapped. Traumatic dislocations of the peroneal tendons are associated with injury to the superior peroneal retinaculum or to its attachment to the fibula. This may occur with forced dorsiflexion or inversion injuries. The tendons subluxate laterally or anteriorly. Radiography may demonstrate small avulsion fractures of the lateral malleolus. Direct observation of the subluxated or dislocated tendons can be accomplished by ultrasonography, CT, or MRI, as well as by peroneal tenography. In some cases, there may be a need for dynamic studies, imaging the tendon while the foot is flexed.

Tears of the peroneal tendons are not rare. These tears may be acute or chronic and do not always cause symptoms. It is believed that in cases of peroneal tendon subluxation, the subluxated peroneus brevis tendon may be compressed between the posteriorly located peroneus longus tendon and the edge of the lateral malleolus, causing longitudinal splits. In addition to the usual increased signal and thickened tendon seen in partial tears of other tendons, portions of the peroneus brevis tendon may separate medially and laterally around the peroneus longus tendon (Rosenberg et al. 1997). Tendon tears and tendinitis not associated with subluxation may be due to direct injury, collagen vascular diseases, or recurrent stresses, as in athletes returning to training. The imaging findings are similar to those discussed previously for other tendons. Acute tears of the peroneus longus tendon are often associated with an avulsion fracture through the os peroneum when this sesamoid bone is present. The posterior migration of bone fragments can be detected on radiographs. For direct visualization of the tendon, both MR imaging (Tjin A Ton et al. 1997) and ultrasonography may be utilized. The findings are similar to those in other tendons discussed previously.

■ Osseous Lesions

Although overt fractures are easily diagnosed with radiography, clinically significant bone injury may be radiographically occult or difficult to assess without imaging. Computed tomography has an important role in complex fractures and in locating small bone fragments. Radionuclide bone scans are sensitive for bone injuries but are often not specific enough, and cannot precisely locate lesions. Magnetic resonance imaging allows direct imaging of the bone marrow and cartilage with precise anatomical location, high sensitivity, and specificity for a variety of osseous abnormalities.

Marrow Imaging

Imaging of abnormalities confined to the bone marrow, or with significant involvement of the marrow, is best accomplished with MRI. CT changes, such as increased or decreased marrow density, can be nonspecific and may appear only after the condition is well established. Radionuclide bone scans are nonspecific in location and appearance. MRI is the most sensitive modality for imaging of bone marrow, has excellent spatial resolution, and may be specific. However, a common finding of different bone marrow lesions is a pattern that has been coined "bone marrow edema." This pattern is manifested by hypointensity on T1 weighted images, hyperintensity on T2 weighted images, and enhancement after administration of contrast agents. Bone contusions are a common source of this pattern, but it is also seen in transient osteoporosis, reflex sympathetic dystrophy, diabetic neuropathy, infection, acute osteonecrosis, and even in nonosseous injuries (Hayes et al. 1993). Diagnosis is often based on other features.

Osteochondral Injuries

Injuries of the articular cartilage and underlying bone of the talus may be associated with a history of trauma or may be secondary to repetitive stress causing microtrauma. When seen on plain radiographs, an osteochondral defect appears as a rounded defect, possibly with a fragment in the defect or with subchondral sclerosis. Stage I lesions in which there is compression of subchondral bone with intact overlying cartilage cannot be seen on radiography. Isolated cartilage lesions are also undetectable. Even transchondral fractures may be undetectable on early radiographs. The role of imaging in osteochondral injury is to confirm the diagnosis, stage the injury, and detect loose bodies (figure 10.9).

Bone scans demonstrate focal increased activity, but it is difficult to assess the severity of the injury. CT is more sensitive than radiographs, but it is unable to demonstrate subtle subchondral and isolated cartilage injuries. MRI is more accurate than CT, although small chondral lesions may be missed (Anderson et al. 1989). Although it can be difficult to differentiate between a fragment that is not detached

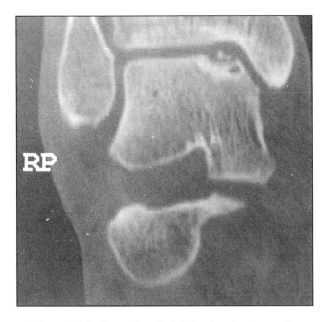

■ **Figure 10.9** Osteochondral defect in talar dome. Coronal CT demonstrates defect in medial dome of the talus containing small bony fragment.

and a detached but nondisplaced fragment, this distinction can be made with MRI (De Smet et al. 1990) and CT arthrography. These techniques are also useful in finding intra-articular loose bodies.

Avascular Necrosis

Osteonecrosis occurs when there is disruption of blood supply, with subsequent necrosis of bone. It may be idiopathic or post-traumatic. In the ankle, it is seen most commonly in the talus, navicular bone, or the distal tibia. Radiographs are negative in the early stages of avascular necrosis. Later, rarefaction and sclerosis may be seen. Bone scans are sensitive for avascular necrosis, except in very early stages in osteopenic patients. However, radionuclide bone scans do not allow assessment of the severity of the lesion, and are nonspecific. MRI is the most sensitive imaging modality for early avascular necrosis and accurately demonstrates the involved area. In the classic description of the MRI appearance of avascular necrosis, T2 weighted images show a serpiginous double line of high and low signal intensity bands surrounding an area of low signal intensity (Mitchell et al. 1987). In the ankle and in early stages, avascular necrosis may appear as a nonspecific bone marrow edema pattern, making the diagnosis more difficult (figure 10.10).

Stress Reaction and Stress Fractures

Stress reactions and fractures, the result of repeated cyclical loading on bones, are often seen in the ankle region. The most common location is the calcaneus. The navicular bone and other sites are less commonly involved. The location of injury is usually closely related to specific activities. Plain radiographs demonstrate a linear radiodense area perpendicular to the

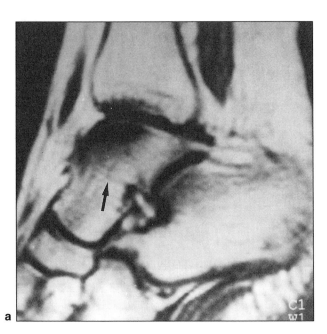 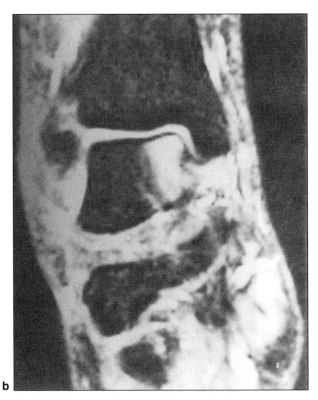

a   b

■ **Figure 10.10** Avascular necrosis of talar dome—MRI. *(a)* T1 weighted spin echo sagittal image demonstrates decreased signal of talar dome. *(b)* Coronal STIR image demonstrates increased signal in the talus without collapse of the cortex.

trabeculae in cancellous bone such as the calcaneus. In cortical stress fractures, there is typically a radiolucent fracture line within an area of cortical thickening and sclerosis. However, there is a lag in time from the first symptoms until positive signs are seen on radiograph. In addition, marked hyperostosis may obscure the fracture line. The role of CT is limited in stress fractures, but it is especially useful in demonstrating a radiolucent fracture line when hyperostosis is marked. Radionuclide bone scans are sensitive, and changes in the study mark the natural history of the stress and healing process. Increased activity is seen on all phases of a bone scan. MRI is as sensitive as bone scan and is more specific in stress fractures. Linear zones of low signal intensity surrounded by poorly defined areas of increased signal intensity are seen on T1 and T2 weighted spin echo and STIR sequences, as well as enhancement after intravenous gadolinium injection.

■ Summary

Imaging has an important role in the diagnosis and assessment of ankle abnormalities. In particular, the tendons, ligaments, bone marrow, and joints can often be studied with the help of different imaging modalities. Each technique has its strengths and disadvantages, and care must be exercised in matching the technique to the clinical abnormality. The role of each modality and of imaging of the ankle is evolving and will change in the future with technological developments and with new clinical insights.

■ References

Anderson IF, Crichton KJ, Grattan-Smith T, et al. Osteochondral fractures of the dome of the talus. J Bone Joint Surg (Am) 1989;70A:1143.

Anzilloti K, Schweitzer ME, Hecht P, Wapner K, Kahn M, Ross M. Effect of foot and ankle imaging on clinical decision making. Radiology 1996; 201:515.

Breitenseher MJ, Haller JH, Kukla C, et al. MRI of the sinus tarsi in acute ankle sprain injuries. J Comput Assist Tomogr 1997;21(2):274.

Breitenseher MJ, Trattnig S, Kukla C, et al. MRI versus lateral stress radiography in acute lateral ankle ligament injuries. J Comput Assist Tomogr 1997;21:280.

Chandnani VP, Harper MT, Ficke JR, et al. Chronic ankle instability: Evaluation with MR arthrography, MR imaging, and stress radiography. Radiology 1994;192:189.

Cheung Y, Rosenberg ZS, Magee T, et al. Normal anatomy and pathologic conditions of ankle tendons: Current imaging techniques. Radiographics 1992;12:492.

De Smet AA, Fisher DR, Burnstein MI. Value of MR imaging in staging osteochondral lesions of the talus (osteochondritis dissecans): Results in 14 patients. Am J Roentgenol 1990;154:555.

Fessell DP, Vanderschueren GM, Jacobson JA, et al. US of the ankle: Technique, anatomy, and diagnosis of pathologic conditions. Radiographics 1998;18:325.

Fordyce AJW, Horn CV. Arthrography in recent injuries of the ligament of the ankle. J Bone Joint Surg (Br) 1972;54:116.

Hayes CW, Conway WF, Daniel WW. MR imaging of bone marrow edema pattern: transient osteoporosis, transient bone marrow edema pattern, or osteonecrosis. Radiographics 1993;13:1001.

Klein MA, Spreitzer AM. MR Imaging of the tarsal sinus and canal: Normal anatomy, pathological findings, and features of the sinus tarsi syndrome. Radiology 1993;186:233.

Link SC, Erickson SJ, Timins ME. MR imaging of the ankle and foot: Normal structures and anatomical variants that may simulate disease. AJR 1993;161:607.

Miller TT, Staron RB, Feldman F, et al. The symptomatic accessory tarsal navicular bone: assessment with MR imaging. Radiology 1995;195:849-853.

Mitchell DG, Rao VM, Dalinka MK, Spritzer CE, Alavi A, Steinberg ME, Fallon M, Kressel HY. Femoral head avascular necrosis: Correlation of MR imaging, radiographic staging, radionuclide imaging, and clinical findings. Radiology 1987;162(3):709-715.

Noto AM, Cheung Y, Rosenberg ZS, Norman A, Leeds NE. MR imaging of the ankle: normal variants. Radiology 1989;170(1 Pt 1):121-124.

Rosenberg ZS, Beltran J, Cheung YY, Colon E, Herraiz F. MR features of longitudinal tears of the peroneal brevis tendon. AJR 1997;168:141-147.

Rosenberg ZS, Cheung Y, Jahss MH, Noto AM, Norman A, Leeds NE. Rupture of posterior tibial tendon: CT and MR imaging with surgical correlation. Radiology 1988;169(1):229-35.

Schneck CD, Mesgarzadeh M, Bonakdapour A, Ross G. MR imaging of the most commonly injured ankle ligaments. Part I. Normal anatomy. Radiology 1992;184:499.

Tjin A Ton ER, Schweitzer ME, Karasick D. MR imaging of peroneal tendon disorders. Am J Roentgenol 1997;168(1):135-140.

Vogl TJ, Hochmuth K, Diebold T, Lubrich J, Hofmann R, Stockle U, Sollner O, Bisson S, Sudkamp N, Maeurer J, Haas N, Felix R. Magnetic resonance imaging in the diagnosis of acute injured distal tibiofibular syndesmosis. Invest Radiol 1997;32(7):401-409.

Zanetti M, De Simoni C, Wetz HH, Zollinger H, Hodler J. Magnetic resonance imaging of injuries to the ankle joint: Can it predict clinical outcome? Skeletal Radiol 1997;26(2):82-88.

Chapter 11

Role of Arthroscopy in Chronic Ankle Sprains

Wolf-Ruediger Dingels, MD, PhD

How often inversion trauma of the upper ankle joint occurs is unknown. Several authors (Brooks et al. 1981; McCulloch et al. 1985; Ruth 1961) report an injury frequency of 1,000 persons per day worldwide. Jackson et al. (1974) found this to be the most common injury at the United States Military Academy, West Point: One-third of the cadets sprain an ankle during their 4 years there. A sprained ankle is the most common injury in sports (Glick et al. 1976; Garrick 1977). In similar studies in Finland (Sandelin 1988) and Norway (Maehlum and Daliord 1984), acute sprains of the ankle represented 21% and 16%, respectively, of all sport-related injuries. The data on epidemiology and incidence are discussed in chapters 1, 5, 20, and 32.

Until the early 1970s, no special diagnostics and therapy were carried out when the prescribed treatment was mainly conservative. After the introduction of radiographs and application of arthroscopy, the industrialized nations began employing differentiated therapy with salve dressing, plaster cast, and surgical repair (Stover 1980). In the 1980s and 1990s in German-speaking countries in Europe, almost every lateral ligament rupture was treated surgically (Tiling et al. 1994), in spite of controlled trials published before 1984 that favored either an operation or conservative treatment. Only after worldwide discussion of this topic did the therapy concept change again in the direction of conservative treatment and particularly toward functional therapy. Current practice, influenced by an increased understanding of anatomy and pathophysiology, emphasizes procedures such as arthroscopy—which had become routine in diagnostics and therapy for other joints—for the sprained ankle.

■ Anatomy and Pathophysiology

For the functional anatomy of the talocrural joint, three facts are significant:

- No muscle inserts on the talus; it is solely guided osseously and by ligaments.

- The trochlea tali is narrower in the back than in the front so that the osseous guiding of the lateral gutter is at its maximum in dorsiflexion of the foot and at its minimum in plantarflexion.

- The ligament's guiding of the talus is at maximum in plantarflexion, at minimum in dorsiflexion.

According to studies by Broström (1964) and Leonard (1949), approximately two-thirds of ankle sprains involve isolated injuries of the anterior talofibular ligament. If the inversion trauma is more severe, the calcaneofibular ligament is also involved. Broström observed that combined rupture of the talofibular and calcaneofibular ligaments occurred in 20% of his patients and that the calcaneofibular ligament was never ruptured alone. According to Niedermann et al. (1981), in 47% of ankle sprains, the lateral ligament capsule apparatus is injured; in 35% of sprains one ligament is ruptured; and in 18% two ligaments are ruptured.

Although 85% of ankle sprains involve inversion injuries, it is the eversion injury that presents a serious problem to the individual in terms of time loss. An inversion injury involves an inversion of the foot on an externally rotating tibia. This results primarily in an avulsion of the anterior talofibular and the anterior tibiofibular ligaments. If the force progresses, the calcaneofibular ligament is also involved in the injury. The mechanism of injury in an eversion sprain is an outward turning of the foot on an internally rotating tibia, resulting in a rupture of the medial ligament. The most important factor in causing a disability is a rupture that damages the interosseus membrane.

In soccer players, there is another category of ankle injury in which a pure external rotation results in an anterior tibiofibular sprain. A mechanism of ankle injury in football players, and perhaps in hockey players, occurs when the athlete has one foot forcefully plantarflexed on the ground and someone falls on the athlete's heel. This causes true forced plantarflexion without any inversion or eversion, resulting in an injury to the anterior syndesmosis. An injury that is unique to dancers occurs when they "go over the top" (extreme plantarflexion) and sprain the front of the ankle.

Currently available imaging procedures, as well as direct viewing of the joint by arthroscopy, show a further damaging of the joint after distortion in all three injuries listed previously. Here we deal with chondral osseous injuries, which have their pathomorphologic source in the anatomy of the ankle and in the pathophysiology of the distortion. The dome of the talus is not a cylinder but is a truncated cone, narrower in the back than in the front (Inman 1976), making the tibiotalar joint potentially unstable in plantarflexion. This laxity disappears in the full pointe position as the posterior lip of the tibia comes to rest against the os calcis. Thus, the subtalar joint is locked in full plantarflexion of the ankle. Gould et al. (1980) pointed out the anatomical analogies between the knee and the ankle:

- Medial knee is analogous to lateral ankle.
- Anterior cruciate ligament is analogous to anterior talofibular ligament.
- Posterior cruciate ligament is analogous to posterior talofibular ligament.

Ruptures of these ligaments lead to analogous anterior-posterior and rotational instabilities. The isolated anterior syndesmosis rupture is a rare injury with a frequency between 3.3% and 5% of all lesions in the upper ankle joint (Cahill 1965; Ferkel and Fischer 1989; Lundeen 1987), which leads to long-term complaints if it is not recognized and treated. The clinical examination for diagnosis of this injury is far more sophisticated than that for the capsule ligament injuries lateral in the ankle. Standardized radiographs are often normal, so it is necessary to use arthrography, computer tomography, and nuclear magnetic resonance tomography to aid in diagnosis (Light and Pupp 1991).

■ Diagnostics

Injuries to the ankle are diagnosed with a detailed history of the accident and a complete clinical examination. Radiographs of the ankle region are necessary to exclude an accompanying fracture. Secondary tests include scans (computed tomography, magnetic resonance imaging) and arthrograms. However, nothing

can surpass direct visualization by diagnostic and operative arthroscopy.

Clinical Diagnostics

An accurate anamnestic evaluation is essential. The description of the exact accident mechanism in the sense of a supination-adduction-inversion-stress, the feeling of something being torn, and the immediate impossibility of weight bearing on the ankle point the way to a diagnosis. The examination of the freshly injured ankle should be carried out with the patient lying down. A comparative examination of the uninjured ankle should be carried out first. A localizable pressure or pain may hint at the ruptured ligament structure. An accompanying rupture of the deltoid ligament should be considered, and an isolated rupture of the anterior syndesmosis ligament should be clinically eliminated. Furthermore, the patient should be examined for injuries of the peroneus tendon, including a luxation or damage of the peroneal nerve.

The stability test of the upper ankle is decisive. This includes assessment of the talus tilt and the talus drawer test. The pathological talus drawer test is normally easier to verify clinically, because the patient rejects this examination less than testing of the talus tilt. To safely release the drawer, the heel should be gripped firmly to enable a backward and forward pushing of the foot while the lower leg is fixed. Clinical evidence of a pathological talus tilt can usually be achieved when the physician distracts the patient during the examination. Only a slight element of surprise is needed so that the patient is unable to hold the talus with the counterreacting pedal flexor. In anxious patients, the clinical and radiological examination can often only be completed under anesthesia. In the clinical examination, sprain mimics, such as Achilles rupture or plantaris rupture, must be excluded.

If a significant period of time has elapsed since the injury has occurred and there is a considerable amount of edema, the diagnosis may not be made on the first examination. Therefore, an additional examination should be made 3 or 4 days later.

Radiological and Extended Imaging Diagnostics

To determine whether the lower ankle is involved, and to exclude a fracture, a survey radiogram of the lower ankle joint in two levels should be made. This is considered standard in documentation. A comparison image of the uninjured ankle is necessary when it is suspected that the fibular epiphysis comes off, as occurs in the ligament rupture in children. If an isolated syndesmosis rupture is suspected, the total fibula must be radiologically imaged to exclude a Maissoneuve fracture. If the condition of the upper ankle is not clear, radiographs of the tarsus should be taken in two levels so that injuries of the total supination line are not overlooked.

In rare cases, a survey radiogram may indicate an osteochondral fracture of the trochlea of the talus edge, the "dome fracture." This can be verified by additional imaging procedures. Old injuries, such as talus cysts or osteophytes of the fibulotalar tibiotalar intra-articular space, point to a chronic relapsing distortion. This category also includes the talus nose, the ventral or dorsal tibia exophytes, as expression of a chronic instability of the upper ankle (soccer player's ankle).

These findings, like evidence of a plump bone shadow subfibular (os subfibular), indicate a chronic clinical condition and must therefore be taken into account as the surgery is planned. When there is a fresh rupture of a chronically scarred and deformed ligament and deformed ligament apparatus, this means that a rupture by stages has occurred.

Sprains are accompanied by fracture <15% of the time, and thus the occurrence of fracture with sprain is relatively rare (Chirls 1973; Schaap et al. 1989). Sixty-two percent of children 8 and older with sprains of the lateral ligament have osseous lateral ligament avulsion associated with the sprains; 80% of children 7 and younger with similar sprains have avulsions associated with the sprains (Reichen and Marti 1974). Prins (1978) put the frequency for the rupture of one ligament in people from the ages of 8 to 57 years at 7%, and the frequency of the rupture of two ligaments at 14%. Zwipp et al. (1987) found a talar dome fracture in 2.4% of 1,235 lateral ligament ruptures. This was located laterally 24 times and medially 5 times. Prins (1978) reports that among 45 ruptures of two ligaments, there were 2 multiple fractures of the lateral talus edge. Zwipp et al. (1987) noted that the frequency of medial malleolus fracture was 1.3%, and the frequency of fracture of the epiphysis malleoli lateralis was 1%.

The radiological clarification of each ankle injury has recently not been considered necessary in every case because of cost factors. According to Stiell et al. (1995), in case of pain in the area of the lateral malleolus, a radiological examination is not necessary if the patient is under 55 years of age, can bear weight after the accident, can walk four steps in the emergency room, and has no bone pressure pain in the posterior edge or top of the malleolus. Under these conditions, no fractures were found in a prospective trial with 847 radiological examinations of the upper ankle joint, or in a validation trial with 385 patients.

Various guidelines have been developed to combat the overuse of radiography in ankle injuries. Stiell et al.'s criteria (1995) have been successful in a multicenter controlled trial, which resulted in significant decreases in ankle radiography (21.9%), waiting times, and costs, without an increased rate of missed fractures.

Acute osteochondral fractures of the talar dome may be radiographically occult in up to 30% of cases. Computed tomography is more sensitive than plain radiography, but it cannot detect early disease and cannot differentiate between stable and unstable fragments. Magnetic resonance imaging (MRI) is accurate in detecting and staging osteochondral lesions and is now the imaging method of choice (Berndt and Harty 1959; Dipaola et al. 1991).

MRI has been used to evaluate ligament injuries around the ankle. In chronic collateral ligament injuries, conventional MRI has shown variable sensitivity, and the best results have been achieved with MR arthrography (Chandnani et al. 1996; Schneck et al. 1992; Erickson et al. 1991).

In one series, an ultrasonic examination showed very clearly the hematoma in the ankle joint (figure 11.1). With recurrent injury, differentiation of tendinosis from partial tear is important, as it may affect management. The ultrasonic criterion for partial tear, discontinuity of the tendon fibers, is the most discriminating feature (Kalebo et al. 1992). MRI is more accurate than ultrasound in detecting partial tears, but the two methods have similar accuracy in detecting tendinosis and complete tears (Neuhold et al. 1992). What, then, is the best strategy for imaging? Because ultrasound is more cost effective than MRI, it would seem that ultrasound should be the initial imaging technique and, where results are inconclusive, MRI should also be performed.

■ Classification of Sprains

For further details see chapters 6 and 7.

Traditionally, in clinical practice, sprains of the ankle have been classified as grade I, or mild; grade II, or moderate; and grade III, or severe (Balduini and Tetzlaff 1982; Balduini et al. 1987; Chapman 1975; Diamond 1989; Lassiter et al. 1989).

- A **grade I** injury involves stretch of the ligament without macroscopic tearing, little swelling or tenderness, slight or no functional loss, and no mechanical instability of the joint.

- A **grade II** injury is a partial macroscopic tear of the ligament with moderate pain, swelling, and tenderness over the involved structures. There is some loss of motion and mild or moderate instability of the joint.

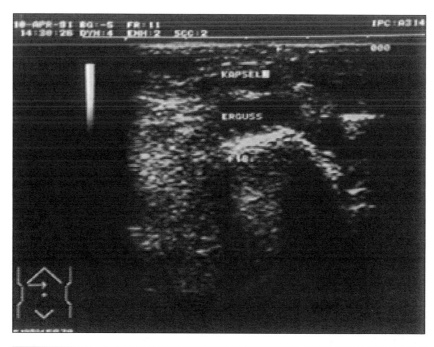

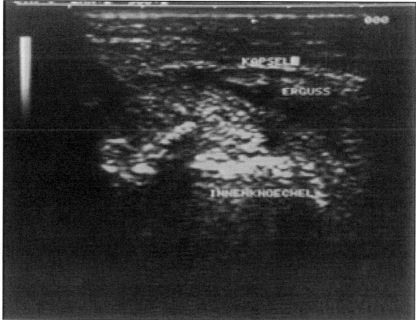

■ **Figure 11.1** Arthroscopic exam showing hematoma in ankle joint.

■ A **grade III** injury is complete rupture of the ligament with severe swelling, hemorrhage, and tenderness. There is loss of function and considerable abnormal motion and instability of the joint.

Establishing Appropriate Treatment Regimens

Once the clinical diagnosis has been made and confirmed by radiographs or other imaging methods, a treatment regimen must be decided.

Almost all of the patients having a grade I or grade II injury recover quickly with nonoperative management (Balduini and Tetzlaff 1982; Balduini et al. 1987; Diamond 1989; Lassiter et al. 1989), and the prognosis is, almost without exception, excellent or good (Balduini and Tetzlaff 1982; Balduini et al. 1987; Diamond 1989; Lassiter et al. 1989; Brooks et al. 1981; Derscheid and Brown 1985; Hamilton 1988; Jackson et al. 1974; Gould et al. 1980; Prins 1978; Schaap et al. 1989). The treatment program, usually called *functional treatment,* includes three phases.

Immediately after the injury, rest, ice (cold), compression, and elevation (RICE) are used. Then a short period of immobilization and protection with supportive bandaging, taping, or bracing (e.g., aircast bracing) is utilized to control pain and swelling. Finally, active range-of-motion exercises are started, followed by weight bearing, appropriate proprioceptive training with a tilt board and other devices (see chapter 22), and strengthening exercises for the peroneus muscle.

The treatment of grade II sprains of the lateral ligament complex is more controversial. Many uncontrolled, nonrandomized studies have suggested that primary repair is the method of choice, because most patients who had operative treatments seemed to have a mechanically stable ankle and satisfactory subjective results (Anderson et al. 1962; Brand et al. 1981; Jaskulka et al. 1988; Korkala et al. 1982; Niethard 1974; Reichen and Marti 1974; Ruth 1961; Staples 1975). However, similar results have been reported after conservative treatment.

Although the cost of operative treatment is, of course, far more than that of conservative treatment, the long-term sequelae of unseen lesions in a sprained ankle can produce even greater costs. Such oversight can be the cause for long-term disability or functional instability, and it may result in the need for a late reconstruction operation, which will have its own morbidity. Thus, although the concept of individualizing treatment after careful injury analysis may seem appealingly straightforward, it is not easy to determine which patients should receive surgical repair and which should be treated by conservative means.

The Role of Arthroscopy in Improving Diagnosis and Treatment

Shea and Manoli (1993) demonstrate that osteochondral lesions have a traumatic etiology and are a common reason for ankle disability. Taga et al. (1993) were able to prove, by arthroscopy, that chondral lesions in freshly injured ankle joints were present in 89% of the cases and in 95% of the ankles with chronic injuries. In our own prospective trial in 1993, we found in 32 of 100 patients (who had undergone arthroscopy during the first 10 days after ankle joint distortion with hematoma as a cardinal symptom) a chondral lesion in the talus and the tibia articular surface. Bobic (1994), in an evaluation of the treatment potential of ankle arthroscopic surgery in sports injuries, found 24 osteochondral lesions out of 76 arthroscopies.

Ancillary tests, such as radiographs, computed tomography, scans, MRI, bone scans, and arthrograms, can also be indicated in determining the cause of the patient's problem. However, the diagnosis of intra-articular lesions of the ankle, as in other major joints, is often made only upon direct visualization. Diagnostic and operative arthroscopy, with its shorter rehabilitation time, has proven extremely beneficial in helping athletes with knee, shoulder, and elbow injuries return to competition. Furthermore, the arthroscope can also assist the surgeon in completing the diagnosis and provide therapeutic treatment for traumatic disorders of the ankle.

Arthroscopic diagnosis and treatment of ankle injuries are similar to the experience with knee arthroscopy. Previously, casts were applied to treat knee ligament injuries, but with terrible results. Then, operative management of the medial collateral ligament was tried, also with terrible results. Now practitioners have realized that a minimally invasive intervention, such as arthroscopy, supports later function and provides very good results. Current practitioners are seeing the same developments in ankle treatment. These developments have led to reassessment of the indications for diagnostics and therapy of the sprained ankle and to a list of the indications for the diagnostic and surgical arthroscopy:

- Hemarthrosis
- Osteocartilaginous lesions
- Instability
- Graduation of ligament rupture
- Blockades

Several authors (Knopp and Neumann 1993; Landsiedel 1991; Gächter and Gerber 1991; Rehm 1985; Parisien 1987) emphasize the necessity of acute arthroscopy when hemarthroses are proved in the ankle joint. In reality, it is only partly true that hemarthrosis in the ankle distributes quickly into the tissue fissure alongside the fibula or rear foot. Corresponding to the pattern of injury, an essential part of hemarthrosis may stay in the ankle and lead to subsequent damage because of enzymatic chondral damage. Rehm (1985) and Knopp et al. (1993) were able to prove that an evaluation of osteochondral lesions and further concomitant injuries of a diastasis of the talofibular syndesmosis, or a rupture of the same structure, could only be determined by arthroscopy and could then be treated by arthroscopically assisted surgery.

Arthroscopy has opened a new dimension of assessment of osteochondral lesions of the medial or lateral talar edge (Landsiedel 1991). According to Anetzberger et al. (1998), an instability of the lateral ligament complex may be recognized, classified, and possibly treated by percutaneous suturing techniques. These techniques involve an elective operation, which must be discussed with the patient. The patient must be informed about the problems of instability resulting from an inadequate treatment and the possibility of conservative treatment. The invasiveness of this surgical intervention should not be ignored. In particular, the danger of damaging nerves and vessels should be mentioned. The patient should be made aware of the postoperative functional treatment in braces.

The indication for arthroscopically controlled ligament suture in the upper ankle in an isolated rupture of the lateral ligament complex exists in patients under 30 years of age, because recurrent luxation followed by chronic instability happens most frequently in this period of life. The arthroscopic method provides two advantages: The hemarthrosis accompanying the rupture can be rinsed out, and the chondral fractures on the lateral talus neck can be recognized and fixed with an adequate therapy.

Blockades, lacerations or scars of the synovial structures, and loose bodies occur as a consequence of the chondral destruction of an ankle sprain and can be avoided with arthroscopy during the initial stage.

■ References

Anderson KJ, Lecocq JF, Clayton ML. Athletic injury to the fibular collateral ligament of the ankle. Din Orthop 23: 146-160, 1962.

Anetzberger H, Hempfling H, Putz R. Sprunggelenk, Chirurgische Operationslehre, 1998. Springer: Berlin.

Balduini FC, Tetzlaff J. Historical perspectives on injuries of the ligaments of the ankle. Clin Sports Med I: 3-12, 1982.

Balduini FC, Vegso JJ, Toro JS, Toro E. Management and rehabilitation of ligamentous injuries of the ankle. Sports Med 4: 364-380, 1987.

Berndt Al, Harty M. Transchondral fractures (osteochondrosis dissecans) of the talus. J Bone Joint Surg (AM), 41-A: 988-1020, 1959.

Bobic V. Ankle Arthroscopy in the Management of Athletic Injuries. Arthroscopy Surgery Research and Training Laboratory, Exeter, 1994.

Brand RL, Collins MDF, Templeton T. Surgical repair of ruptured lateral ankle ligaments. Am J Sports Med 9: 40-44, 1981.

Brooks SC, Potter BT, Rainey, JB. Treatment for partial tears of the lateral ligament of the ankle: a prospective trial. British Med J 282: 606-607, 1981.

Broström L. Sprained ankles. I. Anatomic lesions in recent sprains. Acta Chir Scandinavica 128: 483-495, 1964.

Cahill DR. The anatomy and function of the human tarsal sinus and canal. Anat Rec 153: 1-18, 1965.

Chandnani VP, Harper, MT, Ficke, IR, et al. Chronic ankle instability, evaluation with MRI arthrography, MR imaging, and stress radiography. Radiology 192: 189-194, 1996.

Chapman MW. Part II. Sprains of the ankle. In Instructional Course Lectures. The American Academy of Orthopedic Surgeons Vol. 24, pp. 294-308. St. Louis, C.V. Mosby, 1975.

Chirls M. Inversion injuries of the ankle. J Med Soc New Jersey 70: 751-753, 1973.

Derscheid GL, Brown WC. Rehabilitation of the ankle. Clin Sports Med 4: 527-544, 1985.

Diamond JE. Rehabilitation of ankle sprains. Clin Sports Med 8: 877-891, 1989.

Dipaola JD, Nelson DW, Colville MR. Characterising osteochondral lesions by magnetic resonance imaging. J Arthroscopy Rel Surg 7: 101-104, 1991.

Erickson SI, Smith IW, Ruiz ME, et al. MR imaging of the lateral collateral ligament of the ankle. AJR 156: 131-136, 1991.

Ferkel RD, Fischer SP. Progress in ankle arthroscopy. Clin Orthop 240: 210-220, 1989.

Gächter A, Gerber BE. Arthroskopie des oberen Sprunggelenks in Lokalanaesthesie. Arthroskopie 4: 37-41, 1991.

Garrick JM. The frequency of injury and epidemiology of ankle sprains. Am J Sports Med 5: 241-242, 1977.

Glick JM, Gordon RB, Nishimoto, D. The prevention and treatment of ankle injuries. Am J Sports Med 4: 136-141, 1976.

Gould N, Seligson D, Gassmann I. Early and late repair of lateral ligament of the ankle. Foot Ankle 1: 84-89, 1980.

Hamilton WG. Foot and ankle injuries in dancers. Clin Sports Med 7: 143-173, 1988.

Inman V. The Joints of the Ankle. Baltimore, Williams & Wilkins, 1976.

Jackson DW, Ashley RL, Powell JW. Ankle sprains in young athletes. Relation of severity and disability. Clin Orthop 101: 201-215, 1974.

Jaskulka R, Fischer G, Schedl R. Injuries of the lateral ligaments of the ankle joint. Operative treatment and long-term results, Arch Orthop Traumat Surg 107: 217-221, 1988.

Kalebo P, Allenmark C, Peterson L, et al. Diagnostic value of ultrasonography in partial ruptures of the Achilles tendon. Am J Sports Med 20: 378-381, 1992.

Knopp W, Neumann K. Arthroskopie "kleiner Gelenke," Indikation zur diagnostischen und therapeutischen Arthroskopie. Chirurg 64: 163-169, 1993.

Korkala O, Lauttamus L, Tanskanen P. Lateral ligament injuries of the ankle. Results of primary surgical treatment. Ann Chir Gynaec 71: 161-163, 1982.

Landsiedel F. Die Arthroskopie des oberen Sprunggelenks. Arthroskopie 4: 2-8, 1991.

Lassiter TE Jr, Malone TR, Garrett WE. Injury of the lateral ligaments of the ankle. Orthop Clin N Am 20: 629-640, 1989.

Leonard MH. Injuries of the lateral ligaments of the ankle. A clinical and experimental study. J Bone Joint Surg 31-A: 373-377, April 1949.

Light M, Pupp G. Ganglions in the sinus tarsi. J Foot Ankle Surg 26: 22-25, 1991.

Lundeen RO. Techniques of ankle arthroscopy. J Foot Ankle Surg 30: 350-355, 1987.

Maehlum S, Daliord OA. Acute sports injuries in Oslo: A one-year study. Br J Sports Med 18: 181-185, 1984.

McCulloch JP, Holden P, Robson DJ, Rowley DI, Norris SH. The value of mobilisation and non-steroidal anti-inflammatory analgesia in the management of inversion injuries of the ankle. Br J Clin Pract 39: 69-72, 1985.

Neuhold A, Stiskal, M, Kainberger F et al. Degenerative Achilles tendon disease, assessment by magnetic resonance and ultrasonography. EUR J Radiol 14: 213-220, 1992.

Niedermann B, Andersen A, Andersen SB, Funder V, Jorgensen, JP, Lindholmer, E, Vuust M. Rupture of the lateral ligaments of the ankle: Operation or plaster cast? A prospective study. Acta Orthop Scandinavica 52: 579-587, 1981.

Niethard FU. Die Stabilität des Sprunggelenkes nach Ruptur des lateralen Bandapparates. (The mechanical stability of the ankle joint after rupture of the lateral ligament) (English abstract). Arch Orthop Unfallchir 80: 53-61, 1974.

Parisien IS. Ankle and subtalar joint arthroscopy. An update. Bull Hosp Joint Dis 47: 262-272, 1987.

Prins JG. Diagnosis and treatment of injury of the lateral ligament of the ankle. A comparative clinical study. Acta Chir Scand Suppl 486, 1978.

Rehm KE. Indikation, Technik und Aussagekraft der Sprunggelenksarthroskopie. Arthroskopiekurs Nürnberg, 1985.

Reichen A, Marti K. Die frische fibulare Bandruptur—Diagnose, Therapie, Resultate (Rupture of the fibular collateral ligaments—diagnosis, surgical treatment, results) (English abstract). Arch Orthop Unfallchir 80: 211-222, 1974.

Ruth CJ, The surgical treatment of injuries of the fibular collateral ligaments of the ankle. J Bone Joint Surg 43-A: 229-239, March 1961.

Sandelin J. Acute sports injuries. A clinical and epidemiological study. Dissertation, pp. 1-66, University of Helsinki, Helsinki, Finland, Helsinki, Yllopistopaino, 1988.

Schaap GR, De Keizer G, Marti K. Inversion trauma of the ankle. Arch Orthop Traumat Surg 108: 273-275, 1989.

Schneck GD, Mesgarzadeh M, Bonatedarpour A. MR imaging of the most commonly injured ankle ligaments. Part 2 Ligament injuries. Radiology 184: 507-512, 1992.

Shea MP, Manoli A. Osteochondral lesions of the talar dome. Foot Ankle 14: 48-55, 1993.

Staples OS. Ruptures of the fibular collateral ligaments of the ankle. Result study of immediate surgical treatment. J Bone Joint Surg 57-A: 101-107, Jan. 1975.

Stiell IG, Wells G, Lanpacis A, et al. Multicentre trial to introduce the Ottawa ankle rules for use of radiography in acute ankle injuries. BMI 311: 594-597, 1995.

Stover CN. Air-Stirrup management of ankle injuries in the athlete. Am J Sports Med 8-5: 360-365, 1980.

Taga I, Shino K, Imone M, Nakata K, et al. Articular cartilage lesions in ankles with lateral ligament injury. Am J Sports Med 21: 120-126, 1993.

Tiling TH, Bonk A, Höher I, Klein I. Die akute Aussenbandverletzung des Sprunggelenkes beim Sportler. Der Chirurg 65: 920-933, 1994.

Zwipp H, Reschauer, R. Ergebnisse nach Zugschraubenosteosynthesen bei 62 dislozierten Talusfrakturen und Talusluxationsfrakturen. Unfallheilkunde 81: 324-327, 1987.

Part IV

Complications of Ankle Sprain

Complications of the acute sprain may lead to symptoms that include chronic instability, continuous pain, or both. Subtalar instability may cause symptoms, but it is difficult to diagnose clinically and radiologically.

- **Instability symptoms** may ensue from the ankle itself or from the subtalar joints. Subtalar instability may cause symptoms, but it is difficult to diagnose clinically and radiologically. The chronic instability of the ankle may be divided into two types:

  1. Mechanical, in which there is pathological opening of the ankle joint, either lateral or posterior, in stress radiography.
  2. Functional, in which there are complaints of instability but there is no opening of the joint.

- Chronic pain after acute injury may result from osteochondral fractures, sinus tarsi pain, nerve injuries, tendon injuries, and fractures.

Chapter 12

Chronic Ankle Instability, Mechanical and Functional

Gideon Mann, MD; Meir Nyska, MD; Alex Finsterbush, MD; Naama Constantini, MD; and Joseph Lowe, MD

In the following pages we will discuss the complex subject of mechanical and functional instability of the ankle. Although only about 40% of mechanically unstable ankles are functionally unstable, about 40% of functionally unstable ankles will appear completely stable on a stress radiograph. Many factors could explain this "stable instability," namely, anterior and rotational instability with no instability in the coronal plane, subtalar instability, instability of the mortise, subtalar or ankle post-traumatic adhesions, peroneal tendon tear or subluxation, or peroneal muscle weakness. Although all these are important causes of this phenomenon, it seems that the leading cause for stable instability of the ankle is nerve injury within or proximal to the lateral ligament. This injury could reduce joint and skin sensation, cause weakened peroneal muscles, interfere with joint proprioception, balance, and posture stability, and elongate nerve conduction and reaction times, thus causing repeated ankle injury with or without demonstrable ankle instability.

■ Introduction

Chronic ankle instability is the most frequent and the most disturbing complication of acute ankle sprains (Mann et al. 1993; Peri 1992), occurring in 25 to 50% of acute grade II and III ankle sprains, which make up about one-quarter of all ankle sprains (Lavi 1990). Considering the very high incidence of ankle sprain in most populations (see chapter 1), the extent of permanent disability attributable to this injury may be only imagined.

Chronic lateral instability is manifested by recurrent injuries with pain, tenderness, and possibly bruising repeatedly occurring over the lateral ankle ligament (Broström 1966a, 1966b; Burssens et al. 1988; Good et al. 1975; Leach et al. 1980). Although about one-third (Broström 1966) will be asymptomatic between the events, others may present with chronic lateral pain (Broström 1966; Burssens et al. 1988; Good et al. 1975; McCory & Bladin 1996; van Dijk et al. 1996), tenderness (Anderson & Lecocq 1954; Broström 1966; Leach et al. 1980), swelling (Anderson & Lecocq 1954; Good et al. 1975; Leonard 1949; Ruth 1961), and induration (Broström 1966), causing great difficulties in sports participation and in military service (Anderson & Lecocq 1954; Broström 1966), as well as in daily living.

Diagnosis is made on the basis of a history of insecurity, instability, and giving way (Anderson & Lecocq 1954; Elmslie 1934; Good et al. 1975; Leach et al. 1980; Leonard 1949; Ruth 1961), which outweighs the findings of physical examination (Broström 1966) or the radiograph (Good et al. 1975; Kristiansen 1981; Leach et al. 1980) in defining the diagnosis. The clinical examination in this condition seems to be somewhat unreliable (Orava et al. 1983).

A tear of the lateral ligament complex may cause mechanical instability (Broström 1965; Broström & Sundelin 1966; Broström 1964, 1965, 1966a, 1966b; Evans 1953; Evans et al. 1984; Mann et al. 1993; Peri 1992). Anderson (1954, 1962) reported the measurements of the talar tilt obtained in various anatomic ankle injuries: capsule and ATFL rupture caused a tilt up to 7%. When the CFL was also ruptured, the tilt rose to 12-30%. When the PTFL was also torn, the talus could dislocate out of the mortise (figure 12.1).

We have been running a prospective study on acute ankle sprains with the aim of establishing their prognosis. Our findings have indicated that chronic mechanical instability (CMI) in ankle sprains of grade

In this paper we included material referred by A. Renström and S. Lynch.

II or III would be expected to occur in nearly 20% of injured athletes or soldiers (Mann et al. 1993; Peri 1992). Chronic functional instability (CFI) would be

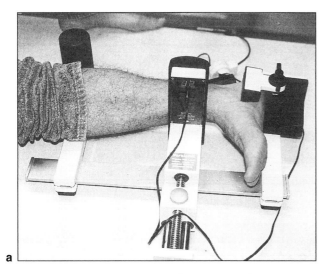

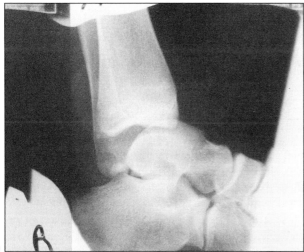

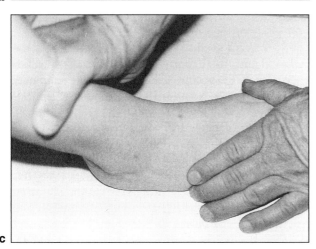

■ **Figure 12.1** *(a)* Performing the draw test using the Telos instrumentation showing mechanical instability on the ankle; *(b)* positive draw test; *(c)* positive tilt test.

expected to occur in approximately 25% of the injured with grade II or III sprains, when CFI is defined as three or more sprains within 6 months after injury (Mann et al. 1993; Peri 1992). This figure rises to near 50% when the definition is changed to one or more sprains in 6 months (Mann et al. 1993; Peri 1992). Of those patients showing CFI, only 30% will be mechanically unstable (Mann et al. 1993; Peri 1992), and of the mechanically unstable ankles 20% to 30% may not show signs of CFI (Mann et al. 1993; Peri 1992). Our findings also determined that after an ankle sprain of grade II or III, about 40% of patients with stable ankles (without CMI) suffered CFI, and about 70% of patients now suffering from CFI showed neither acute nor chronic mechanical instability.

Other investigators showed somewhat different numbers, with about 40% of patients suffering from CMI demonstrating CFI (Bosien et al. 1955; Coutts & Woodward 1965; Freeman et al. 1965; Freeman 1965a, 1965b; Good et al. 1975), and approximately the same percentage of patients suffering repeated ankle sprains (CFI) demonstrated no roentgenographic mechanical instability (no CMI) (Kristiansen 1981; Rechtime et al. 1982).

It could be summarized that even though there may be some disagreement on the exact figures, there is an unsatisfactory correlation between the mechanical stability as demonstrated on stress roentgenography or by physical examination, and the functional instability presenting as recurrent ankle sprains perceived by the injured athlete (Anderson & Lecocq 1954; Freeman 1965a, 1965b; Good et al. 1975; Leonard 1949; Park 1982; Ruth 1961).

■ Possible Causes of Stable Instability

Many hypotheses have been offered to explain this so-called stable instability (Mann et al. 1994, 1998).

Various Hypotheses

For years, investigators have been intrigued by the loose correlation between mechanical and functional instability. Various hypotheses regarding the cause or causes have been suggested, some convincing, some less so. These causes may often be combined.

■ Normal rotation of the ankle may reach 25°, half of which may take place in the tibiofibular joint (McCollugh & Burge 1980). Anteroposterior instability (Hicks 1961) or rotational talar instability (McCollugh & Burge 1980; Rasmussen & Jensen 1981; Sefton et al. 1979) could be easily missed when only talar tilt is examined, as these measures will not be demonstrated on stress inversion and yet could cause the giving way typical of CFI.

■ The subtalar joint enables walking or running on uneven surfaces, and its controlled motion is important in balancing the body during physical activity (Perkins 1964). Subtalar instability (Freeman et al. 1965; Freeman 1965a, 1965b; Laurin et al. 1968; Meyer et al. 1988; Rubin & Witten 1962) may occur following damage to the stabilizing structures, the calcaneofibular and talocalcaneal ligaments (Gillespie & Boucher 1971; Staples 1975). Subtalar instability has been claimed in the past to underlie 10-20% of ankle instabilities (Rechtime et al. 1982).

■ Restricted mobility of the subtalar joint due to post-traumatic adhesions (Freeman 1965a, 1965b; Hicks 1961) may be perceived as a sense of insecurity during physical activity.

■ Peroneal tendon tear (Abraham & Stirnaman 1979) or direct mechanical damage could cause functional instability due to insufficiency of the dynamic stabilizing structures.

■ Diastasis or damage of the tibiofibular syndesmosis (Hicks 1961; Renström & Konradsen 1997) could be perceived as giving way. This injury is assumed to occur in 10% of acute sprains (Katznel et al. 1984).

■ Adhesions at the ankle joint, leading to decreased mobility, especially in dorsiflexion (Renström & Konradsen 1997), may give a sense of instability.

■ It is possible that CFI by repeated sprains may eventually cause CMI, the latter being the result rather than the cause, as discussed by Freeman in 1965.

Nerve Injury

The most likely, and probably the most common, cause of functional instability when no mechanical instability exists is neurological damage resulting from damage to nerve fibers within or proximal to the lateral ligaments, causing what could be termed **proprioceptive detachment** (Freeman et al. 1965; Renström & Konradsen 1997). In 1965, Freeman and colleagues introduced the concept, which involved the elasticity of the nerve endings being inferior to that of the collagen fibers in the lateral ligaments of the ankle. Thus, an ankle sprain would cause detachment of the nerve endings from the mechanoreceptors demonstrated by anatomical studies in the joint ligament and capsule (Renström & Konradsen 1997), and it would inactivate the reflex arc that normally enables dynamic preservation of ankle stability (Freeman et al. 1965). The modified Romberg test (figure 12.2) was demonstrated by Freeman to demonstrate diminished proprioceptive capacity (Freeman et al. 1965). This test was later developed to measurable figures using stabilometry (Tropp 1985). These find-

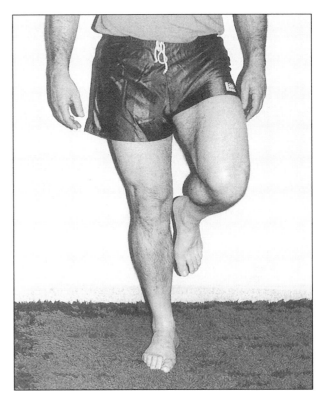

■ **Figure 12.2** Performing the modified Romberg test.

ings were claimed to explain the superior results of functional treatment for acute sprains (Freeman 1965; Hughes 1945), as discussed in detail elsewhere in this text (chapters 5, 20, and 21).

Nerve injuries caused by ankle sprains have been demonstrated by many authorities (Acus & Flanagan 1991; Bullock-Saxton 1995; Gauffin et al 1988; Isakov et al. 1986; Jerosch et al. 1995b; Konradsen et al. 1993; Konradsen & Ravn 1990; Lotem et al. 1987; Nitz et al. 1985; Shapira et al. 1992; Tropp et al. 1984; Tropp & Odeninck 1988). These may lead to reduction of superficial sensation (Bullock-Saxton 1994, 1995; Shapira et al. 1992, 1995), weakness of the peroneal muscles (Tropp & Odeninck 1988), interference with proprioception (Elmslie 1934; Freeman et al. 1965; Garn & Newton 1988; Jerosch et al. 1995; Kleinrensink et al. 1994; Leanderson et al. 1996), and interference of detection of passive motion (Gross 1987; Garrick & Requa 1988). Disturbance of postural sway (Leanderson et al. 1996; Gauffin et al 1988; Tropp et al. 1984; Tropp & Odeninck 1988) has been documented as seen after an ankle sprain (Brunt et al. 1992) and slowing of nerve conduction and reaction time (Beckman & Buchanan 1995; Brunt et al. 1992; Bullock et al. 1994; Bullock & Saxon 1995; Karlsson & Anderson 1992; Karlsson et al. 1989; Konradsen & Ravn 1990; Lofvenberg et al. 1995), although this was not a constant finding (Donahue et al. 1997; Kaminski 1997). The latency of the peroneal muscles has been found to be significantly slower in functionally unstable ankles (Karlsson & Lansinger 1992; Konradsen et al. 1993; Lofvenberg et al. 1995; Renström & Konradsen 1997), although this also was not determined by others (Brunt et al. 1992; Isakov et al. 1986; Johnson & Johnson 1993). Interrupted peripheral sensation would interfere with postural static stability (Brunt et al. 1992; Chrintz et al. 1991; Clark et al. 1985; Lord et al. 1991), which would be enhanced by reduced joint position sense, plantar and dorsiflexion strength, and depressed reaction time (Kaikkonen et al. 1994).

An unresolved debate continues between those advocating that reaction time could not possibly prevent an ankle sprain, as the injury occurs at such a speed that the peronei will not have sufficient time to contract (Isakov et al. 1986; Lotem et al. 1987), and those claiming that in consideration of the whole and complex combined reaction reflex, the body would have ample time to prevent the ligament injury (Konradsen & Ravn 1990).

■ Diagnosis

Definition of mechanical instability is not universally agreed on. The wide range of normal variation, with the various radiograph techniques and different forces used during diagnostic testing, makes the evaluation of the cutoff point for "pathology" rather unclear. Rubin and Witten (1984) found a normal range of talar tilt (figure 12.3) up to 23°, although over 20° was unusual. Seldin (1960) found a normal range of up to 14° with a side-to-side difference of 10°. Berridge and Bonnin (1944) confirmed a talar tilt of up to 25° in 5% of the population. Bonnin (1940, 1970) classified the uninjured patients with a talar tilt of 5° to 15° as having a *hypermobile ankle*. Clanton and Schon (1993) showed a normal anterior translation (figure 12.4) ranging from 2 to 9 mm. Although some would define a mechanically unstable ankle as an ankle showing on a stress roentgenorgram a talar tilt of 9° on one side or a side-to-side difference of 3° (Renström & Konradsen 1997), others would accept a side-to-side difference in the talar tilt of up to 5° (Rechtime et al. 1982; Silver & Deutsch 1982) or 6° (Freeman 1965), and some would even accept a side-to-side difference of up to 10° (Canale 1980; Evans & Frenyo 1979). And although some would consider an anterior talar translation of 10 mm or a side-to-side difference of 3 mm as pathologic (Broström et al. 1965; Karlsson & Anderson 1992; Renström & Konradsen 1997), others point out a normal variation of 2 to 9 mm and would consider a translation over 5 mm to indicate a torn ATF ligament (Clanton & Schon 1993).

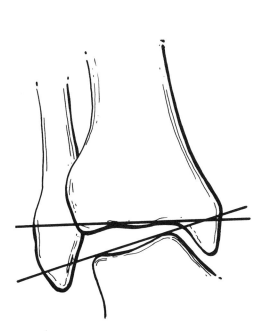

■ **Figure 12.3** The talar tilt stress radiograph. The talar tilt angle refers to the angle between the two lines drawn on the tibial plafond and the talar dome. During the stress, the ankle is in neutral position, but is internally rotated 10° to 20°.

Adapted from Renström and Lynch.

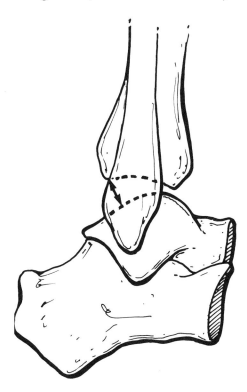

■ **Figure 12.4** The principle for the anterior drawer stress radiographs. Anterior talar displacement is recorded by measuring the shortest distance from the posterior articular surface of the tibia to the talar dome.

Adapted from Renström and Lynch.

In our own clinical work and research, we consider a 5° side-to-side difference in the tilt test, and a 4-mm side-to-side difference in the drawer test, to be the upper limit of normal (Mann et al. 1993; Peri 1992).

The accuracy of the physical examination (figures 12.5 and 12.6) is dependent on the stage of injury, and is generally more accurate in the longstanding case and less accurate in the recently injured ankle. In addition, because the accuracy of the physical examination is also dependent on the examiner's personal skill and experience, its results should be accepted with caution.

In pure CFI, both the physical examination (Broström 1966) and the radiographic diagnosis (Good et al. 1975; Kristiansen 1981; Leach et al. 1980) have no practical importance, as the diagnosis is based solely on the history of insecurity, instability, and giving way as described by the athlete (Anderson & Lecocq 1954; Elmslie 1934; Good et al. 1975; Leach et al. 1980; Leonard 1949; Ruth 1961).

The cutting line for the presence of CFL is not well defined. We use the definition suggested by

Nyska et al. in 1993 of three or more ankle sprains in the last six months.

Treatment is based on reestablishing the functional stability by means of physical therapy assisted

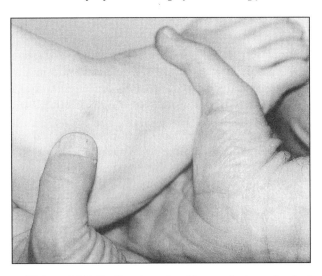

■ **Figure 12.5** Performing the tilt test during physical examination of the ankle.

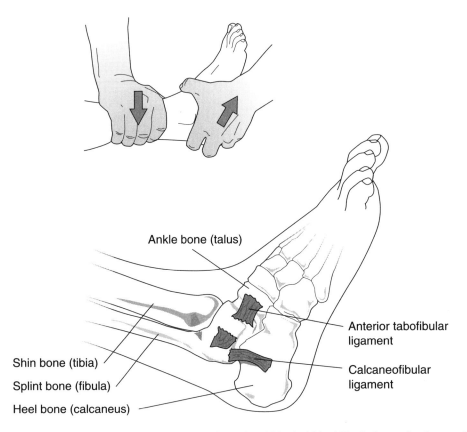

Ankle bone (talus)

Anterior tabofibular ligament

Calcaneofibular ligament

Shin bone (tibia)

Splint bone (fibula)

Heel bone (calcaneus)

■ **Figure 12.6** The anterior drawer test of the ankle. The foot should be held in 10° of plantarflexion, and the foot should be pulled forward with a counter pressure against the tibia. (For further detail, see chapter 30.)

Adapted from Renström and Lynch.

by mechanical supports (Jerosch 1995a), which both enhance proprioception and lend mechanical assistance. This treatment is dealt with in detail in chapters 5, 21, and 22.

■ References

Abraham E, Stirnaman JE. 1979. Neglected ruptures of the peroneal tendons causing recurrent sprains of the ankle: a case report. J Bone Joint Surg Am 61:1247-1248.

Acus RW, Flanagan JP. 1991. Perineural fibrosis of superficial peroneal nerve complicating ankle sprain: a case report. Foot Ankle Int 11:233-235.

Anderson KJ, Lecocq JF. 1954. Operative treatment of injury to the fibular collateral ligament of the ankle. J Bone Joint Surg Am 36:825-832.

Anderson KJ, Lecocq JF, Clayton ML. 1962. Athletic injury to the fibular collateral ligament of the ankle. Clin Ortho Rel Res 23:146-160.

Beckman SM, Buchanan TS. 1995. Ankle inversion injury and hypermobility: effect on hip and ankle muscle electromyography onset latency. Arch Phys Med Rehabil 76(12):1138-1143.

Berridge FR, Bonnin JG. 1944. The radiographic examination of the ankle joint including arthrograph. Surg Gynecol Obstet 79:383-389.

Bonnin JG. 1940. The hypermobile ankle. Proc Roy Soc Med 37:282-286.

Bonnin JG. 1970. Injuries to the ankle. Darien, CT: Hafner. p. 109-118.

Bosien WR, Staples OS, Russel SW. 1955. Residual disability following acute ankle sprains. J Bone Joint Surg Am 37:1237.

Broström L. 1964. Sprained ankles I. Anatomic lesions in recent sprains. Acta Chir Scand 128:483-495.

Broström L. 1965. Sprained ankles III. Clinical observations in recent ligament ruptures. Acta Chir Scand 130-560-569.

Broström L. 1966a. Sprained ankles V. Treatment and prognosis in recent ligament ruptures. Acta Chir Scand 135:537-550.

Broström L. 1966b. Sprained ankles VI. Surgical treatment of ligament ruptures. Acta Chir Scand 132:551-565.

Broström L, Liljedahl SO, Lindvald N. 1966. Sprained ankles II. Arthrographic diagnosis of recent ligament ruptures. Acta Chir Scand 129:485-499.

Broström L, Sundelin P. 1966. Sprained ankles IV. Histologic changes in recent and chronic ligament ruptures. Acta Chir Scand 132(3): 248-253.

Brunt D, Andersen JC, Huntsman B, Reinhert LB, Thorell AC, Sterling JC. 1992. Postural responses to lateral perturbation in healthy subjects and ankle sprain patients. Med Sci Sports Ex 24(2):171-176.

Bullock-Saxton JE, Janda V, Bullock MI. 1994. The influence of ankle sprain injury on muscle activation during hip extension. Int J Sports Med 15(6):330-334.

Bullock-Saxton JE. 1994. Local sensation changes and altered hip muscle function following severe ankle sprain. Phys Ther 74(1):17-28.

Bullock-Saxton JE. 1995. Sensory changes associated with severe ankle sprain. Scand J Rehabil Med 227(3):161-167.

Burssens P, Destoop N, Classens H. 1988. Unexplained post-traumatic lateral ankle pain: a new syndrome? In Mann G, editor. Sports injuries: proceeding of the fourth Jerusalem Symposium. London: Freund Publishing House Ltd. p. 195-201.

Chrintz H, Faister O, Roed J. 1991. Single leg postural equilibrium test. Scand J Med Sci Sports 1:244-246.

Clanton TO, Schon LC. 1993. Athletic injuries to the soft tissues of the foot and ankle. In Mann RA, Coughlin MJ, editors. Surgery of the foot and ankle. Vol 2. 6th ed. London: Mosby. p. 1125-1126.

Clark FJ, Burgess RC, Chapin JW, Lipcombs WT. 1985. Role of intramuscular receptors in the awareness of limb position. J Neurophysiol 54(6):1529-1540.

Coutts B, Woodward PE. 1965. Surgery and sprained ankles. Clin Ortho Rel Res 42:81-90.

Donahue M, Sandry MA, Kuhlman JS, Edwards JE. 1997. The effect of semi-rigid ankle braces on peroneus longus pre-motor time during sudden ankle inversion. J Athl Train 32(2):39.

Elmslie RC. 1934. Recurrent dislocation of the ankle joint. Ann Surg 100:364-367.

Evans DL. 1953. Recurrent instability of the ankle. A method of surgical treatment. Proc Roy Soc Med 46:343-344.

Evans GA, Hardcastle P, Frenyo AD. 1984. Acute rupture of the lateral ligament of the ankle. To suture or not to suture? J Bone Joint Surg 66B(2):209-212.

Freeman MAR. 1965a. Instability of the foot after injuries to the lateral ligament of the ankle. J Bone Joint Surg 47(B):669-677.

Freeman MAR. 1965b. Treatment of ruptures of the lateral ligament of the ankle. J Bone Joint Surg 47(B):661-668.

Freeman MAR, Dean MRE, Hanham IWF. 1965. The etiology and prevention of functional instability of the foot. J Bone Joint Surg (Br) 47(B):678-685.

Garn SN, Newton RA. 1988. Kinesthetic awareness in subjects with multiple ankle sprains. Phys Ther 68(11):1667-1671.

Garrick JG, Requa RK. 1988. The epidemiology of foot and ankle. Injuries in sports. Clin Sports Med 7(1):29-36.

Gauffin H, Tropp H, Odenrick P. 1988. Effect of ankle disk training on postural control in patients with functional instability of the ankle joint. (2):141-4

Gillespie HS, Boucher P. 1971. Watson Jones repair of lateral instability of the ankle. J Bone Joint Surg 53(A):920-924.

Good CJ, Jones MA, Livingstone BN. 1975. Reconstruction of the lateral ligament of the ankle. Injury 7:63-65.

Gross MT. 1987. Effects of recurrent lateral ankle sprains on active and passive judgment of joint position. Phys Ther 67:1505-1509.

Hicks JH. 1961. The three weight-bearing mechanisms of the foot. In Gaynor Evans, editor. Biomechanical studies of the musculo-skeletal system. Illinois: Charles C Thomas.

Hughes JR. 1945. The frequency significance and treatment of tilting of the talus in the tibiofibular mortise. M.D. thesis, University of Liverpool, Liverpool, England 1945 (quoted by Freeman 1960).

Isakov E, Mizrachi J, Solzi P, Susak Z, Lotem M. 1986. Response of the peroneal muscles to sudden inversion of the ankle during standing. Int J Sports Biomech 2:100-109.

Jerosch J, Hoffstetter I, Bork H, Bishof M. 1995a. The influence of orthoses on the proprioception of the ankle joint. Knee Surg Sports Trauma Arthro 3(1):39-46.

Jerosch J, Reer R, Bork H, Bischof M. 1995b. Post-traumatic proprioception deficit of the ankle joint. Isr J Sports Med 2:195-199.

Johnson MB, Johnson CL. 1993. Electromyographic response of peroneal muscles in surgical and nonsurgical injured ankles during sudden inversion. Journal Orthopaedic Sports Physical Therapy 18:497-501.

Kaikkonen A, Kannus P, Jarvinen M. 1994. A performance test protocol and scoring scale for the evaluation of ankle injuries. Am J Sports Med 22(4):462-469.

Kaminiski TW. 1997. Modified Romberg balance test scores between uninjured and functionally unstable ankles J Athl Train 32(2):25.

Karlsson J, Anderson GO. 1992. The effect of external ankle support in chronic lateral ankle joint instability. An electromyographic study. Am J Sports Med 20:257-261.

Karlsson J, Bergsten T, Lansinger O, et al. 1989. Surgical treatment of chronic lateral instability of the ankle joint. Am J Sports Med 17:268-274.

Karlsson J, Lansinger O. 1992. Lateral instability of the ankle joint. Clin Ortho Rel Res 276:253-261.

Katznelson A, Lin E, Militiano J. 1983 . Ruptures of the ligaments about the tibiofibular syndesmosis. Injury 25:170-172.

Kleinrensink GJ, Stoeckart R, Meulstee J, et al. 1994. Lowered motor conduction velocity of the peroneal nerve after inversion trauma. Med Sci Sports Ex 26(7):877-883.

Konradsen L, Ravn JB. 1990. Ankle instability caused by prolonged peroneal reaction time. Acta Ortho Scand 61(5):388-390.

Konradsen L, Ravn JB, Sorensen AI. 1993. Proprioception at the ankle: The effect of anesthetic blockade of ligament receptors. J Bone Joint Surg (Br) 75(3):433-436.

Kristiansen B. 1981. Evans' repair of lateral instability of the ankle joint. Acta Ortho Scand 52:679-682.

Lassiter TE, Malone TR, Garret WE. 1989. Injury to the lateral ligament of the ankle. Ortho Clin N Am 20:629-640.

Laurin CA, Quellet R, St. Jacques S. 1968. Talar and subtalar tilt: an experimental investigation. Can J Surg 11(3):270-279.

Lavi O. 1990. A prospective study of risk factors for lateral ankle sprains, and the effect of training with 3/4 high shoe on the incidence of ankle sprains among recruits. M.D. Thesis, Hebrew University School of Medicine.

Leach RE, Namiki O, Paul ER, Stockel J. 1980. Secondary reconstruction of the lateral ligaments of the ankle. Clin Ortho Rel Res 160:201-211.

Leanderson J, Eriksson E, Nilsson C, Wykman A. 1996. Proprioception in classical ballet dancers. A prospective study of the influence of an ankle sprain on proprioception in the ankle joint. Am J Sports Med 24(3):370-374.

Leonard MH. 1949. Injuries of the lateral ligaments of the ankle. J Bone Joint Surg 32(A):373-377.

Lofvenberg R, Karrholm J, Sundelin G, Ahlgren O. 1995. Prolonged reaction time in patients with chronic lateral instability of the ankle. Am J Sports Med 23(4):414-417.

Lord SR, Clark RD, Webster IW. 1991. Postural stability and associated physiological factors in a population of aged persons. J Gerontol 4:69-76.

Lotem M, Isakov E, Mizrachi J, Solzi P, Susak Z. 1987. Response of the peroneal muscles to sudden inversion of the ankle during standing. Proc Israel Ortho Assn 13: 13.

Mack RP. 1982. Ankle injuries in athletes. Clin Sports Med 1:71-84.

Mann G, Elishuv O, Perry C, Finsterbush A, Frankl U, Nyska M, Matan Y. 1994. Recurrent ankle sprain: literature review. Israeli J Sports Med 104-113.

Mann G, Elishuv O, Lowe J. 1998. Repeated ankle sprain revisited - pathology and pathogenesis. In Chan KM, Fu F, Maffulli N, Rolf C, Kurosaka M, Liu S, editors. Controversies in orthopedic sports medicine. New Territories, Hong Kong: Williams & Wilkins. 445-459.

Mann G, Perry H, Nyska M, Matan Y, Frankl U, Finsterbush A. 1993. Ankle sprain: occurrence of chronic functional instability and its chronic relation to mechanical instability. A prospective study. Presented at the 9th International Jerusalem Symposium on Sports Injuries, January, Jerusalem, Israel.

McCollugh CJ, Burge PD. 1980. Rotary stability of the load bearing ankle. J Bone Joint Surg 62(B):460-464.

McCory P, Bladin C. 1996. Fractures of the lateral process of the talus: a clinical review. "Snowboarders Ankle." Clin J Sports Med 6(2):124-128.

Meyer JM, Garsia J, Hoffmeyer P, Fritshy D. 1988. The subtalar sprain— a roentgenographic study. Clin Ortho 226:169-173.

Nitz AJ, Dobner JS, Kersey D. 1985. Nerve injury and grade II and III ankle sprains. Am J Sports Med 13:177-182.

Nyska M, Porat A, Howard CB, Matan Y, Mann G, Dekel S. 1993. Radiological assessment of chronic instability of the ankle. J Sports Traumatol 15:193-8.

Orava S, Jaroma H, Suvela M. 1983. Radiological instability of the ankle after Evans' repair. Acta Ortho Scan 54:734-738.

Peri H. 1992. Recurrent ankle sprains: mechanical stability vs functional stability M.D. thesis. Directed by Mann G, Finsterbush A. Presented to the Hadassah Hebrew University Medical School, Jerusalem, Israel.

Perkins G. 1964. Orthopaedics. London: The Athlone Press. 607 pp.

Rasmussen O, Tovborg-Jensen I. 1981. Rotational instability after strains. Acta Ortho Scand 52:99-102.

Rechtime GR, McCarrol JR, Webster DA. 1982. Reconstruction for chronic lateral instability of the ankle: A review of twenty-eight surgical patients. Ortho 5:51-56.

Renström AFH, Konradsen L. 1997. Chronic ankle instability. Proc Isr Soc Sports Med October pg 10.

Rubin G, Witten M. 1962. The subtalar joint and symptoms of turning over on the ankle. A new method of evaluation using tomography. Am J Ortho 4:16-19.

Rubin G, Witten M. 1984. The talar-tilt angle and the fibular collateral ligaments. A method for the determination of talar tilt. J Bone Joint Surg 66:336-339.

Ruth CJ. 1961. The surgical treatment of injuries of the fibular collateral ligaments of the ankle. J Bone Joint Surg 43(A):229-239.

Sefton GK, George J, Fitton JM, McMullen H. 1979. Reconstruction of the anterior talofibular ligament for the treatment of the unstable ankle. J Bone Joint Surg 61(B):352-354.

Shapira A, Lin E, Gordin A, Peshin J, Hiss Y, Herness D. 1992. Damage of the cutaneous nerves about the ankle following ankle sprain. Presented at the 8th International Jerusalem Symposium on Sports Injuries, January, Jerusalem, Israel.

Silver CM, Deutsch SD. 1982. Evans repair of lateral instability of the ankle. Ortho 5(1):51-56.

Staples OS. 1975. Ruptures of the fibular collateral ligaments of the ankle. J Bone Joint Surg 57A:101-107.

Tropp H. 1985. Functional instability of the ankle joint. Linkoping, Sweden: University Press.

Tropp H, Ekstrand J, Gillquist J. 1984. Stabilometry in functional instability of the ankle and its values in predicting injury Med Sci Sports Exerc 16:64-66.

Tropp H, Odeninck P. 1988. Postural control in single limb stances. J Ortho Res Rel 6:883-939.

van Dijk CN, Bossuyt PM, Marti RK. 1996. Medial ankle pain after lateral ligament rupture. J Bone Joint Surg (Br) 78(4):526-527.

Chapter 13

Osteochondral Fractures of the Talus

Chaim Zinman, MD; Meir Nyska, MD; and Gideon Mann, MD

Osteochondral fracture of the talar dome (OCD) is an uncommon lesion occurring after inversion ankle injury. The reported incidence in the literature ranges from 0.11% to 6.5% of all ankle sprains. The etiology and pathogenesis of osteochondral lesions of the talar dome are the result of a fracture that failed to heal or are due to subchondral necrosis of unknown etiology. They have been described in the past with a variety of terms: osteochondritis dissecans (Roden et al. 1954), transchondral fractures (Davidson et al. 1967), dome fractures (Coltrat 1952; Mukherjee and Young 1973), and flake fractures (Biedert 1989). Lesions identical in characteristics have been called fractures by some and osteochondritis by others (Berndt and Harty 1959). By definition, this is a fracture through that part of the talus that is lined with articular cartilage (Davidson et al. 1967). Most authors agree that trauma is the common etiology.

The age of presentation is adolescent or older age but usually the injury occurs from middle of the second decade to the third decade. Madhok (1987) presented a child limping due to OCD of the talus. Higuera et al. (1998) recently presented a series of OCD in the child and adolescent and suggested that the lesion occurs more frequently during childhood than previously thought.

■ Pathology and Etiology

The talar dome lesions can be medial or lateral. The medial are rounded lesions in the posteromedial shoulder of the talus. The lateral are waferlike shapes at the anterolateral border of the talus. The etiology of talar dome lesions usually, but not always, involves trauma:

■ **Non-traumatic etiology.** The medial talar dome lesion is the one generally recognized as osteochondritis dissecans (Ray and Coughlin 1947). At the medial lesion, history of trauma may be lacking and then the lesion will be attributed to ischemic necrosis, hormonal factors, or hereditary contributions. Bauer and Ochsner (1987) reviewed 56 patients with OCD of the talus. In 33 patients there was no history of trauma, and the lesion was medial. Deep osteolysis close to the margin indicated the cases were not the result of trauma. Woods and Harris (1995) presented OCD occurring in identical twins. Anderson and Lyne (1984) presented three medial lesions in two siblings. In both publications there was no history of trauma. In 10-25% of patients, the occurrence of the lesion is bilateral, and therefore the medial lesion may occur as a result of ischemia and not as a result of trauma.

■ **Traumatic etiology.** In most of the cases of talar dome lesions, a history of trauma can be presented, usually after inversion injury of the ankle, mainly in the lateral OCD (Campbell & Ranawat 1966). Scharling (1978), in a review of 19 patients, found that five out of six cases of lateral dome lesions were due to trauma, whereas 5 of 13 medial lesions had a history of trauma. Naumetz and Schweigel (1980), in a review of 31 patients, found that the talar dome had traumatic etiology. Flick and Gould (1985), in a review of 22 patients, found that 100% of the lateral dome lesions had a history of trauma, and 80% of the patients with medial lesions had a history of trauma. Brendt and Harty (1959), in a detailed biomechanical evaluation of the lesions, demonstrated the lesion to occur in inversion injury. The medial side is affected during inversion injury with plantarflexion of the foot, and lateral lesion occurs in inversion-dorsiflexion injuries. Bruns et al. (1992) demonstrated in a cadaveric study that even without dissection of the lateral ligaments, the peak pressures were located at the medial rim of the talus. They concluded that supination, overweight, and lax ankle ligaments have an important influence on the development of OCD at least at the medial rim of the talus. In a biomechanical topography study, Athanasiou et al. (1995) found that tibial cartilage was stiffer than talar cartilage, and the softest cartilage was found at the most medial and lateral areas of the talus. They concluded that cartilage lesions in a repetitive overuse process in the ankle joint may be related to a disparity of mechanical properties between articulating surfaces of the tibial and talar regions. In a follow-up study of athletes suffering from osteochondritis of the talus, Bruns and Rosenbach (1992) found that sports activities with sprained ankle or recurrent microtrauma of the ankle could be found in most of the cases.

In summary, most authors agree that medial talar lesions are mainly due to trauma, with a significant role for idiopathic origin, and that the lateral dome lesions are due to trauma, usually inversion trauma of the ankle.

■ Clinical Presentation, Diagnosis, and Classification

Pain in the ankle following inversion injury is not unusual. Osteochondral fractures are important in the differential diagnosis. Recognition is enabled by a high incidence of suspicion.

Clinical Presentation

Persistent pain, especially between the talus and the tibiofibular syndesmosis, should be suspect. Tenderness, crepitation, recurrent swelling, clicking sensation, antalgic gait, pain aggravated by ambulation, and painful range of motion all raise the possibility of

a fracture of the dome of the talus (Naumetz and Schweigel 1980). The history of ankle trauma, mainly inversion injury of the ankle followed by persistent pain that is increased in physical activity, leads to a suspicion of OCD. On physical examination, there is no definite sign for the presence of OCD, and there can be diffuse tenderness, usually as a result of widespread synovitis of the ankle, or localized tenderness on the medial or lateral side of the ankle. The tenderness is not necessarily due to medial lesions on the medial side of the ankle. Most probably, the pain is not due to the defect itself, since articular cartilage has no nerve endings. However, the pain might come from the synovitis. In arthritic changes, there will be painful limitation of ankle range of motion. However, arthritic changes are found infrequently in OCD, even in long-term follow-up, and then only to a minor degree (Bruns 1993).

Diagnosis

The definite diagnosis is based on imaging the lesion. Other modes of imaging, such as CT, MRI, and bone scintigraphy, may evaluate the presence of OCD and its definite character, its exact location, and its activity (figures 13.1 and 13.2). Following is a discussion of each of these imaging modes.

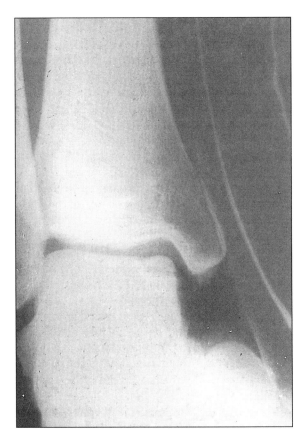

■ **Figure 13.1** Medial osteochondritic lesion of the talus, probably in stable position.

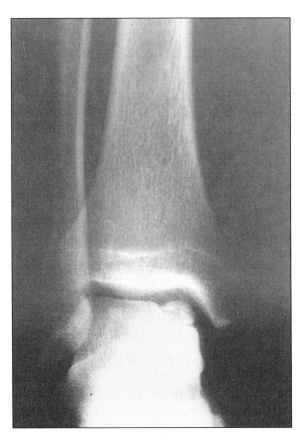

■ **Figure 13.2** Medial osteochondritic lesion of the talus, probably loose and mobile.

■ **Plain radiography** is still the key for diagnosis. AP and lateral radiographs of the ankle are not adequate for the diagnosis (Roden et al. 1954). Ten to fifteen AP internal oblique views (mortise) are mandatory in ankle trauma. In the mortise view, the lateral and medial malleolus are parallel and the talofibular joint is open. This view enables one to see even a small flake of bone or crescent-shaped defect. Flick and Gould (1985) found that the initial diagnosis, seen retrospectively on radiographs, was missed 43% of the time by emergency room physicians.

■ **CT scan** should be performed for any persistent pain after trauma when OCD is suspected, even with negative routine ankle radiographs (figure 13.3). We have shown in 12 patients that the use of CT confirmed the diagnosis (when in doubt) and determined the precise location and extent of the lesion, assisting in the decision for treatment (Zinman and Reis 1982). In another series, plain radiography led to the diagnosis of OCD in two-thirds of the patients, and the rest were diagnosed by CT. The CT was superior to plain radiography in 20 patients in showing healing of the lesion (Zinman et al. 1988). In order to improve the accuracy of the CT, it was shown that baseline CT exams accurately depicted all the lesions except for early (grade I) lesions. The administration of intra-articular contrast agent (CT arthrography) increased the diagnostic accuracy in articular cartilage studies (Ragozzino et al. 1996). Heare et al. (1988) demonstrated that coronal CT after double contrast arthrography clearly shows the state of attachment of the osteochondritic fragment to the talus. Davies and Cassar-Pullicino (1989) found similar results. CT arthrography identified the precise location in each case, and consistently revealed the extent of the lesion to be greater than that apparent on plain radiographs. The talar cartilage over the lesion was shown to be thinned in four cases and was shown to be deficient in two cases. Fissuring of the cartilage was demonstrated in four cases. Subarticular cysts were identified in all but two cases, and contrast medium was shown to enter the cysts in two cases, indicating communication with the ankle joint. CT studies of OCD have become the standard way of evaluating these patients.

■ **MRI** may evaluate the extent of the lesions mainly if there are no definite bony changes. De Smet et al (1990), in a prospective study, found there was an excellent correlation between the stages in MRI and arthroscopy, showing correct prediction of stable and unstable fragments in 92% of cases. In contrast, fragment stability could not be efficiently assessed by conventional radiology, as fragments could be lying stable in their crater in cases of bony separation (Jurgensen et al. 1996). Dipaola et al. (1991) also

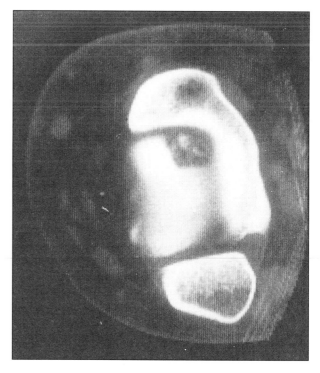

■ **Figure 13.3** A computerized tomogram in the horizontal view showing an osteochondritic lesion with a loose body in the crater.

found good correlation of MRI findings to arthroscopic findings.

■ **Bone scintography** can demonstrate bone activity at the OCD location. If there are no bony changes on plain radiography, it can evaluate the suspicion of a fracture when there is increased uptake in the late phase. If there is increased activity in the early phase, it may indicate synovitis.

Classification

The radiographic classification suggested by Brendt and Harty some 40 years ago is still the main classification used in most of the studies. Their classification is based on the anatomical changes of the fragment as related to the trauma. In grade I, there is only compression of the cartilage, and usually there are no radiographic findings because the injury is cartilaginous in character. In grade II, there is partial avulsion of osteochondral fragment, but the main fragment is still not detached from the talus. In grade III, there is complete detachment from the talus and failure of healing of the fragment, but without displacement of the fragment. Grade IV is when the fragment is displaced or there are arthritic changes. CT studies can verify the grades more accurately than plain radiographic classification. Magnetic resonance studies will demonstrate grade I lesion when the CT does not demonstrate any bony changes. Therefore, we suggest that in cases of suspected OCD, plain radiography and CT should be performed. If these studies are negative, then a positive bone scan can indicate a possibility of grade I lesions. Then MR studies can verify the presence of grade I lesions.

■ Treatment

The management of OCD depends on the symptomatology and grade of the lesion. The treatment can be conservative or operative:

■ **Conservative treatment** includes measures to reduce the synovitis and consequently the pain. These measures include local or systemic nonsteroidal anti-inflammatories and physiotherapy. In early stages, nonweightbearing or immobilization in a cast can be utilized.

■ **Surgical treatment** is indicated when conservative treatment fails or the patient presents with an unstable fragment. The long-term results of operative management are still questionable. The preferred surgical procedure is still under debate, and there are few operative approaches.

Surgical vs Conservative Treatment

In a series of long-term follow-ups over about 15 years, in 5 of 6 patients treated conservatively, radiological assessment showed that the lesion had failed to heal but the joint was relatively asymptomatic. Ankle osteoarthrosis developed in only two ankles and was considered to be an uncommon complication (McCullough and Venugopal 1979). Bruns found that osteoarthritis of the ankle is not a common sequela and it occurs only in a mild degree in adult patients (1993). Flick and Gould (1985) found that surgical treatment yields superior results to conservative therapy. O'Farrell and Costello (1982) found that early operation gives the best results, 12 months being the critical delay time. In another series, drilling and curettage gave good results in 22 patients, fair results in two patients, and poor results in one patient (Alexander and Lichtman 1980). Naumetz and Schweigel demonstrated that excision or excision with curretage gave good results in 63% of patients and fair results in 30% (1980). Biedert (1989), in a short-term follow-up, also found disappointing results of operative treatment. Among patients, 46% had good results, 33% had fair results, and 20% had poor results. Angermann and Jensen (1989), in a long-term follow-up, showed that drilling and curretage had poor initial results, which deteriorated in time. More than half of the patients had some degree of pain and swelling of the ankle during activity.

Higeura et al. (1998), after reviewing 18 children and adolescents, recommended that the preliminary treatment should be conservative. Bruns and Rosenbach (1992) advocated that adolescents without any loose bodies should first be treated conservatively. The older the patient, the shorter the nonsurgical treatment should be.

Operative Approach

The main approaches are through anteromedial or anterolateral arthrotomy, but in the case of large fragments on the posteromedial area, there is a need for osteotomy of the medial or lateral malleolus. Zinman et al. (1988) also used medial malleolar osteotomy in their series (figure 13.4). Wallen and Fallat (1989) advocated crescentic medial malleolar osteotomy. Approach to the medial lesion using medial osteotomy leads to local osteoarthritis and less favorable clinical outcome (Gaulrapp et al. 1996). Gepstein et al. (1986) demonstrated percutaneous drilling through the medial malleolus using an image intensifier. Ankle arthroscopy is an effective procedure for evaluation and management of OCD (Baker et al. 1986). Arthroscopic excision, curretage, and drilling can be performed using a transmalleolar approach or a standard cruciate drill guide. Bryant and Siegel (1993) advocated using the meniscal repair instrumentation.

Surgical Technique

The basic operative treatment is surgical removal of a loose fragment if the fragment is small, as well as curretage and drilling to the subchondral bone (Brandt and Harty 1959; O'Farrell and Costello 1982). Retrograde drilling is an option using a small guide pin with a bone biopsy needle and insertion of a cancellous

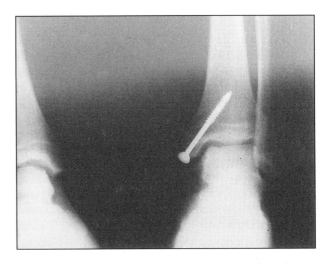

■ **Figure 13.4** After removal of an osteochondritic lesion by a transmalleolar approach.

bone graft. Bruns (1993), in his study that resulted in good results in nearly 70% of the patients, performed removal of the subchondral sclerosis and autologous bone transplantation. Gaulrapp et al. (1996) reviewed operative management of 58 patients who had been operated on using different procedures, which included excision of the lesion, drilling, and bone grafting. No significant difference was noted for size of the lesion or the applied operative technique. Kristensen et al. (1990) demonstrated an arthroscopic technique of fixation of a grade IV lesion using Biofix—a biodegradable fixation with excellent results. Hangody et al. (1997) described a new technique of treatment of OCD, the mosaicplasty, in which one stage autogenous osteochondral graft taken from the knee was inserted into a lesion after its curretage. This led to good results in 1-year follow-up.

■ References

Alexander AH, Lichtman DM. Surgical treatment of transchondral talar-dome fractures (osteochondritis dissecans). Long-term follow-up, J Bone Joint Surg [Am] 1980;62(4):646-652.

Anderson DV, Lyne ED. Osteochondritis dissecans of the talus: case report on two family members, J Pediatr Orthop 1984;4(3):356-357.

Angermann P, Jensen P. Osteochondritis dissecans of the talus: long-term results of surgical treatment. Foot Ankle 1989;10(3):161-163.

Athanasiou KA, Niederauer GG, Schenck RC Jr. Biomechanical topography of human ankle cartilage, Ann Biomed Eng 1995;23(5):697-704.

Baker CL, Andrews JR, Ryan JB. Arthroscopic treatment of transchondral talar dome fractures, Arthroscopy 1986;2(2):82-87.

Bauer RS, Ochsner PE. Nosology of osteochondrosis dissecans of the trochlea of the talus, Z Orthop 1987;125(2):194-200.

Biedert R. Osteochondral lesions of the talus, Unfallchirurg 1989;92(4):199-205.

Brendt AL, Harty M. Transcondral fractures (osteochondritis dissecans) of the talus. J Bone Joint Sureg 1959;41A:988-1020.

Bruns J, Rosenbach B, Kahrs J. Etiopathogenetic aspects of medial osteochondrosis dissecans tali, Sportverletz Sportschaden 1992;6(2):43-49.

Bruns J, Rosenbach B. Osteochondrosis dissecans of the talus. Comparison of results of surgical treatment in adolescents and adults, Arch Orthop Trauma Surg 1992;112(1):23-27.

Bruns J. Osteochondrosis dissecans tali. Results of surgical therapy, Unfallchirurg 1993;96(2):75-81.

Bryant DD III, Siegel MG. Osteochondritis dissecans of the talus: a new technique for arthroscopic drilling, Arthroscopy 1993;9(2):238-241.

Campbell CJ, Ranawat CS. Osteochondritis dissecans: the question of etiology, J Trauma 1966;6(2):201-221.

Coltart WD. Aviatior's astragalus, J Bone Joint Surg 1952;34B:546-566

Davidson AM, Steele HD, MacKenzie DA. A review of twenty-one cases of transchondral fracture of the talus, J Trauma 1967; 7:378-413.

Davies AM, Cassar-Pullicino VN. Demonstration of osteochondritis dissecans of the talus by coronal computed tomographic arthrography, Br J Radiol 1989;62(744):1050-1055.

De Smet AA, Fisher DR, Burnstein MI, Graf BK, Lange RH. Value of MR imaging in staging osteochondral lesions of the talus (osteochondritis

dissecans): results in 14 patients, Am J Roentgenol 1990;154(3):555-558.

Dipaola JD, Nelson DW, Colville. Characterizing osteochondral lesions by magnetic resonance imaging, MR Arthroscopy 1991;7(1):101-104.

Flick AB, Gould N. Osteochondritis dissecans of the talus (transchondral fractures of the talus): review of the literature and new surgical approach for medial dome lesions, Foot Ankle 1985;5(4):165-185.

Gaulrapp H, Hagena FW, Wasmer G. Postoperative evaluation of osteochondrosis dissecans of the talus with special reference to medial malleolar osteotomy, Z Orthop Ihre Grenzgeb 1996;134(4):346-353.

Gepstein R, Conforty B, Weiss RE, Hallel T. Closed percutaneous drilling for osteochondritis dissecans of the talus. A report of two cases, Clin Orthop 1986;213:197-200.

Hangody L, Kish G, Karpati Z, Szerb I, Eberhardt R. Treatment of osteochondritis dissecans of the talus: use of the mosaicplasty technique—a preliminary report, Foot Ankle Int 1997;18(10):628-634.

Heare MM, Gillespy T III, Bittar ES. Direct coronal computed tomography arthrography of osteochondritis dissecans of the talus, Skeletal Radiol 1988;17(3):187-189.

Higuera J, Laguna R, Peral M, Aranda E, Soleto J. Osteochondritis dissecans of the talus during childhood and adolescence, J Pediatr Orthop 1998;18(3):328-332.

Jurgensen I, Bachmann G, Siaplaouras J, Cassens J. Clinical value of conventional radiology and MRI in assessing osteochondrosis dissecans stability, Unfallchirurg 1996;99(10):758-763.

Kristensen G, Lind T, Lavard P, Olsen PA. Fracture stage 4 of the lateral talar dome treated arthroscopically using Biofix for fixation, Arthroscopy 1990;6(3):242-244.

Madhok R. Limping child—osteochondritis dissecans of the talus. A case report, Orthop Rev 1987;16(10):757-759.

McCullough CJ, Venugopal V. Osteochondritis dissecans of the talus: the natural history, Clin Orthop 1979;144:264-268.

Mukherjee SK, Young AB. Dome fracture of the talus. J Bone Joint Sureg 1973;55B:319-326.

Naumetz VA, Schweigel JF. Osteocartilagenous lesions of the talar dome, J Trauma 1980;20(11):924-927.

O'Farrell TA, Costello BG. Osteochondritis dissecans of the talus. The late results of surgical treatment, J Bone Joint Surg [Br] 1982;64 (B):494-497.

Ragozzino A, Rossi G, Esposito S, Giovine S, Tuccillo M. Computerized tomography of osteochondral diseases of the talus dome, Radiol Med (Torino) 1996;92(6):682-686.

Ray RB, Coughlin EJ. Osteochondritis dissecans of the talus. J Bone Joint Surg 1947;29:697-706.

Roden S, Tillegard P, Unander-Scharin L. Osteochondritis dissecans and similar lesion of the talus: a report of fifty-five cases with special reference to etiology and treatment, Acta Orthop Scand 1954;23:51-66.

Scharling. Osteochondritis dissecans of the talus, Acta Orthop Scand 1978 Feb;49(1):89-94.

Wallen EA, Fallat LM. Crescentic transmalleolar osteotomy for optimal exposure of the medial talar dome, J Foot Surg 1989;28(5):389-394.

Woods K, Harris I. Osteochondritis dissecans of the talus in identical twins, Bone Joint Surg Br 1995;77(2):331.

Zinman C, Reis ND. Osteochondritis dissecans of the talus: use of the high resolution computed tomography scanner, Acta Orthop Scand 1982;53(4):697-700.

Zinman C, Wolfson N, Reis ND. Osteochondritis dissecans of the dome of the talus. Computed tomography scanning in diagnosis and follow-up. J Bone Joint Surg [Am] 1988;70(7):1017-1019.

Chapter 14

Sinus Tarsi Syndrome

Meir Nyska, MD; Gideon Mann, MD; and Cobi Lidor, MD

Sinus tarsi syndrome is a clinical entity related to an abnormal tarsal sinus and tarsal canal. It is induced by inversion injury of the ankle and is characterized by chronic pain over the lateral ankle, which is increased by physical activity. O'Connor first noted in 1958 that this is an unusual but not rare condition and that it frequently follows an ankle sprain. Clinical examination discloses localized tenderness over the sinus tarsi; this tenderness is increased by inversion or eversion of the hindfoot. Plain radiographic examination is normal, and there remains no diagnostic standard of reference. Subtalar arthrography demonstrates complete disappearance of the microrecesses along the interosseous ligament. MRI studies demonstrate pathology in the soft tissue of the sinus tarsi, and there is close association to injury of the lateral ligaments of the ankle. The initial treatment is conservative, including local injections and physiotherapy. In case of failure of conservative treatment, surgical debridement is recommended, and good results can be expected. O'Connor (1958) presented 14 patients of 45 who were amenable to conservative treatment. In these patients, he cleaned out the fat pad in the sinus tarsi and resected the superficial ligamentous floor, which was part of the anterior annular ligament (cervical ligament). He described complete recovery in 9 patients and some improvement in 5 patients. Since then, although our understanding of the syndrome has increased dramatically, there has been no change in the treatment or the prognosis.

■ Anatomy

The tarsal canal and the tarsal sinus form a boundary between the posterior subtalar joint and the anteriorly located talocalcaneonavicular joint. The sinus tarsi and tarsal canal course from posteromedial to anterolateral. Wood Jones (1944) emphasized the difference between the sinus tarsi, which is more superficial, and the tarsal canal. The long axis is approximately 45° to the calcaneus (Cahill 1965). The tarsal canal is the portion that extends to the medial aspect of the foot posterior to the sustentaculum tali. The tarsal sinus is cone-shaped and widens laterally. The sinus tarsi contains ligaments, nerves, and blood vessels, all embedded in fibrofatty tissue.

Ligaments of the Sinus Tarsi

There are five distinct ligaments: medial, intermediate, and lateral roots of the inferior extensor retinaculum; the cervical ligament; and the interosseous ligament, which lies deep between the talus and the calcaneus (Schmidt 1978) (see chapter 2). All these ligaments are extracapsular. Closely related structures, which can also be injured in inversion injury and are difficult to differentiate, are the bifurcate ligament (midfoot sprain), lateral talocalcaneal ligament, and extensor digitorum brevis (Klein and Spreitzer 1993). The inferior extensor retinaculum is a Y-shaped structure. The upper limb arises from the medial malleolus, and the lower limb extends from the first cuneiform and the sole of the foot. The upper limb splits to form a separate canal for the tibialis anterior tendon and courses laterally, joining with the lower segment at the extensor digitorum longus tendons. These segments converge and split into superficial and deep components around the extensor digitorum longus tendons and the peroneus tertius. The inferior extensor retinaculum subsequently divides into medial, intermediate, and lateral roots, which insert to the sinus tarsi and tarsal canal. The lateral root of the inferior extensor retinaculum attaches to the calcaneus at the external aspect of the sinus tarsi. The medial root extends deep within the tarsal sinus and attaches to the

We would like to thank Dr. Elisha Freund for his help in finalizing this chapter.

calcaneus just anterior to the calcaneal attachment site of the interosseous ligament. The intermediate root attaches to the calcaneus within the tarsal sinus, just posterior to the cervical ligament. The cervical ligament lies in the anterior tarsal sinus, extending from the neck of the talus to the lateral aspect of the calcaneus. The ligament lies at 45°, extending from superomedial to inferolateral. The interosseous ligament (ligament of the tarsal canal) is the most posteromedial and is the medial border of the sinus tarsi (Harper 1991). It is located just anterior to the posterior subtalar joint, and is also angulated from the calcaneus to the talus superomedial to inferolateral (figure 14.1).

The Blood Vessels

The sinus tarsi artery is the principal supplier of intrasinus structures and of the talus. It is formed from anastomoses between various arteries of the lateral region of the foot. These usually include the anterior lateral malleolar and proximal lateral tarsal arteries. Schwarzenbach et al. (1997) found that in 70% of cadaveric specimens there was a branch from the distal lateral tarsal artery, and in 30% a branch from the peroneal artery to form the sinus tarsi artery. He found in all cadaveric specimens that there were anastomoses within the sinus tarsi be-

tween the sinus tarsi artery and the canalis tarsi artery, derived from the tibialis posterior artery. The major blood supply to the body of the talus is the canalis tarsi artery, and only a minor part of the talus is supplied by the sinus tarsi artery (Gelberman and Mortensen 1983). There is also a large venous plexus in the sinus tarsi, which drains particularly the venous outflow from the talus and the anterior part of the capsule of the posterior talocalcaneal joint to the lateral and medial venous systems of the foot (figure 14.2).

The Nerves

Apart from free nerve endings, which lie in the fibrofatty tissue, and mechanoreceptors in the lateral ligaments of the ankle, there are branches of the sural nerve that cross the outer surface of the sinus tarsi. During inversion injury, these might stretch and give rise to neuralgic pain. The sural nerve usually has three branches in the retromalleolar region, which are known as the lateral calcaneal nerves. In the malleolar area there are several small articular twigs to the inferior tibiofibular, tibiotalar, and talocalcaneal joints that traverse medially from the main trunk of the sural nerve. About 14 mm distal and posterior to the tip of the lateral malleolus, the sural nerve curves distally and bifurcates to give rise to an

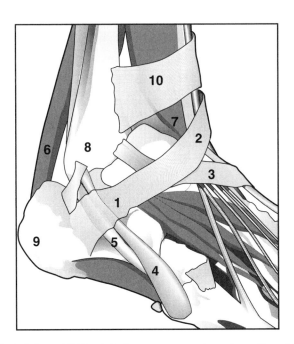

■ **Figure 14.1** Lateral view of the left foot: *(1)* The inferior extensor retinaculum; *(2 and 3)* upper and lower divisions of the retinaculum; *(4 and 5)* peroneus longus and brevis tendons; *(6)* Achilles tendon; *(7)* extensor digitorum longus tendons; *(8)* fibula; *(9)* calcaneum; *(10)* superior extensor retinaculum.

anastomotic branch and to the lateral dorsal cutaneous nerve. The anastomotic branch supplies the area of the sinus tarsi and then disappears in the fibrofatty tissue, or anastomoses with a branch of the superficial peroneal nerve. The lateral dorsal cutaneous nerve lies horizontally compared to the oblique peroneal tendons at that area, and it crosses them at the base of the fifth metatarsal bifurcate to form dorsomedial and dorsolateral branches (Lawrence and Botte 1994) (figure 14.3).

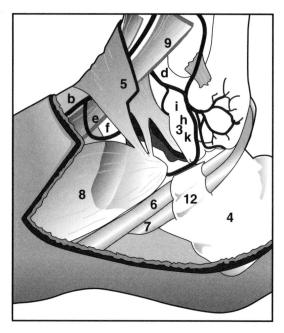

■ **Figure 14.2** Arteries of the lower lateral foot region supplying the sinus tarsi (perforating branch of peroneal artery): *(a)* anterior tibial artery; *(b)* dorsal artery of the foot; *(c)* anterior lateral malleolar artery; *(d)* proximal lateral tarsal artery; *(e)* distal lateral tarsal artery, from which a branch *(f)* runs retrogradely into the sinus tarsi; *(g)* sinus tarsi artery with *(h)* proximal branch and *(i)* distal branch; *(j)* site of passage of perforating branch of the peroneal artery for *(1)* tibia; *(2)* fibular; *(3)* talus; *(4)* calcaneous; *(5)* inferior extensor retinaculum; *(6 and 7)* tendon of peroneous brevis and longus muscles; *(8 and 9)* extensor digitorum longus and brevis muscles; *(10)* extensor hallucis longus muscle; *(11)* tibialis anterior (TA) muscle; and *(12)* inferior peroneal retinaculum.

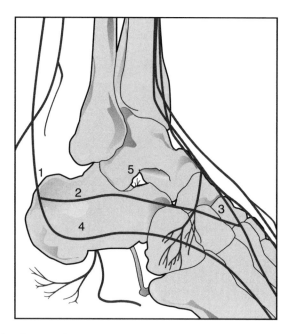

■ **Figure 14.3** Nerve supply to the sinus tarsi region: *(1)* sural nerve; *(2)* upper and lower divisions of the retinaculum; *(3)*

■ Biomechanics

The superficial layer of the inferior extensor retinaculum is consistently found to be a thick, strong, well-defined layer readily accessible for repairs of lateral ankle instability, as was suggested by Gould (Harper 1991; Gould 1987). However, because it is the most superficial layer, is easily distensible, and contains a large proportion of elastic fibers, it cannot be a major mechanical stabilizer of the hindfoot.

Kjaersgaard-Anderson et al. (1988) suggested that the main stabilizers of the hindfoot are the interosseous talocalcaneal ligaments and the cervical ligament, which are thick and strong. Both connect the talus and the calcaneus deep in the sinus tarsi and tarsal canal, and both consist primarily of collagen fibers. In a biomechanical study, they found that an isolated lesion of the cervical ligament or the interosseous ligament resulted in minor increases in movement of the total hindfoot joint complex and the talocalcaneal joint. However, the resultant instability is considerable when these increases in movements are compared to the total range of movement, especially at the talocalcaneal joint. Therefore, they suggested that the demonstrated minor instability apparent in these lesions might have a clinical role in sinus tarsi syndrome.

■ Histopathology

Histological findings usually indicated chronic inflammation. Tailard et al. (1981) demonstrated, in 13 cases in which the sinus tarsi was resected, changes compatible with old injury, such as hyperplasia of the synovium, proliferation of the fibrous tissue, obliteration of all the synovial recesses, and slight deposition of hemosiderin, indicative of old hemorrhage. In several cases, remnants of ligaments embedded in the scar tissue were found. Meyer and Lagier (1977) found synovial hyperplasia and cicatricial remodeling of ligament tissue. Lowy et al (1985) also demonstrated chronic synovitis to be the most common pathological finding. Other findings included fibrosis, focal fat fibrosis, neovascularization, thickened blood vessels, synovial cysts, and inflammatory cell infiltrates.

■ Diagnosis

Pain on the lateral side of the ankle following ankle sprain is not unusual, and often differential diagnosis is difficult and demanding. Knowledge of the clinical presentation as well as of diagnostic techniques is mandatory.

Clinical Presentation and Evaluation

Although there are no established diagnostic criteria for post-traumatic sinus tarsi syndrome, it is a well-defined entity of foot pathology. It is induced by supination trauma of the hindfoot. The clinical presentation includes localized pain in the sinus tarsi that is increased by hindfoot motion, supination, or pronation. Pain is increased in physical activity such as walking or running, especially on uneven ground. The patient feels "giving way" of the ankle but there are no signs of mechanical instability. Of approximately 220 cases of the sinus tarsi reported in the literature, 70% were caused by inversion injury of the ankle (Klein and Spreitzer 1993). Consequently, there is a high association of tarsal sinus and canal ligament tears with tears of the lateral collateral ligaments. The association between subtalar and ankle ligamentous injuries has been stressed by Meyer et al. (1988), who found that 32 out of 40 patients had ruptures of components of the talar and the subtalar capsuloligamentous structures after inversion injury of the ankle. Patients with that syndrome rarely present objective hindfoot instability, although a major complaint is the feeling of hindfoot instability.

A more severe variant of this syndrome is one in which the patient complains of pain on the medial aspect of the hindfoot as well. The medial symptom complex has been identified as the canalis tarsi syndrome (Zwipp et al. 1991). The etiology of the chronic pain is most probably damage to the ligaments, or scarring of the fibrofatty tissue in the canal. Post-traumatic fibrotic changes in the wall and surrounding tissue of the large venous plexus in the sinus tarsi may cause disturbance of venous outflow, which would lead to increased intrasinusal pressure, which may in turn be the cause for chronic pain (Schwarzenbach et al. 1997). The superficial nerves in that area—mainly the anastomotic branch by itself, or with its communication to a branch of the superficial peroneal nerve—may stretch during the injury, giving rise to neuralgic pain. Tailard et al. (1981) showed abnormalities in electromyographic recordings of the function of the peronei during walking in patients presenting with medial hindfoot neuralgic pain. In such cases, the pain may be localized, causing hyperesthesia or radiating pain. Differential block is one of the hallmarks of the diagnosis. Injection of steroids, and local anesthesia to the sinus tarsi or tarsal canal, will relieve the pain. In cases of neuralgic pain, the injection must be directed to the maximal point of tenderness, superficial to the area of the nerve itself.

Imaging Techniques in Sinus Tarsi Syndrome

Because the major injury is to the soft tissue, plain radiographs are helpful only in excluding any fracture. The early phase of triphasic bone scan may demonstrate increased uptake but it is nonspecific. Computed tomography should be used in order to exclude occult fractures such as those of the lateral process of the talus and posterior body of the talus, mainly in patients with chronic pain and normal plain radiography. Arthrography of the subtalar joint in a patient with a confirmed sinus tarsi syndrome demonstrates a sac-like anterior bulge of the capsule. Performed on a nonpathologic tarsal sinus, this procedure would demonstrate a corrugated appearance of the capsule, without this anterior protrusion (Zwipp et al. 1991). Tailard et al. (1981) also demonstrated specific abnormalities in arthrography of the subtalar joint. In fresh lesions, he found blood mixed with synovial fluid in the subtalar joint. The contrast material dispersed, indicating a tear of the capsule and the disappearance of small synovial recesses. In old lesions, the contrast material in the posterior subtalar joint abruptly stopped when it reached the sinus tarsi, and there was complete disappearance of the microrecesses along the interosseous ligament. The latter is believed to be the most important sign. Meyer and Lagier (1977) found in subtalar arthrography that there was obliteration of synovial recesses on the posterior subtalar joint, and explained that this resulted from synovial hyperplasia and cicatricial remodeling of ligament tissue. We are unaware of imaging of the pathological sinus tarsi using ultrasound, although the use of ultrasound appears logical because of its accuracy in imaging soft tissue pathologies.

In the past decade, there have been detailed studies on the anatomy of the sinus tarsi using MRI in cadavers and normal subjects, then comparing them to patients having sinus tarsi syndrome (Trattnig et al. 1995; Breitenseher et al. 1997; Mabit et al. 1997; Beltran et al. 1990; Beltran 1994; Klein and Spreitzer 1993). Klein and Spreitzer (1993) evaluated MRI studies of cadaveric, normal, and pathological images of the sinus tarsi and demonstrated the normal anatomy of the ligaments in the sinus tarsi. In evaluation of 123 MRI images of 116 patients with confirmed sinus tarsi syndrome, chronic synovitis and nonspecific inflammatory changes were seen in 33% of cases, fibrosis in 52% of cases, and synovial cysts in 15% of the patients with sinus tarsi syndrome. There was a high association of tarsal sinus and tarsal canal ligament tears (79%) with lateral collateral ligament tears. The MRI appearance of the abnormal tarsal sinus and tarsal canal correlated well with the symptoms of the sinus tarsi syndrome. Breitenseher et al. (1997) also found that acute ankle sprain injuries, when evaluated by MRI, show acute abnormalities of the sinus tarsi in 43% of patients and correlate with the extent of lateral ankle ligament tearing. Trattnig et al. (1995) also found that MRI demonstrated characteristic findings with obliteration of normal fat and lack of visualization of the ligaments. They found as well that the syndrome is associated in about 70% of the patients with lateral collateral ligament and tibialis posterior tendon injuries.

Differential Diagnosis

Because there are no objective criteria of sinus tarsi syndrome, the diagnosis is based on elimination. The reasons for lateral ankle localized pain after inversion injury may be numerous. Common locations for fractures on that area after inversion injury include the tip of the fibula, the lateral process of the talus, and the articular cartilage of the lateral talus. Avulsion fractures of the insertions of the bifurcate ligament, the lateral side of the navicularis, the anterior tuberosity of the calcaneus, and the dorsolateral area of the cuboid also occur. Bone scan and CT should be sufficient to exclude any fracture on these areas. The main ligamentous injuries around the sinus tarsi include tears of midsubstance of the bifurcate ligament and tears of the lateral ligaments of the ankle, which may accompany the ligamentous injury of the sinus tarsi. Light and Pupp (1991) found that formation of ganglions in the sinus tarsi may cause chronic pain. One case in a series studied by Lowy et al. (1985) had ganglion in the sinus tarsi as a result of gout (1985). Recently we encountered an ice-skating dancer who had developed sinus tarsi pain and limitation of subtalar motion. Clinical examination revealed soft, painful bulging in the sinus tarsi, which was confirmed by ultrasound to be a ganglion cyst. Conservative treatment, including injection, failed, but resection of the ganglion cyst led to full recovery.

■ Treatment

Treatment may be conservative or operative. The main treatment is conservative.

Conservative Treatment

Conservative treatment includes physiotherapy, injections, orthotics, immobilization in cast, local anti-inflammatory gels, local irritants such as capsaicin (Zostrix), and systemic drugs aimed at reducing neuralgic pain. Physiotherapy, including mobilization, friction massage, and deep massage using ultrasound, soft laser, TENS, or any other method of deep massage, may be helpful. When there is ankle instability or a sensation of "giving way," physiotherapy should first be tried. It is aimed at muscle strengthening and improving the reaction time conducted by the peroneal nerve. Zwipp et al. (1991) treated 95 patients during a 10-year period with injections of steroids and local anesthetic to the sinus tarsi, with recovery from the symptoms in most of the patients. Tailard et al. (1981) found that conservative treatment was successful in about two-thirds of patients. Biomechanical evaluation of the function of the foot, with application of corrective shoe inserts, may alleviate the symptoms. Shear et al. (1993) reported successful treatment of sinus tarsi syndrome using corrective orthotics after biomechanical evaluation of a patient. Because the pathologic basis of the syndrome is post-traumatic inflammation, measures to decrease the inflammation, such as local or systemic anti-inflammatory drugs, immobilization in a cast, or a splint, such as Aircast, can be used. The splint stabilizes the subtalar joint, enabling recovery of the ligaments while reducing the inflammatory process.

Surgical Treatment

In case of failure of conservative treatment, surgical treatment is suggested. The surgical procedure includes resection of the fibrofatty tissue from the sinus tarsi, including the ligaments. The operation can improve 90% of the patients (Tailard et al. 1981). Lowy et al. (1985) reviewed 22 cases of sinus tarsi syndrome that underwent decompression of the sinus tarsi. They concluded that the operation is successful and offers little chance of postoperative complications. Brunner and Gachter (1993) reviewed 42 feet in 41 patients who underwent debridement of the sinus tarsi because of persistant pain, despite local infiltration with steroids. Fifteen patients had some persistent problems or inadequate results. In 60% of the patients, hindfoot instability required a ligamentous reconstruction as well. Kuwada (1994) reviewed his 15-year follow-up on conservative and surgical treatment of chronic sinus tarsi syndrome. Most of his patients eventually required surgical intervention after conservative treatment failed to alleviate their symptoms. The surgical treatment proved to be effective in relieving the sinus tarsi pain. Kjaersgaard-Anderson et al. (1989) demonstrated seven cases in which only one patient had good results with conservative treatment. Three patients underwent a procedure of stabilization of ankle ligaments, with limited results, except for one patient who had complete pain relief after subtalar fusion.

■ References

Beltran J. Sinus tarsi syndrome. Magn. Reson. Imaging Clin. N. Am. 1994;2(1)65-69.

Beltran J, Munchow AM, Khabiri H, Magee DG, McGee RB, Grossman SB. Ligaments of the lateral aspects of the ankle and sinus tarsi: an MR imaging study. Radiology. 1990; 177(2) 455-458.

Breitenseher MJ, Haller J, Kukla C, Gaebler C, Kaider A, Fleschmann D, Helbich T, Trattnig S. MRI of the sinus tarsi in acute ankle sprain injuries. J. Comput. Assist. Tomogr. 1997;21(2)274-279.

Brunner R, Gachter A. Sinus tarsi syndrome. Results of surgical treatment. Unfallchirurg. 1993;96(10)534-537.

Cahill DR. The anatomy and function of the contents of the human tarsal sinus and canal. Anat. Rec. 1965;153:1-18.

Gelberman RH, Mortensen WW. The arterial anatomy of the talus. Foot Ankle 1983;4(2) 64-72.

Gould N. Lateral approach to sinus tarsi. Foot Ankle. 1983;3(4)244-246.

Gould N. Repair of lateral ligament of ankle, Foot Ankle 1987; 8:55.

Harper MC. The lateral ligamentous support of the subtalar joint. Foot Ankle 1991;11(6)354-358.

Kjaersgaard-Andersen P, Andersen K, Soballe K. Pilgaard S. Sinus tarsi syndrome: presentation of seven cases and review of the literature. J. Foot Surg. 1989;28(1) 3-6.

Kjaersgaard-Andersen P, Wethelund JO, Helmig P, Soballe K. The stabilizing effect of the ligamentous structures in the sinus and canalis tarsi on movements in the hindfoot. An experimental study. Am. J. Sports Med. 1988;16(5)512-516.

Klein MA, Spreitzer AM. MR imaging of the tarsal sinus and canal: normal anatomy, pathologic findings and features of the sinus tarsi syndrome, Radiology 1993;186(1):233-240.

Kuwada GT. Long term retrospective analysis of the treatment of sinus tarsi syndrome. J. Foot Ankle Surg. 1994;33(1) 28-29.

Lawrence SJ, Botte MJ. The sural nerve in the foot and ankle: an anatomic study with clinical and surgical implications, Foot Ankle Int. 1994;15(9)490-494.

Light M, Pupp G. Ganglions in the sinus tarsi. J. Foot Surg. 1991;30(4) 350-355.

Lowy A, Schilero J, Kanat IO. Sinus tarsi syndrome: a postoperative analysis. J. Foot Surg. 1985;24(2)108-112.

Mabit C, Boncoeur-Martel MP, Chaudruc JM, Valleix D, Descottes B, Caix M. Anatomy and MRI study of the subtalar ligamentous support. Surg. Radiol. Anat. 1997;19(2)111-117.

Meyer JM, Lagier R. Post-traumatic sinus tarsi syndrome. An anatomical and radiological study. Acta Orthop. Scand. 1977;48(1) 121-128.

Meyer JM, Garcia J, Hoffmeyer P. Subtalar pain: a radiological study. Paper presented at the American Orthopaedic Foot and Ankle Society Annual Meeting, Atlanta, February 1988.

O'Connor D. Sinus tarsi syndrome. A clinical entity. J. Bone Joint Surg. 1958;40A-720.

Schmidt HM. Gestalt und befestigung der bandsysteme im sinus und canalis tarsi des menchen. Acta Anat. (Basel) 1978;102:184-194.

Schwarzenbach B, Bora C, Lang A, Kissling RO. Blood vessels of the sinus tarsi and the sinus tarsi syndrome. Clin. Anat. 1997;10(3)172-82.

Shear MS, Baich SP, Shear DB. Sinus tarsi syndrome: the importance of biomechanically based evaluation and treatment. Arch. Phys. Med. Rehabil. 1983;74(7)777-781.

Tailard W, Meyer JM, Garcia J, Blanc Y. The sinus tarsi syndrome. Int. Orthop. 1981;5(2)117-130.

Trattnig S, Breitenseher MJ, Haller J, Heinz-Peer G, Kukla C, Imhof H. Sinus tarsi syndrome. MRI diagnosis, Radiloge. 1995;35(7)463-467.

Wood Jones F. The talocalcaneal articulation, Lancet. 1944;241-242.

Zwipp H. Swoboda B, Holch M, Maschek HJ, Reichelt S. Sinus tarsi and canalis tarsi syndromes. A post-traumatic entity. Unfallchirurg. 1991;94(12)608-613.

Chapter 15

Tendon Injuries in Acute Ankle Sprains

Lew C. Schon, MD, and Claude D. Anderson, MD

Ankle sprains are the most common specific injury in sport. The concept of a "simple" ankle sprain can be misleading. The literature documents many additional injuries that can occur at the time of an ankle sprain, such as damage to ligaments, muscles, bone, cartilage, nerves, arteries, and tendons, and which may be unrecognized initially. This chapter focuses on tendon injuries associated with acute ankle sprains.

Tendons are not all created equal. Their blood supply, excursion, and course vary. Histologically, a tendon consists of densely packed type-I collagen fiber bundles that are oriented in line with the axis of the tension (Clancy 1990). Between the bundles are spindle-shaped fibroblasts that create and maintain the matrix. Surrounding the entire tendon is a connective tissue sheath (the peritenon) that has an inner (visceral) and an outer (parietal) layer. Mesotenon provides connections between the two layers. Peritenon is called tenosynovium if synovial fluid exists between the two layers (Teitz et al. 1997; Woo et al. 1994). Tendons of the digital flexors and extensors are very stiff, and their length changes very little when muscle forces are applied through them. In contrast, tendons involved in locomotion, such as the Achilles, are elastic. During the late stance phase of gait, energy is stored in the Achilles tendon as it is stretched. This energy is returned during the pushoff phase, but not without a price. Tendons that transmit large loads under eccentric and elastic conditions are more subject to injury (Teitz et al. 1997).

Traditionally, *tendinitis* is the term given to an area within a tendon that is inflamed and painful. However, when surgical specimens are examined histologically, there are usually few inflammatory cells, such as macrophages or polymorphonuclear leukocytes. Instead, the pattern seen is more suggestive of a degenerative condition: The collagen matrix is random, without the typical axial alignment, fibroblasts are more numerous, and there is an increase in vascularity. The degenerative nature of the tendon can be fatty, mucoid, or hyaline in character. This condition is more correctly termed tendinosis (Clancy 1990; Puddu et al. 1976). The inflammatory process tends to affect the well-vascularized peritendinous structures rather than the tendon itself. *Peritendinitis* is inflammation that affects the paratenon, and *tenosynovitis* (tendovaginitis) refers to inflammation in the synovium of the tendon (Jozsa & Kannus 1997a).

The tendons injured with acute ankle sprains, in order of frequency, are the peroneal tendons, followed by the posterior tibial tendon (PTT), Achilles tendon, anterior tibial tendon (ATT), and (rarely) the flexor and extensor tendons of the hallux and toes. In all cases, the patient may present with findings similar to those of an uncomplicated medial or lateral ankle sprain. History of an inversion or eversion event with or without the sensation of a "pop" is characteristic for both. In the setting of an acute ankle sprain, the instigating event is a small tear in the tendon, ligament, or retinaculum that leads to hemorrhage in the sheath. Tenosynovitis may then develop over several weeks. When the process involves the tendon itself, then the diagnosis of tendinosis is appropriate. Physical examination may be comparable to an ankle sprain except for tenderness over the specific tendon injured. Resistive testing should elicit pain and/or weakness. With the exception of a complete rupture, acute treatment is dictated by symptoms and is followed by therapy to enhance strength and address any abnormal mechanics.

■ Peroneal Tendons

Peroneal tendons may be injured by the same mechanisms of an ankle sprain. This problem may manifest with peroneal tendinitis, peroneal tendon partial or complete rupture, or subluxation/dislocation of the tendons.

Anatomy

The peroneal tendons originate from the posterolateral fibula in the lateral compartment of the lower leg and proceed to a common synovial sheath approximately 4 cm proximal to the lateral malleolus. At the distal extent of the lateral malleolus, a groove (the retromalleolar sulcus) is present. This groove is lined with fibrocartilage and, along with the thickened peroneal sheath, lends increased stability as the tendons course behind the fibula. Edwards (1928) showed that the sulcus is shallow in 82% of anatomic specimens, and not well formed in 18%. In the general population, the average dimensions of the sulcus range from 5 to 10 mm in width and 2 to 4 mm in depth. A lateral ridge of bone further enhances the sulcus in 70% of cadavers. The bony ridge and overlying cartilaginous cap add 3 to 6 mm lateral height to the sulcus (Edwards 1928), and the sheath is augmented medially by the calcaneofibular ligament and laterally by the superior and inferior peroneal retinacula. The sheath and the groove together form a fibro-osseous tunnel, with the brevis lying anterior to the longus tendon. Just inferior to the lateral malleolus, each tendon enters a separate sheath. The brevis tendon inserts on the fifth metatarsal styloid, and the longus tendon continues to the cuboid. There it enters a second tunnel that brings the tendon to the plantar aspect of the foot, where it traverses under the tarsometatarsal joints to the medial side and inserts onto the first metatarsal (McGarvey & Clanton 1996).

There exist additional peroneal muscles as described by Sobel et al. (1991). Of note is the peroneus quartus present in 21% of cadavers. It has variable anatomy, but in most cases it originates from the peroneus brevis musculotendinous junction and inserts on the peroneal tubercle of the calcaneus (Plattner & Mann 1993).

Tenosynovitis

Tenosynovitis, or peritendinitis, is defined as inflammation of the peritenon or paratenon that envelops the tendon, and/or inflammation of the synovial lining of the tendon sheath (figure 15.1) (Clanton & Schon 1993). Stenosing tenosynovitis of the peroneals has been described as a resultant thickening of the tendon sheath and subsequent constriction of the enclosed tendons. These processes usually occur at three anatomic sites: the retromalleolar sulcus, the peroneal tubercle on the calcaneus, and the cuboid tunnel. Trauma is believed to be the cause in most cases. Not only inversion ankle sprains, but also fibula fractures, calcaneal fractures, and direct trauma can lead to tenosynovitis. Tendon rupture may result from any one of the previously mentioned conditions, or rupture can occur without preexisting symptoms (see "Treatment," page 123).

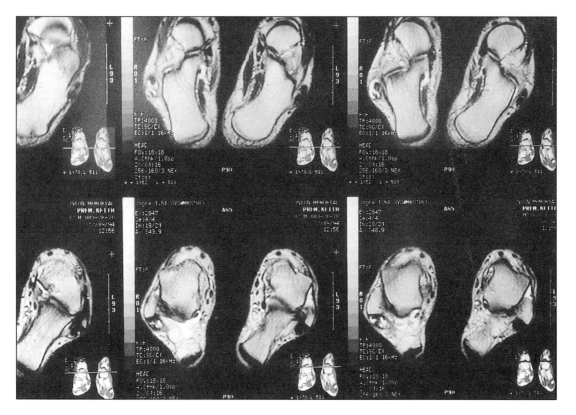

■ **Figure 15.1** MRI demonstrating tenosynovitis of left peroneal tendons.

Clinical Findings

Patients often describe a history of ankle weakness or repeated ankle sprains. They may describe a specific event at the time of injury, or they may be unable to recall the exact mechanism or event. Acutely, symptoms include pain and swelling along the lateral aspect of the ankle. One can often detect some warmth and even crepitus during movement of the tendon. Moving the foot into plantarflexion and inversion, or resisted eversion on a supinated foot, can elicit pain. Strength of the peroneals is usually good. Diagnosis can be confirmed with an injection of local anesthetic into the peroneal sheath: Relief of symptoms strongly suggests peroneal pathology.

Radiographic examination is necessary to exclude other sources of pain such as an exostosis, osteochondroma, or hypertrophic peroneal tubercle. Additionally, a ruptured peroneus longus tendon may present radiographically with a proximally migrated os perineum or a fractured os (figure 15.2). Tenography has been described by some authors; however, magnetic resonance imaging (MRI) or ultrasound scanning is recommended in those patients who present a diagnostic dilemma (figure 15.3).

Treatment

Recommended nonoperative management involves rest, ice, compression, and elevation. Anti-inflammatory medication is a valuable adjunct. The earlier the treatment is instituted, the more rapid is the recovery. A brief period of immobilization using a cast, boot, or brace may be necessary. In chronic cases, nonoperative management may include one steroid injection into the sheath and a medial heel wedge to roll calcaneus away from peroneals. We generally recommend avoiding or minimizing these injections because of soft tissue atrophy or tendon ruptures. It is extremely rare that a tenosynovitis will progress to the point where surgery is necessary, but if the symptoms continue or recur immediately after the resumption of activity, surgery is recommended (Clanton & Schon 1993).

Surgery involves exploration with tenolysis or debridement. The superior and inferior peroneal retinacula should be preserved, if at all possible, and meticulously repaired if released (Plattner & Mann 1993). The surgeon should look for any longitudinal tears or fraying and repair them as described above.

Rupture

Peroneal tendons may undergo complete or partial rupture in conjunction with an inversion injury.

Diagnosis

Ruptures of the peroneus longus and brevis are uncommon and may be longitudinal or transverse, acute or chronic. When a complete transverse tear occurs, the patient presents with demonstrable weakness and possibly a palpable gap or nodule. The peroneus

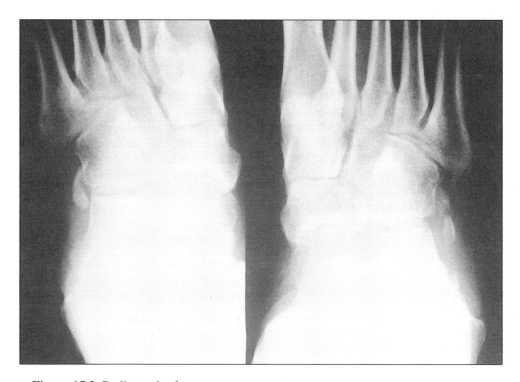

■ **Figure 15.2** Radiograph of an os peroneum rupture.

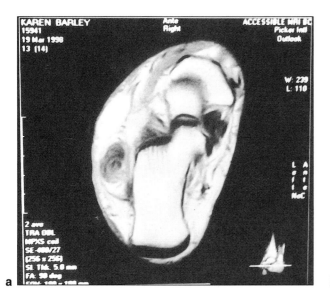 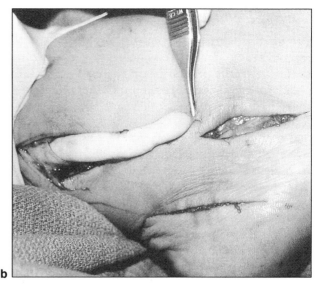

■ **Figure 15.3** A 35-year-old woman with a history of pain and swelling of the lateral ankle experienced a "pop" during ankle sprain. *(a)* MRI demonstrates peroneal tenosynovitis and abnormal tendon signal. *(b)* Intraoperative photograph demonstrating complete rupture.

longus functions as a depressor of the first ray and secondarily as an everter of the foot. Complete rupture of the peroneus longus could result in loss of pushoff power, and may compromise the ability to balance on one foot because the tendon would be unable to depress the first metatarsal head. Physical examination would demonstrate diminished first-ray plantarflexion. The peroneus brevis is the primary everter of the foot. Physical examination would demonstrate weakness with resisted eversion (Schon & Bell 1996). In the setting of a twisting injury to the ankle, such a history and physical is unusual.

More commonly, a longitudinal split in one of the peroneal tendons (usually the brevis) results from an ankle sprain. Autopsy studies have shown attritional tears of the peroneus brevis in 11% of ankles examined (Sobel et al. 1990). These tears commonly occur in the retromalleolar sulcus. With repeated inversion events, the superior peroneal retinaculum becomes attenuated. The peroneus brevis can become trapped between the sharp posterior edge of the fibula anteriorly and the peroneus longus tendon posteriorly, resulting in a splaying out of the brevis or the formation of one of more longitudinal attritional tears (figure 15.4). With time, it is reasonable to assume that the longus can develop longitudinal tears from the same mechanism. A history of chronic lateral ankle pain, swelling, or instability may indicate an attritional tear of the peroneus brevis and longus tendons. With a longitudinal tear, the tendon may be thickened and tender on examination, but not significantly weak. In a clinical series of 47 ankle ligament reconstructions, peroneus brevis tendon lesions were observed in 11 ankles of 10 patients (Soma & Mandelbaum 1994). All patients had a history of chronic recurrent ankle sprains, with symptoms of pain being more disabling than instability. The causative factor in most cases was a history of significant trauma to the ankle with abnormal repetitive stress to the peroneus brevis tendon (Soma & Mandelbaum 1994).

Ruptures of the peroneus longus tendon through a fracture of the os peroneum sesamoid, or distal to the sesamoid bone adjacent to the cuboid tunnel, have been surgically documented only a few times. Careful radiographic examination with multiple views and comparison views can help differentiate between a cuboid avulsion fracture, a multipartate os peroneum, and an os perineum fracture or migration of an os perineum.

In general, the diagnosis of peroneal pathology is a clinical one. If, however, the diagnosis is in doubt, an MRI or ultrasound evaluation may be helpful in determining the status of the peroneals, although the latter technique is dependent on the skill of the operator.

Treatment

Initially, nonoperative treatment is warranted for incomplete tears, but for complete tears, surgical intervention should be considered.

General Comments
Complete transverse ruptures should be treated surgically when the injury is suspected. A whip stitch with 2-0 or 3-0 nonabsorbable suture is usually sufficient.

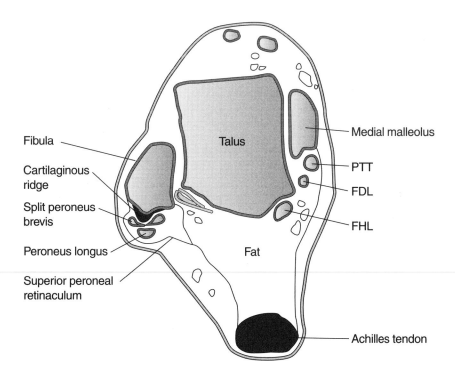

■ Figure 15.4 Cross-section at the level of the fibular groove showing the mechanism of injury. Peroneus brevis is split, with the longus lying within the fissure.

Weight bearing may be begun in 2 weeks. Postoperatively, the foot should be immobilized in a position of slight eversion and equinus to remove tension from the repair. The patient should be maintained in a nonweightbearing status for approximately 2 weeks, after which the foot can be recast in a neutral position or the brace can be adjusted for an additional 2 weeks. Six weeks after surgery, gentle, passive, and assisted active range-of-motion exercises are instituted. Functional bracing for at least 3 months in a device to control inversion stress is warranted. The repair must be protected from inversion or resistive forces for 12 weeks (Bell & Schon 1996).

Patients with attritional tears usually present with chronic lateral ankle pain and swelling and have most likely undergone previous nonoperative treatment for an ankle sprain. In those patients suspected of having a longitudinal tear of either tendon, further nonoperative management beyond 8 weeks from the time of injury is generally nonproductive, and surgery may be recommended. If no treatment has been instituted in patients with suspected attritional tears, nonoperative management may include 6 to 8 weeks of immobilization. Failing this, surgery is considered. Longitudinal tears can be directly repaired 6 weeks after an acute episode. The area surrounding the immediate tear should be ellipsed out and then internally sutured with 4-0 braided, nonabsorbable material (figure 15.5). Similarly, peroneal tendon pathol-

ogy must be considered in any patient undergoing operative intervention for chronic lateral ankle pain or instability (McGarvey & Clanton 1996).

Specific Technical Points Regarding Surgery
Surgery should be performed in the lateral decubitus position or in the supine position with a roll under the ipsilateral hip to assist in internally rotating the leg. A thigh tourniquet may be applied if the surgery is to be performed under general anesthesia, but it is not routinely necessary because the surgery is usually relatively bloodless. The incision follows the course of the peroneal tendons, beginning approximately 5 cm proximal to the distal fibula and extending to the tip of the fibula; it occasionally curves anteriorly and distally along with the tendons 2 cm distal to the fibula (figure 15.6, p. 127). Care should be taken to avoid injury to the sural nerve, which should be in the posterior flap. An occasional nerve branch may traverse the operative field and should be preserved if at all possible. The superior peroneal retinaculum will be encountered and it should be inspected for any evidence of attenuation. To minimize scarring, we always attempt to leave at least 1 cm of the retinaculum intact by the tip of the fibula.

If the retinaculum needs to be incised, a cuff of tissue should be left for closure at the end of the repair. Just underneath the superior peroneal retinaculum is the peroneal sheath. It should be incised in line with the skin incision. The peroneal tendons

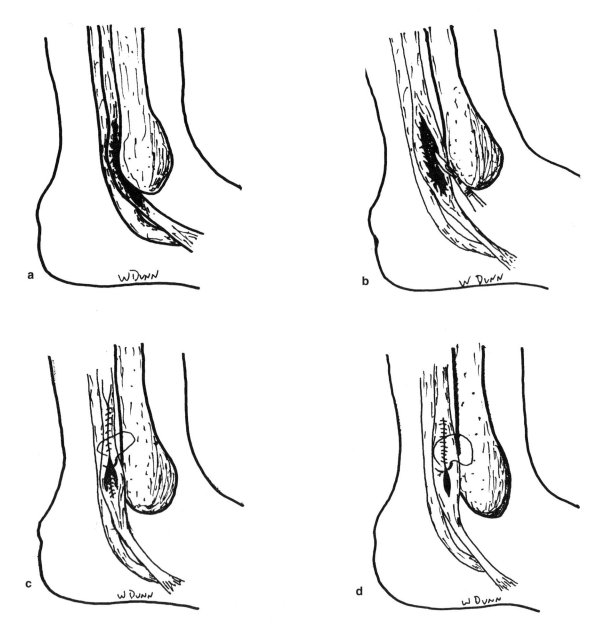

■ **Figure 15.5** *(a)* Longitudinal tear in peroneal brevis tendon. *(b)* Tear elliptically excised. *(c)* and *(d)* Tear repaired with 4-0 braided, nonabsorbable suture.

will be evident, with the longus more lateral and posterior to the brevis. Each tendon should be examined for evidence of tears. Any proliferative synovium should be removed. If a peroneus quartus is encountered or if excessive peroneal muscle fibers exist distal to the superficial peroneal retinaculum, they should be excised (Mizel et al. 1996).

Where there is no reconstructible tendon, but the sheath is intact, then a free graft can be interposed between the proximal and distal ends of the tendon (figure 15.7). If there is no salvageable tendon, then the flexor digitorum longus (FDL) tendon can be transferred as follows: The FDL is harvested through a transverse 4-cm incision in line with the skin creases

in the arch of the foot over the master knot of Henry. The plantar fascia is incised, the medial plantar nerve is reflected medially, and the FDL and flexor hallucis longus (FHL) are sutured together. The FDL is then cut proximal to the tenodesis, and a suture is placed in the end of the transected FDL. A 3-cm incision is made just proximal to the tip of the medial malleolus over the FDL, and the tendon is withdrawn through this incision. If the tendon is not free, the plantar wound and the FHL should be examined. There is usually a tendon bundle of the FDL that fuses with the FHL; cutting this portion of the FHL will free the FDL. A third 3-cm medial incision is made beginning 8 to 9 cm proximal to the medial malleolus over the

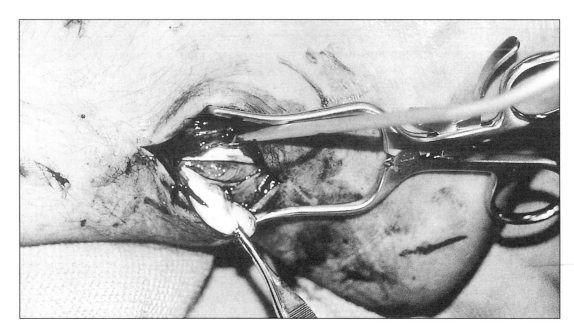

■ **Figure 15.6** Eight months previously, this patient felt a pop in his posterolateral ankle after an ankle sprain. The intraoperative photograph shows the ruptured peroneus longus tendon and os peroneum retracted proximally behind distal fibula.

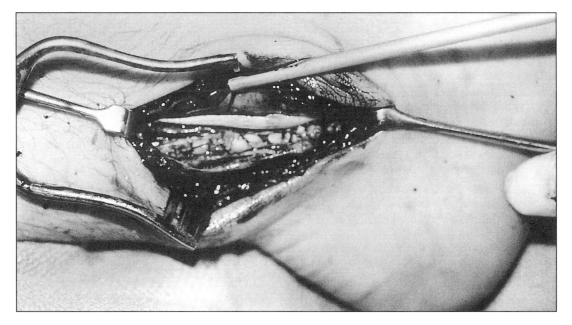

■ **Figure 15.7** Intraoperative photograph of a split peroneus longus free graft interposed between proximal and distal ends of the peroneus brevis.

FDL. The tendon is pulled through this incision, and the deeper fascia lateral to this tendon is incised to permit transfer from medial to lateral. The FDL is drawn through the peroneal sheath and attached distally to the fifth metatarsal or the remaining peroneal tendon end.

When there is no tendon and no sheath, a Hunter rod can be placed in the first stage of a two-stage procedure. Mizel et al. (1996) recommended a staged procedure by which a Hunter rod is initially placed where the peroneus brevis previously existed. The second stage is performed 3 months later, at which time the FHL or FDL is harvested, transferred, and sutured to the distal stump of the peroneus brevis.

The postoperative course is the same as that for complete transverse ruptures (described previously).

Traumatic Subluxation and Dislocation

Subluxation or dislocation of the peroneal tendons occasionally occurs with ankle injuries. The injury usually results from a twisting event, and it is frequently misdiagnosed as an ankle sprain. The same mechanism of injury that causes a lateral ankle sprain may also cause the peroneals to dislocate or tear; however, the exact position of the ankle at the time of injury to the peroneals may vary. Typically, there is a sudden reflex contracture of the peroneals in response to a traumatic event necessary to produce the injury. In a review of the literature, 71% of these injuries have occurred in alpine snow skiers and 7% occurred in football players (Alm et al. 1975; Beck 1981; Clanton & Schon 1993; Davies 1979; Earle et al. 1972; Edwards 1928; Escalas et al. 1980; Martens et al. 1986; McLennan 1980; Micheli et al. 1989; Slatis et al. 1988; Stein 1987; Stover & Bryan 1962) In skiers, it has been described as resulting from the tips of the skis digging into the snow. This sudden deceleration force, combined with the fixed dorsiflexed position of the ankle in the ski boot, allows the peroneals to rupture their sheath and dislocate anteriorly; they may also tear when they reflexively and violently contract (Stover & Bryan 1962).

Other etiologies have been noted (Sobel et al. 1991). Kojima et al. (1991) noted that a small percentage of neonates had clinically demonstrable peroneal tendon subluxation that spontaneously resolved. Huber and Imhoff (1988) found that most patients with peroneal tendon dislocation could not recall a history of trauma. Frey and Shereff (1988) divided subluxing peroneal tendons into two varieties: (1) traumatic and (2) habitual or voluntary. This information, along with anatomical studies by Edwards (1928), suggests that a congenital anatomical deficiency of the peroneal retinaculum or retromalleolar sulcus may be one cause for atraumatic peroneal subluxation (McGarvey & Clanton 1996).

Diagnosis

According to Clanton and Schon (1993), Monteggia was the first to report on peroneal subluxation in 1803. By 1895, peroneal subluxation and dislocation was considered a "well-recognized condition." However, despite this well-documented past, peroneal tendon dislocations are often misdiagnosed as lateral ankle sprains because ankle sprains are one of the most common injuries seen by orthopedic surgeons in the emergency room, and peroneal tendon dislocations are relatively rare. The presentation for both injuries is similar, and they may occur together. Nevertheless, there are findings that can allow one to separate the two diagnoses.

With chronic, recurrent dislocation, there is a history of a snapping sensation over the distal fibula with or without pain. Patients may also describe a "giving way" of the ankle. Unlike patients who present with a purely lateral ankle sprain, patients with peroneal dislocations will frequently be unable to describe a mechanism of injury. Physical examination demonstrates swelling and tenderness about the peroneal tendon sheath behind the lateral malleolus. Pain may be elicited with resisted dorsiflexion and eversion of a plantarflexed and inverted foot. Demonstrating subluxation or straightforward dislocation of the tendons is difficult in the clinical setting. The absence of clinically palpable dislocations or subluxations of the tendon should not lead the clinician away from the diagnosis. The key to diagnosis is having a suspicion that the entity of peroneal subluxation might exist; testing will reveal pain and, possibly, peroneal instability.

Routine radiographs are indicated in any patient with a suspected peroneal tendon dislocation. Rarely, an avulsion of the distal posterior border of the distal fibula may be seen, indicating a dislocation event. However, most radiographs are normal. In cases where the diagnosis is in doubt, other studies may be used. Peroneal tenogram has been described by McLennan (1980), but its usefulness has been questioned with the advent of less invasive studies. Computed tomography (CT) is helpful in evaluating the bony morphology of the retromalleolar sulcus in relation to the tendons. Magnetic resonance imaging (MRI) and ultrasound scanning are excellent studies for evaluating soft tissue injury and, therefore, peroneal tendon pathology (Sobel et al. 1991; Zeiss et al. 1989). However, peroneal tendon subluxation and dislocation can usually be determined based on clinical grounds.

Classification

Eckert and Davis (1976) investigated 73 cases of acute peroneal dislocation and described three types of injury, and Oden (1987) described a rare fourth type of injury.

■ In **grade I** injuries, the retinaculum and its attachment to the periosteum are stripped away but not torn free from the posterolateral border of the distal fibula. The peroneal tendons dislocate anteriorly into the pouch formed between the raw lateral border of the fibula and the stripped periosteum and retinaculum.

■ In **grade II** injuries, the cartilaginous rim, to which the retinaculum and periosteum are attached, is avulsed off the fibula. This injury is likened to a Bankart lesion in the shoulder.

■ In **grade III** injuries (the least common), the bone to which the cartilaginous rim is attached is avulsed (figure 15.8). The findings of a grade III injury with a rim avulsion fracture of the lateral malleolus are considered to be pathognomonic of tendon dislocation.

In the rare **fourth type of injury,** the peroneals dislocate through a tear in the peroneal retinaculum.

Treatment of Acute Injury

If the diagnosis is made acutely, then it is quite reasonable to attempt nonoperative treatment. The optimal nonoperative treatment of an acute peroneal dislocation is controversial. The best results have been seen with well-molded nonweightbearing cast immobilization for 6 weeks. The foot should be placed in 10° to 15° of plantarflexion and slight *inversion* to relax the peroneal tendons, yet keep them in a reduced position. This approach can lead to good results in more than 50% of the cases; however, a shorter period of immobilization can result in a high rate of recurrence (Stover & Bryan 1962). A nonarticulating walking boot is a reasonable alternative to a cast. However, with a near 50% recurrence rate even with optimal nonoperative treatment, there

is a strong argument to proceed directly to surgical repair. For those patients who have an active lifestyle, our recommended treatment for an acute injury is surgery.

Surgical treatment in the acute injury setting is best performed with the patient in the lateral decubitus position, with or without a tourniquet. The anesthesia may be general, regional, or local. We usually use a beanbag to secure a lateral decubitus position and perform the surgery with an ankle block, including the superficial peroneal and sural nerves, and intravenous sedation. The incision is made over the posterior border of the distal fibula, beginning approximately 4 cm above the tip and extending down to just inferior to the tip of the fibula. Careful sharp dissection is carried out through the subcutaneous tissues, avoiding any branches of the sural nerve. The retinaculum is identified, and the retinaculum is incised approximately 1 to 2 mm off the posterior border of the fibula. Although this incision may bring the surgeon directly over the peroneal tendon, care must be exercised not to injure the tendons. Once the retinaculum is incised, the anterior flap, which may be separate from or contain the cartilaginous rim, is dissected continuously more anteriorly off the fibula with a sleeve of periosteum. The peroneal tendons are

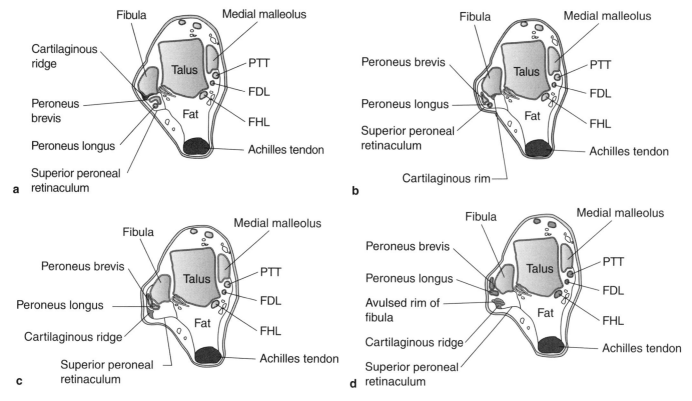

■ **Figure 15.8** Peroneal tendon dislocation classification. *(a)* Normal. *(b)* Grade I (supination of the superior retinaculum from the fibula). *(c)* Grade II (avulsion of the fibrous cartilaginous rim off the posterolateral aspect of the fibula). *(d)* Grade III (avulsion of the posterolateral aspect of the fibula by the superior peroneal retinaculum).

inspected for damage (figure 15.9). Small tears are excised, and any intrasubstance tears are ellipsed and then repaired. The tendons are reduced back into their groove. Next, three to four drill holes are made, approximately 1 cm apart, from the tip of the fibula, extending more proximally. Drill holes are made with 0.045-inch Kirshner wires (K-wires). The K-wires are cut while in the hole to permit ease of subsequent identification. Next, using 2-0 Ethibond sutures, the posterior flap of the retinaculum is reattached to the roughened surface of the fibula and tied over its lateral border. The K-wire is removed from the hole just before the passage of the suture through the tunnel, thereby ensuring that the hole does not get "lost." Next, the anterior portion of the retinaculum/periosteum is sutured over the repair using 2.0 and 4.0 Vicryl sutures. If an Eckert grade III lesion is noted preoperatively, then the fragment can be reduced back to the fibula with sutures or K-wires. This is closed with nylon sutures.

Postoperatively, patients are kept in a well-padded, nonweightbearing splint holding the foot in neutral for 10 to 14 days. A weightbearing cast or boot can then be placed and is worn for an additional 4 weeks. Return to preinjury activity depends on regaining full range of motion and strength, which usually occurs approximately 3 to 4 months after surgery.

Treatment of Chronic Injury

In most cases, patients will usually present well beyond the acute phase, after they have suffered repeated dislocation episodes. In such cases, nonoperative management is of little benefit. Chronic recurrent subluxations that are symptomatic are best treated with surgery. The real dilemma involves deciding which of the more than 20 surgical treatments

is best. These procedures may be classified into five categories:

1. Direct repair by reattachment of the peroneal retinaculum with reinforcement from local tissue
2. Reconstruction of the peroneal retinaculum with transferred tissue
3. One block procedures
4. Groove-deepening procedures with osteoperiosteal flaps
5. Rerouting procedures of the peroneal tendons under the calcaneofibular ligaments

Each method has advantages and disadvantages; however, our experience is that the best results are seen with peroneal groove deepening. This procedure allows for a near-anatomic, isometric reconstruction, and permits the fullest range of motion with the least sacrifice to any nearby structures. The procedure is rather straightforward and simple to do.

The patient is positioned on a bean bag in the lateral decubitus position. A local block with lidocaine and bupivacaine of the sural nerve and superficial peroneal nerve is administered with sedation. Next, an incision is made just posterior to the tip of the fibula over the posterior and distal fibula, ranging for approximately 4 cm. Careful sharp dissection is carried out through the subcutaneous tissues down to the retinaculum. The retinaculum is then opened to approximately 1 to 2 mm off the posterior and distal aspect of the fibula. The anterior flap is dissected sharply off the fibula, extending dissection anteriorly, lifting off the periosteum of the fibula for approximately 1.5 cm. Next, the tendons are inspected and any tendon pathology is addressed. A chisel is then inserted at the junction of the back lip of the fibrocartilage and the lateral aspect of the fibula. With this chisel, an osseous fibrocartilaginous flap is raised, approximately 2 mm thick. This flap is continued from the tip of the fibula proximally up the back of the posterior fibula until the medial cortex of the posterior fibula is cut. Next, using a burr, the cancellous bone is removed. Approximately 5 to 8 mm of deepening is preferable. Once this has been achieved, three to four drill holes are made in the lateral aspect of the fibula. As each drill hole is made, the 0.045-inch K-wire that is used is clipped to permit easy identification of the holes in the bone. Next, the bone tamp is used to gently compress the osseous fibrocartilaginous posterior surface of the fibula down into the newly created trough. The peroneal tendons are put in place and the tendons are inspected to make sure that there is no tendency to sublux or dislocate. Using the 2.0 Ethibond suture, the posterior retinaculum is sutured to the fibula and the knots are tied over the bone. Next, the anterior flap is secured over the repair to reinforce

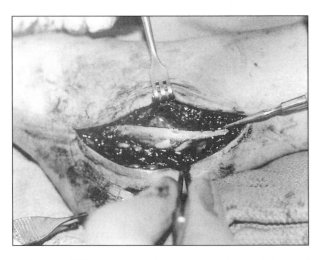

■ **Figure 15.9** Intraoperative photograph of a dislocated peroneus brevis.

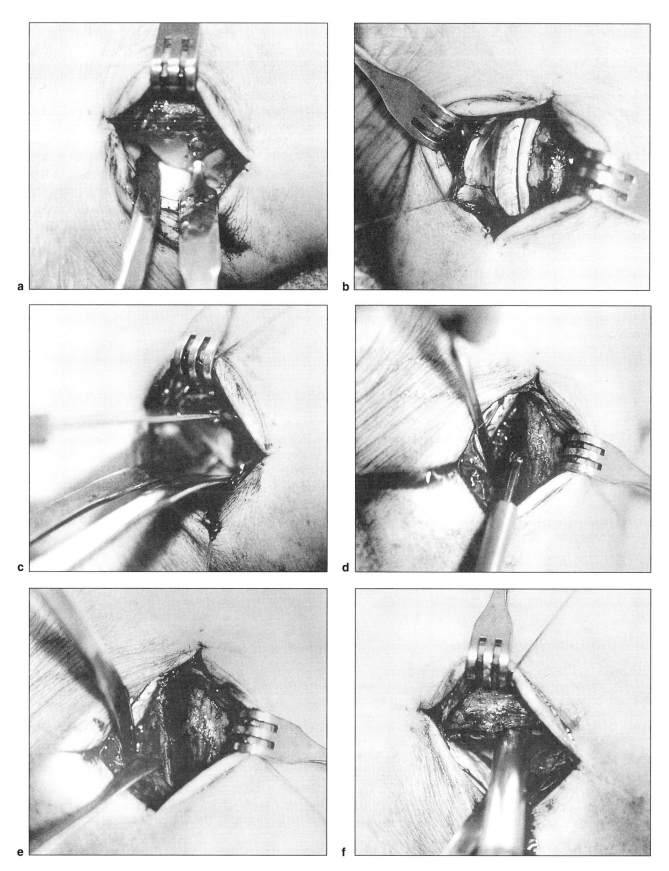

■ **Figure 15.10** *(a)* Retromalleolar sulcus with peroneals reflected posteriorly. *(b)* Lateral photograph of peroneal tendons exposed through an incision made just posterior to the posterior border of the fibula. *(c)* A chisel is inserted against the fibula to raise the fibrocartilaginous flap. *(d)* Burring of cancellous bone to deepen the groove. *(e)* Flap of fibrocartilage before tamping. *(f)* Tamping flap into position.

the initial repair. The subcutaneous tissues are closed with 4.0 Vicryl. The skin is closed with a nylon suture (figure 15.10).

Postoperatively, the patient is placed in a U and posterior splint for 10 days to 2 weeks, nonweightbearing in a neutral position. The patient is allowed to bear weight in a boot brace at 2 weeks and is advanced to full weight bearing and increasing walking as tolerated by 6 weeks. The patient may be converted to a stirrup brace (AirCast, AirCast Inc., Summit, NJ) between the second and sixth week, as tolerated (figure 15.11). The patient is to avoid plantarflexion and inversion beyond 15° but may dorsiflex as much as possible. The patient should also avoid supination and pronation in conjunction with dorsiflexion, plantarflexion, or circumduction of the foot for approximately 3 months. A stationary bike may be used at 2 or 3 weeks, but the patient should wear the air stirrup brace. The patient may also begin using stair-stepper equipment at 6 weeks and thereafter may wean out of the brace for straightforward walking (after which time the risk of an inversion injury is low). For more rigorous or prolonged activity, the brace should be worn from 6 to 12 weeks postoperatively. The patient may begin active

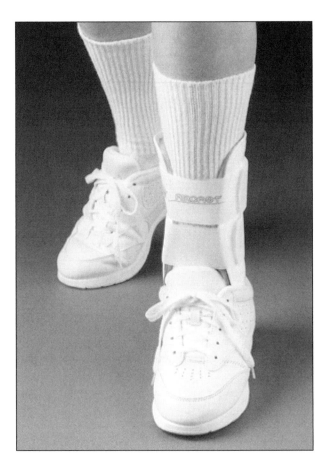

■ **Figure 15.11** Example of a stirrup brace (AirCast) for PTT tenosynovitis.

plantarflexion and inversion beyond 10° to 15° progressively between 6 and 12 weeks. Peroneal tendon, posterior tibial, dorsiflexion, and plantarflexion strengthening are begun at 2 weeks, as long as there is avoidance of plantarflexion beyond 15° to 20° for the first 6 weeks. Between 6 and 12 weeks, range of motion and strengthening can proceed progressively. The patient may use a stair stepper at 6 weeks. Return to sport may occur at 8 weeks for runners and at 12 weeks for cutting sports (e.g., soccer, lacrosse). When playing sports, the patient should wear a stirrup brace or a sleeve brace for 3 to 5 months after the reconstruction.

■ Posterior Tibial Tendon

Other than overuse-related tenosynovitis, the vast majority of PTT problems, particularly ruptures, occur in middle-aged women. Although PTT injuries do occur in young athletes, most of the literature focuses on chronic dysfunction. In the younger group, disorders include symptomatic accessory navicular, tenosynovitis, longitudinal tearing, complete rupture, or avulsion with arch collapse. Several studies of sport injury series mention tendinitis of the PTT among overuse problems. In one series, acute tenosynovitis was reported in 58 (6%) of 974 runners (Cavanagh 1980). Twisting injuries can produce avulsions off the navicular or accessory navicular. Acute rupture of the PTT before the age of 30 can occur but has been reported in only a few series (Henceroth & Deyerle 1982; Kettelkamp & Alexander 1969; Marks & Schon 1998; Trevino et al. 1981; Woods & Leach 1991). It is also extremely rare to find a subluxing or dislocating PTT (Biedert 1992; Larsen & Lauridsen 1984). Thus, despite the vast literature discussing chronic dysfunction of the PTT, there are few reports that focus on injury of this tendon during inversion or eversion ankle sprains.

Anatomy

The PTT originates from the posterior tibial, medial fibula, and the interosseous membrane in the proximal deep posterior compartment of the calf. The tendinous portion forms at the distal third of the leg and is contained in a sheath under the posteromedial flexor retinaculum. The tendon courses through the tarsal tunnel along with the FDL, neurovascular bundle, and the FHL. At the tunnel's distal extent, the PTT becomes intimately associated with the posterior aspect of the medial malleolus, where it is held in a groove by the overlying flexor retinaculum. Distal to the medial malleolus, the tendon courses toward the navicular, where it divides into two slips. The anterior slip inserts onto the tuberosity of the navicular, the inferior aspect of the capsule of the medial naviculocuneiform joint, and the inferior surface of the medial cuneiform. The posterior slip attaches to the plantar surfaces of the middle and lateral cuneiforms, the cuboid, and the bases of the second through fourth metatarsals (Myerson 1996).

The vascular supply of the PTT is derived from branches of the posterior tibial artery proximally, and the distal supply is shared by the branches of the posterior tibial and dorsalis pedis arteries. Recent studies have demonstrated a 14-mm zone of relative hypovascularity approximately 40 mm proximal to the tendon insertion site on the navicular. This section of tendon is thought to be vulnerable to degeneration and tears. Another anatomic factor that is important to tendon viability is that the PTT is contained within a mesotenon in its proximal portion beneath the flexor retinaculum, but that distally, no such sheath exists. This lack of synovial lining may also contribute to a deficiency of synovial nutritional supply and may be a factor in healing. Biomechanically, the proximity of the PTT to the medial malleolar sulcus puts the tendon at this location in jeopardy during acute trauma. The bony prominence may act as a fulcrum over which the tendon is stretched. Another potential weak point is between the os navicular and navicular. This synostosis may be more vulnerable to rupture than the broad tendon bone junction that is reinforced by Sharpie's fibers.

Posterior Tibial Tendon Dysfunction

Posterior tibial tendon dysfunction may result from overuse related to tenosynovitis or may follow an acute injury.

Staging

The presentation of PTT dysfunction is varied, ranging from tenosynovitis in a normal-appearing foot to a fixed, rigid, planovalgus deformity. In 1989, Johnson and Strom described three clinical stages of PTT dysfunction, and Myerson (1996) described a fourth one.

■ **Stage I** is characterized by pain and swelling of the medial aspect of the foot and ankle. At this stage, the length of the tendon is normal, but the tendinitis may be associated with mild degeneration. Pain is more clinically significant than is mild weakness, and minimum deformity is present.

■ In **stage II**, the tendon is ruptured and the patient is unable to perform a single-stance heel rise on the affected side. Secondary deformity begins as the midfoot pronates and the forefoot supinates and abducts at the transverse tarsal joint. These deformities, as well as the subtalar joint, remain flexible.

■ In **stage III**, the deformity is more severe, and the hindfoot is rigid. Severe degeneration is present in the tendon.

■ **Stage IV** is characterized by valgus angulation of the talus and early degeneration of the ankle joint.

Diagnosis

Most patients with PTT dysfunction have an insidious onset of unilateral flatfoot deformity. Only 50% recall a history of trauma. An intact PTT requires a fairly substantial force to cause it to rupture; however, in the presence of preexisting disease, the injuring force may be trivial. When acute trauma plays a role in rupture of the PTT, patients recall a specific history of a sprain or other injury of the foot and ankle that is associated with clinical deterioration. Thus, if the injury was mild, the surgeon should search for historical evidence that the patient suffered from clinical or subclinical PTT dysfunction. A patient with an acute ankle sprain and PTT injury will usually present with swelling and pain but, unlike a standard ankle sprain, the symptoms will be greater medially than laterally. If the PTT is intact, the patient will have both tenderness along the course of the tendon and pain with resisted inversion, but the strength of the tendon should be adequate. In the case of a rupture, there will be weakness to resisted inversion of the plantarflexed foot. The surgeon should be alert for the patient who compensates for a ruptured or weakened PTT by substituting the FHL/FDL during resisted inversion testing. The PTT may be isolated during resisted inversion testing by having the patient extend the toes during inversion. Compensators will instinctively curl their toes during the test. In addition, patients with ruptured or severely degenerated PTTs will be unable to perform a single-leg heel rise. The clinician should also compare the degree of heel inversion in both feet during this test. There will be less varus on the injured side.

If the patient is seen several months to years after an acute event, then a pes planovalgus deformity may be evident. When viewed from behind, such patients demonstrate excessive heel valgus or the too-many-toes sign—an increased abduction of the forefoot when viewed from the posterior aspect of the leg while the patient is standing. The subtalar joint may be rigid, the arch may be collapsed, and the forefoot may be abducted and fixed in supination.

Weightbearing anteroposterior, lateral, and oblique radiographs of the foot should be obtained. In the acute setting, the radiographs may be normal except for soft-tissue swelling. The clinician should look for an avulsion fracture of the navicular or a displaced accessory navicular. An external oblique view of the foot can permit better visualization of an accessory navicular. In more long-standing dysfunction, the anteroposterior view can reveal subluxation of the talonavicular joint with uncovering of the talar head. Sagging of the first metatarsocuneiform, talonavicular, or naviculocuneiform joint may be evident on the lateral radiograph.

Although the single most critical tool in diagnosing a PTT injury is the physical examination, there may be cases in which the diagnosis is in doubt. In cases where the information will alter treatment, an MRI or ultrasound scan should be obtained.

Treatment

Treatment of mild acute tenosynovitis after sprain involves modification of activity, use of nonsteroidal anti-inflammatory medications, an AirCast stirrup brace, and possibly an arch support with minimal medial heel posting. If the symptoms do not resolve in 4 to 6 weeks, or if they are severe on initial presentation, immobilization in a weightbearing boot or cast for 4 to 6 weeks may be necessary. If symptoms still persist after immobilization, then tenosynovectomy is considered. The tendon should be explored from the medial malleolus to its navicular insertion. The tendon should be inspected for any longitudinal tears, which should be repaired at the time of surgery. Postoperatively, a nonweightbearing cast holding the foot in slight plantarflexion and inversion is worn for 2 to 3 weeks, followed by an AirCast brace for 6 to 12 weeks. If there appears to be a partial rupture at the navicular insertion, then the tendon is advanced through a drill hole or suture anchor. If the tendon shows degenerative changes, the repair should be augmented with an FDL transfer to the navicular. Such patients should be kept nonweightbearing for 6 weeks in mild equinovarus; then they may progressively increase weight bearing in a neutral position between 6 to 12 weeks.

The treatment for PTT longitudinal or transverse ruptures is surgical, assuming the diagnosis has been made acutely and there is no collapse of the arch. The rupture usually occurs between the medial malleolus and the navicular (figure 15.12). The rupture in the PTT is repaired with nonabsorbable sutures, and the repair should be augmented with the FDL even in the setting of an acute rupture, unless the rupture was due to penetrating trauma (Conti 1994; Teitz et al. 1997).

Patients with chronic tenosynovitis after sprain may be able to be treated with an orthosis made with a varus heel wedge and a medial forefoot post with intermittent or frequent use of a stirrup brace. When such patients have good PTT strength and mild flexible valgus deformity but symptoms persist, reconstruction with the FDL transfer is indicated. When there is a moderate, flexible valgus deformity (>5° on side-to-side comparison or a baseline valgus of >15°), a calcaneal osteotomy is indicated.

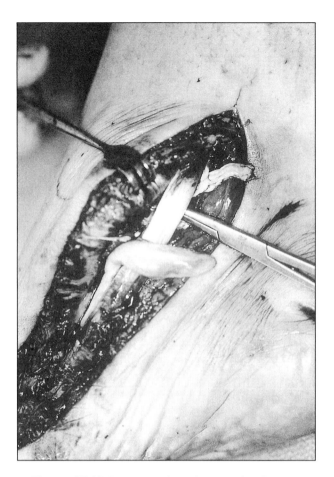

■ **Figure 15.12** Intraoperative photograph of an acute rupture of the PTT.

A patient with a chronic rupture, long-standing dysfunction, and fixed valgus deformity requires a fusion if nonoperative measures fail. A patient with a moderate or severe (15° to 20° of valgus or a >15° side-to-side difference) partially flexible valgus deformity may require either a calcaneocuboid distraction bone block arthrodesis with or without a medial column arthrodesis (depending on the degree of residual supination) or a triple arthrodesis. The rigid, severe valgus deformity with fixed forefoot supination typically requires a triple arthrodesis (Teitz et al. 1997).

■ Anterior Tibial Tendon

The ATT is considered the third most frequently ruptured tendon in the lower limb. The rupture site is usually at, or distal to, the extensor retinaculum of the ankle (Jozsa & Kannus 1997b). ATT injuries usually result from attrition in elderly individuals. Subclinical ruptures occur most frequently in men between the ages of 60 and 80 (Mankey 1996). Lacerations may result at the ankle where the tendon is immediately subcutaneous. Tendinitis of the ATT may develop after an ankle sprain, but it is rare. Typically injury results from a powerful contraction of the ATT against a hyperplantarflexion force of the ankle. Tendinitis usually follows hemorrhage, which results from microtears within the tendon sheath. Stenosing tenosynovitis is the result of repetitive dorsiflexion movement of the foot, such as occurs in running, cross-country skiing, or swimming with fins. The most common stenotic site is in the upper edge of the superior extensor retinaculum. In some cases, direct irritation from the anterior edge of a shoe or boot may cause inflammation (Jozsa & Kannus 1997a). The senior author (LCS) has treated one case of a chronic incomplete rupture secondary to a sprain in an athlete, compared with 10 cases of subclinical ruptures, all occurring in the middle-aged and elderly. Ouzounian and Anderson (1995) reported a complete rupture in a 65-year-old man that resulted from an ankle-twisting injury.

Anatomy

The ATT is the most medial of the four main extensors of the foot and ankle. It originates from the lateral aspect of the proximal tibia and intermuscular septum in the anterior compartment of the leg. It passes under the superior and inferior extensor retinaculi in a tight, fibro-osseous canal. A synovial lining is present where the tendon traverses under the inferior extensor retinaculum. It inserts into the medial and plantar aspects of the medial cuneiform bone and into the adjacent base of the first metatarsal. The tibialis anterior muscle is the largest dorsiflexor of the foot; it also adducts and inverts (supinates) the foot.

Anterior Tibial Tendon Pathology

Anterior tibial tendon pathology may occur as an overuse injury in work or sport or as a degenerative process in older patients.

Diagnosis

Patients with pathology to the ATT may be unable to recall a specific mechanism of injury or any trauma at all, as is often the case in an attritional rupture in the elderly. In the older population, the presentation is usually slowly progressive, with a foot drop as well as swelling and pain in the anterior ankle. Because there are no symptoms until the foot drop is complete, diagnosis is often delayed. Patients with stenosing tenosynovitis complain of pain and swelling, but their strength is good. Peritendinitis can present with a painful rubbing or cracking sensation overlying the anterior ankle. This "peritendinitis crepitans" occurs most frequently in young men as an overuse injury of sport and work, but we have noted this finding in

dancers and military recruits as well. Occasionally it will occur after an ankle sprain. The sensation of crepitus is caused by fibrin exudates within the ATT sheath (Jozsa & Kannus 1997a). The crepitus can be easily palpated when the patient actively flexes the ankle.

Treatment

Treatment is the same as for an ankle sprain. In addition, an ankle-foot orthosis or posterior splint is recommended in the acute setting. With an intact tendon, acute inflammatory conditions should be treated with a dorsiflexion splint for 2 weeks or until the acute symptoms have subsided. Night splinting can be effective because it avoids the resting equinus position that stretches the tendon. Physical therapy can begin, initially emphasizing range of motion and strengthening. Full eversion against resistance and 20° of plantarflexion against resistance may be performed, but dorsiflexion against resistance should be avoided. Walking and Achilles stretching is also encouraged for 3 months after the pain has subsided. Lidocaine/bupivacaine injection into the tendon sheath to distend the sheath and relieve the adhesions may be helpful for athletes with chronic tendinitis.

Complete ruptures should be operatively repaired. One must be mindful of establishing the proper length during the repair. Postoperatively, weight bearing can begin immediately in an ankle/foot orthosis or boot brace. Achilles stretching is important, and a night splint should be used for the first 3 months to avoid inadvertently stretching the repair at night. If the rupture is chronic, it is recommended that it be repaired with augmentation using the extensor hallucis longus. A night splint that holds the ankle in slight dorsiflexion for 6 months postoperatively may be necessary.

■ Achilles Tendon

Direct Achilles tendon injuries secondary to ankle sprains are rare. Achilles tendon problems may rarely occur directly or indirectly secondary to ankle sprains. Occurrence is rare because the mechanism of injury for Achilles tendon ruptures is an eccentric load applied to the triceps surae with the ankle forcibly dorsiflexed (Cetti 1997). In this position, the talus is stabilized in the ankle mortise, preventing an inversion or eversion event necessary for a sprain to occur. In fact, there are no known reports in the literature of a rupture secondary to an ankle sprain. Achilles tendinitis or tendinosis typically occurs from repetitive ankle motion, but can occur indirectly as a result of an acute ankle sprain. If there is no physical therapy instituted after an ankle sprain, and the patient uses nonweightbearing crutches while holding the ankle in equinus, then Achilles contraction may result. Nonoperative treatment—that is, weightbearing stretches and physical therapy—is recommended. If a peritendinitis or tendinitis of the Achilles results, then surgery to release the peritenon and debridement of any tendinosis is considered.

Anatomy

The Achilles tendon is the strongest and thickest tendon in the body, averaging approximately 15 cm in length. It is formed by the confluence of the gastrocnemius and soleus muscles, also known as the triceps surae, in the middle third of the lower leg in the superficial posterior compartment. The gastrocnemius is the more superficial of the two muscles and originates from the popliteal fossa and the posterior knee joint capsule. Its two muscular heads pass distal to the knee joint and unite in a tendinous raphe that subsequently becomes an aponeurosis. This aponeurosis joins with that of the soleus. The soleus lies anterior to the gastrocnemius and originates from the proximal posterior surfaces of the tibia, fibula, and interosseous membrane. Its muscle fibers converge into a separate aponeurosis that joins with the gastrocnemius aponeurosis to form the Achilles tendon. The fibers of the Achilles tendon rotate externally approximately 90° before inserting on the posterior tuberosity of the calcaneus. This results in the soleus fibers primarily inserting medially and the gastrocnemius fibers inserting laterally. This insertion is roughly 1.5 cm distal to the superior calcaneal tuberosity. Occasionally, the plantaris tendon may insert primarily into the Achilles tendon itself (Perry 1997). Together, the gastrocnemius and soleus are the primary plantarflexors of the ankle. During running activities, the Achilles tendon is subject to tensile loads of up to eight times body weight (Soma & Mandelbaum 1994).

The Achilles tendon is enclosed by a paratenon that is not lined with synovial tissue. The paratenon allows for approximately 1.5 cm of tendon glide. The least vascular area of the Achilles tendon is approximately 4 cm proximal to its calcaneal insertion. As a result, the area of the Achilles tendon most prone to injury lies 2 to 6 cm proximal to the calcaneal insertion, where the tendon's blood supply is poorest.

Achilles Tendon Rupture

Even though an ankle sprain is an unlikely mechanism for a rupture, one should be aware of it as a remote possibility in the examination of an acute ankle injury.

Diagnosis

Patients with an acute rupture during a sporting event will present with a typical history of feeling as if they were struck or shot in the back of the ankle or calf. They present with pain and inability to push off forcefully. On physical examination, a defect can often be seen and palpated. There is an inability to perform a heel rise on the affected limb. A positive Thompson's test will reveal the lack of ankle plantarflexion when the calf musculature is squeezed (Cetti 1997).

As mentioned earlier, the patient with Achilles tendinitis is also unlikely to present with a recent or remote history of an ankle sprain. A recent change in activity, training technique, athletic surface, or shoe gear usually precedes the onset of pain. On examination, the patient will be tender to palpation along the distal 5 cm of the tendon, and swelling in this area may be seen acutely. Typically, no weakness is seen. As the symptoms become more chronic, pain can become more generalized. The tendon can become thickened and nodular. If the thickening is in the paratenon, the mass will not move with ankle motion. However, nodules in the tendon itself will move with ankle motion and can result in palpable crepitus (Clancy & Heiden 1997).

Treatment

Athletic patients with acute ruptures who are even moderately active should undergo operative repair. We perform an open repair with a whip stitch. Postoperatively, after 7 to 10 days, we allow full weight bearing in a brace in equinus. The patient is instructed to walk with the injured leg in front, the foot plantarflexed, and the knee and hip flexed (like a fencer's front leg). Range-of-motion exercises are begun at 2 weeks. The patient is full weight bearing in neutral by 6 weeks but remains in a brace until 12 weeks.

Patients who present acutely with Achilles tendinitis should be splinted in a neutral position at the ankle. Gentle, active, assistive range-of-motion exercises should be instituted early. Once the acute symptoms have subsided (in approximately 2 to 6 weeks), aggressive rehabilitation and conditioning are begun. A pneumatic Achilles wrap may provide symptomatic relief and edema reduction in the acute, subacute, or chronic phases (figure 15.13). Adjusting the amount of air in the system will alter the magnitude of compressive force; this adjustment must be individualized.

In patients with chronic tenovaginitis, injecting the sheath with lidocaine/bupivacaine to distend the tendon sheath may release adhesions and reduce

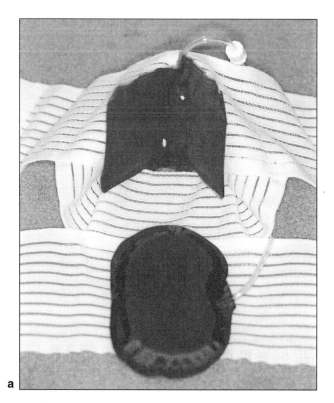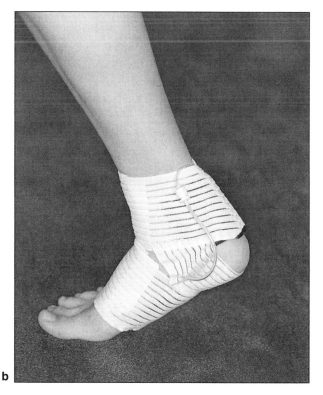

■ Figure 15.13 AirCast wrap for Achilles tendinitis. *(a)* Internal view shows air bladder underneath the arch connected to bladders that intermittently compress the Achilles tendon. *(b)* Wrap in place.

symptoms. Patients who have a tendinosis or who have nodules should be placed in a boot brace for 6 weeks. However, if no relief is obtained, local debridement of the tendon with stripping of the paratenon is recommended.

■ Conclusion

Tendon injuries may occur in association with ankle sprains. Inversion or eversion forces are more likely to affect the peroneals and the PTT then the ATT or the Achilles tendon. Achilles tendon pathology may be seen when it is secondary to improper rehabilitation after sprain. Overall, treatment of these associated tendon injuries is largely nonoperative unless a tendon has ruptured or there is subluxation dislocation of the peroneal tendons. However, operative intervention is required for the athletic population.

■ References

Alm A, Lamke LO, Liljedahl SO: Surgical treatment of dislocation of the peroneal tendons. Injury 7:14-19, 1975.

Beck E: Operative treatment of recurrent dislocation of the peroneal tendons. Arch Orthop Trauma Surg 98:247-250, 1981.

Bell W, Schon LC: Tendon lacerations in the toes and foot. Foot Ankle Clin 1:355-372, 1996.

Biedert R: Dislocation of the tibialis posterior tendon. Am J Sports Med 20:775-776, 1992.

Cavanagh PR: The Running Shoe Book, p 270. Mountain View, CA: Anderson World, 1980.

Cetti R: Rupture of the Achilles tendon. Operative vs. nonoperative options. Foot Ankle Clin 2:501-519, 1997.

Clancy WG Jr. Tendon trauma and overuse injuries. In Ledbetter WB, Buckwalter JA, Gordon SL (eds): Clinical and Basic Science Concepts, pp 609-617. Park Ridge, IL: American Academy of Orthopaedic Surgeons, 1990.

Clancy WG, Heiden EA: Achilles tendonitis treatment in the athlete. Foot Ankle Clin 2:429-438, 1997.

Clanton TO, Schon LC: Athletic injuries to the soft tissues of the foot and ankle. In Mann RA, Coughlin MJ (eds): Surgery of the Foot and Ankle, 6th ed, pp 1095-1224. St. Louis, MO: Mosby-Year Book Inc, 1993.

Conti SF: Posterior tibial tendon problems in athletes. Orthop Clin North Am 25:109-121, 1994.

Davies JAK: Peroneal compartment syndrome secondary to rupture of the peroneus longus. A case report. J Bone Joint Surg 61A:783-784, 1979.

Earle AS, Moritz JR, Tapper EM: Dislocation of the peroneal tendons at the ankle: an analysis of 25 ski injuries. Northwest Med 71:108-110, 1972.

Eckert WR, Davis EA, Jr. Acute rupture of the peroneal retinaculum. J Bone Joint Surg 58A:670-672, 1976.

Edwards ME: The relations of the peroneal tendons to the fibula, calcaneus, and cuboideum. Am J Anat 42:213-253, 1928.

Escalas F, Figueras JM, Merino JA: Dislocation of the peroneal tendons. Long-term results of surgical treatment. J Bone Joint Surg 62A:451-453, 1980.

Frey CC, Shereff MJ: Tendon injuries about the ankle in athletes. Clin Sports Med 7:103-118, 1988.

Henceroth WD, II, Deyerle WM: The acquired unilateral flatfoot in the adult: some causative factors. Foot Ankle 2:304-308, 1982.

Huber H, Imhoff A: [Habitual peroneal tendon dislocation]. Z Orthop 126:609-612, 1988.

Johnson KA, Strom DE: Tibialis posterior tendon dysfunction. Clin Orthop 239:196-206, 1989.

Jozsa LG, Kannus P: Overuse injuries of tendons. In Human Tendons. Anatomy, Physiology, and Pathology, pp 164-253. Champaign, IL: Human Kinetics, 1997a.

Jozsa LG, Kannus P: Spontaneous rupture of tendons. In Human Tendons. Anatomy, Physiology, and Pathology, pp 254-325. Champaign, IL: Human Kinetics, 1997b.

Kettelkamp DB, Alexander HH: Spontaneous rupture of the posterior tibial tendon. J Bone Joint Surg 51A:759-764, 1969.

Kojima Y, Kataoka Y, Suzuki S, Akagi M: Dislocation of the peroneal tendons in neonates and infants. Clin Orthop 266:180-184, 1991.

Larsen E, Lauridsen F: Dislocation of the tibialis posterior tendon in two athletes. Am J Sports Med 12:429-430, 1984.

Mankey MG: Anterior tibial tendon ruptures. Foot Ankle Clin 1:315-324, 1996.

Marks RM, Schon LC: Posttraumatic posterior tibialis tendon insertional elongation with functional incompetency: a case report. Foot Ankle Int 19:180-183, 1998.

Martens MA, Noyez JF, Mulier JC: Recurrent dislocation of the peroneal tendons. Results of rerouting the tendons under the calcaneofibular ligament. Am J Sports Med 14:148-150, 1986.

McGarvey WC, Clanton TO: Peroneal tendon dislocations. Foot Ankle Clin 1:325-342, 1996.

McLennan JG: Treatment of acute and chronic luxations of the peroneal tendons. Am J Sports Med 8:432-436, 1980.

Micheli LJ, Waters PM, Sanders DP: Sliding fibular graft repair for chronic dislocation of the peroneal tendons. Am J Sports Med 17:68-71, 1989.

Mizel MS, Michelson JD, Wapner KL: Diagnosis and treatment of peroneus brevis injury. Foot Ankle Clin 1:343-354, 1996.

Myerson MS: Adult acquired flatfoot deformity. Treatment of dysfunction of the posterior tibial tendon. J Bone Joint Surg 78A:780-792, 1996.

Oden RR: Tendon injuries about the ankle resulting from skiing. Clin Orthop 216:63-69, 1987.

Ouzounian TJ, Anderson R: Anterior tibial tendon rupture. Foot Ankle Int 16:406-410, 1995.

Perry JR: Achilles tendon anatomy. Normal and pathologic. Foot Ankle Clin 2:363-370, 1997.

Plattner P, Mann R: Disorders of tendons. In Mann RA, Coughlin MJ (eds): Surgery of the Foot and Ankle, 6th ed, pp 805-835. St. Louis, MO: Mosby-Year Book, Inc, 1993.

Puddu G, Ippolito E, Postacchini F: A classification of Achilles tendon disease. Am J Sports Med 4:145-150, 1976.

Schon LC, Bell W: Fusions of the transverse tarsal and midtarsal joints. Foot Ankle Clin 1:93-108, 1996.

Slatis P, Santavirta S, Sandelin J: Surgical treatment of chronic dislocation of the peroneal tendons. Br J Sports Med 22:16-18, 1988.

Sobel M, Bohne WH, Levy ME: Longitudinal attrition of the peroneus brevis tendon in the fibular groove: an anatomic study [see comments]. Foot Ankle 11:124-128, 1990.

Sobel M, Bohne WH, Markisz JA: Cadaver correlation of peroneal tendon changes with magnetic resonance imaging. Foot Ankle 11:384-388, 1991.

Soma CA, Mandelbaum BR: Achilles tendon disorders. Clin Sports Med 13:811-823, 1994.

Stein RE: Reconstruction of the superior peroneal retinaculum using a portion of the peroneus brevis tendon. A case report. J Bone Joint Surg 69A:298-299, 1987.

Stover CN, Bryan DR: Traumatic dislocation of the peroneal tendons. Am J Surg 103:180-186, 1962.

Teitz CC, Garrett WE, Jr., Miniaci A, Lee MH, Mann RA: Tendon problems in athletic individuals. Instr Course Lect 46:569-82:569-582, 1997.

Trevino S, Gould N, Korson R: Surgical treatment of stenosing tenosynovitis at the ankle. Foot Ankle 2:37-45, 1981.

Woo SL-Y, An K-N, Arnoczky SP, Wayne JS, Fithian DC, Myers BS: Anatomy, biology, and biomechanics of tendon, ligament and meniscus. In Simon SR (ed): Orthopaedic Basic Science, pp 45-87. Rosemont, IL: American Academy of Orthopaedic Surgeons, 1994.

Woods L, Leach RE: Posterior tibial tendon rupture in athletic people. Am J Sports Med 19:495-498, 1991.

Zeiss J, Saddemi SR, Ebraheim NA: MR imaging of the peroneal tunnel. J Comput Assist Tomogr 13:840-844, 1989.

Chapter 16

Posterior Ankle Impingement

C. Niek van Dijk, MD, PhD; A.B. Stibbe, MD; and R.K. Marti, MD, PhD

Posterior ankle pain can be derived from intra- or extra-articular pathology. The most important mechanical cause of articular posterior ankle pain is the posterior impingement syndrome. Posterior ankle impingement is a pain syndrome. It is characterized by pain in the posterior aspect of the ankle joint. This pain is predominantly present on (forced) plantarflexion. The syndrome can result from acute or chronic injury. The presence of an anatomic anomaly such as an os trigonum possibly facilitates the occurrence of this pain syndrome. Overuse injuries associated with posterior impingement syndrome often occur in ballet or running, while acute injuries causing the syndrome are more commonly reported to occur in contact sports such as soccer. In plantarflexion, the posterior distal edge of the tibia and superior border of the calcaneus are only separated by the capsule of the posterior ankle joint. In the presence of a prominent posterior part of the talus, this joint capsule can become compressed between these bony structures. Especially in the presence of an os trigonum, this "nutcracker phenomenon" can lead to inflammation of the involved structures (Hedrick & McBryde 1994).

■ Anatomy

The talus has no muscular insertions. Any movement of the talus in regard to the tibia is realized by passive transmission of motion by means of the ligamentous guiding system (van Dijk 1994). Active motion is realized by the long foot muscles, which insert onto the midtarsal and metatarsal bones. The posterior joint capsule envelops the posterior joint space. It is attached to the posterior surface of the tibia and to the talus at the border between bone and cartilage. The outer fibrous layer of the capsule is continuous with the fibrous layer of the periosteum. The posterior capsule is lax in plantarflexion, and tight in dorsiflexion. The posterior talofibular ligament (PTFL) passes almost horizontally from a groove at the inside of the

posterior margin of the lateral malleolus to the posterior prominence of the talus (figure 16.1). Frequently, a separate bundle of fibers originates from the same groove on the inside of the posterior part of the lateral malleolus and runs below the posterior tibiofibular ligament to the posterior surface of the tibia (Ludolph & Hierholzer 1986). Both structures are incorporated in the joint capsule. In plantarflexion and neutral position, the ligament is relaxed, while in dorsiflexion the ligament is tensed. The posterior tibiofibular ligament is a flat fibrous band, with the distal fibers being the longest. The fibers originate from the posterior tubercle of the tibia and run at an approximate angle of 45° distally and laterally, where they attach to the posterior aspect of the fibula. Sometimes the ligament consists of a double structure. The proximal

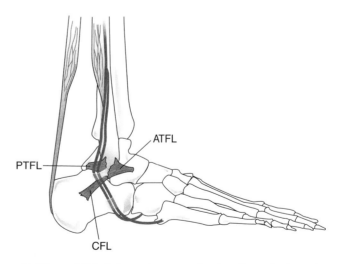

■ **Figure 16.1** Schematic anatomic view from the lateral side. The three lateral ligaments—the anterior talofibular ligament (ATFL), calcaneofibular ligament (CFL), and the posterior tibiofibular ligament (PTFL)—can be seen. The PTFL attaches to the posterior prominence of the talus. This posterior prominence can be palpated between the Achilles tendon and peroneal tendons. In this plantigrade position, the posterior prominence of the talus is located just cranially from the distal tip of the lateral malleolus.

part crosses directly from the tibia to the posterior part of the fibula, whereas the distal section is part of the joint capsule and runs to a groove on the inner side of the posterior margin of the lateral malleolus. It can be recognized as a ligament structure when observing the posterior joint capsule from the inside of the joint as is done in arthroscopy (van Dijk et al. 1990).

The most prominent posterior part of the talus is located posterolaterally. Apart from the posterior joint capsule, the posterior talofibular ligament attaches to this posterior talar process. Medial from this prominent bony process is the flexor hallucis longus. The flexor hallucis longus tendon thus separates the posterior talar process from the medial talar tubercle. The posterior talar process forms the roof of the posterior facet of the subtalar joint. Embryologically, the body of the talus and posterior talar process are separate ossification centers. The posterior talar process appears as a separate ossicle, which is called "os trigonum," between the 8th and 10th years of life. The body of the talus is usually visible on radiographs around 7 months. The os trigonum may be considered as a secondary ossification center, similar to the calcaneal apophysis. The os trigonum usually fuses with the talus within a year of its appearance. In about 7% of the normal adult population, however, it is still present as an accessory bone (Salyers & Fu 1989). It can be present bilaterally or unilaterally.

■ Etiology

Posterior ankle impingement can be caused by overuse or trauma. It is important to distinguish between these two, because posterior impingement resulting from overuse has a better prognosis (Stibbe et al. 1994).

Overuse

A posterior ankle impingement syndrome resulting from overuse is mainly found in ballet dancers and runners (van Dijk et al. 1990; Hamilton et al. 1996; Hedrick & McBryde 1994). Running that involves forced plantarflexion, such as downhill running, can put repetitive stress on the posterior aspect of the ankle joint (Hedrick & McBryde 1994). The forceful plantarflexion that occurs during the "en pointe" position or the "demi-pointe" position produces compression at the posterior aspect of the ankle joint. Either of these situations can put extreme pressure on the anatomical structures that are normally present between the calcaneus and the posterior part of the distal tibia (figure 16.2). Through exercise, the joint mobility and range of motion in the joint gradually increase, gradually reducing the distance between the calcaneus and the posterior part of the distal tibia still further. Thus, if abnormal structures, such as an os trigonum, hypertrophic posterior talar process, a thick-

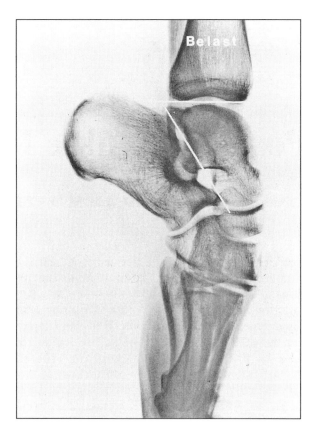

■ **Figure 16.2** The forceful plantarflexion during the "demi-pointe" position produces compression at the posterior aspect of the ankle joint. Through exercise, the joint mobility and range of motion in ballet dancers gradually increase. In the presence of a prominent posterior talar process, this can lead to compression of the posterior located structures.

ened posterior joint capsule, post-traumatic scar tissue, post-traumatic calcifications of the posterior joint capsule, a loose body in the posterior part of the ankle joint, or an osteophyte of the posterior distal tibia, are present in this region, they may be compressed.

The presence of a prominent posterior talar process or os trigonum in itself, however, is not sufficient to produce the syndrome (figure 16.3). In 1995 we reported on a group of 19 retired dancers and examined their ankle and subtalar joints (van Dijk et al. 1995). The mean length of the ballet dancers' professional careers was 37 years. All of the dancers had been dancing "on pointe." The mean dance time per week was 45 hours. The mean age of the dancers was 59 years (range 50 to 66). None of the ballet dancers had been free from injuries, but no macrotrauma had occurred. None of the dancers had experienced a posterior ankle impingement syndrome. In 18 of the 38 investigated ankle joints, a hypertrophic posterior talar process or an os trigonum was present. In most cases, the os trigonum was relatively large (van Dijk et al. 1995). The presence of an os trigonum or prominent talar process in itself, therefore, does not seem to be relevant. This anatomic anomaly must be combined with a traumatic event such as supination trauma, dancing on hard surfaces, or pushing beyond anatomic limits. The pain is caused by an abnormal movement between os trigonum and talus, compression of thickened joint capsules or scar tissue between the os trigonum and tibia, or compression between os trigonum and calcaneus (known as "dancers' heel").

Trauma

Forced plantarflexion causes compression of the posterior talar prominence between tibia and calcaneus.

In the presence of an os trigonum, this can lead to a displacement of the os trigonum (figure 16.4). In the case of a prominent posterior talar process, a fracture can occur. Compression of the posterior joint capsule can lead to calcification. Combined supination and plantarflexion (leading to a lateral ankle ligament lesion) also leads to compression of posteromedial joint structures in some patients. The post-traumatic calcifications in these cases most often are located posteromedially (figure 16.5). Hyperplantarflexion can result from an automobile or motorcycle accident, but can also result from sporting activities such as soccer.

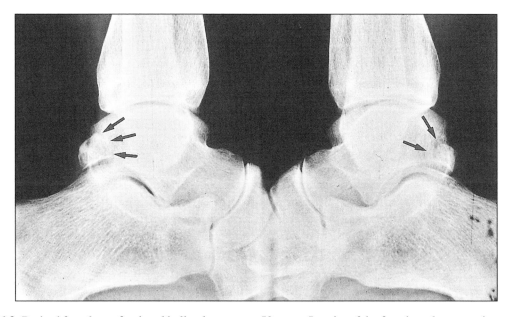

■ **Figure 16.3** Retired female professional ballet dancer, age 58 years. In spite of the fact that a large os trigonum is present in both ankles, she never developed a posterior impingement syndrome.

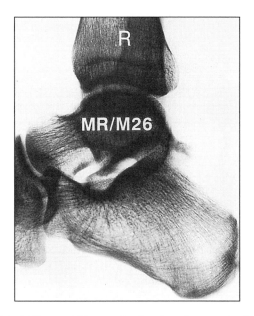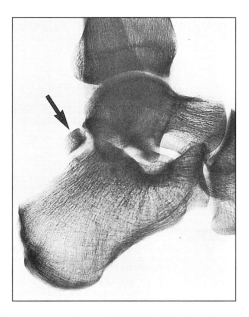

■ **Figure 16.4** A 27-year-old man who developed a posterior impingement syndrome of the left ankle after a hyperplantarflexion trauma 2 years before. After resection of the displaced os trigonum through a posterolateral approach, the patient became symptom-free.

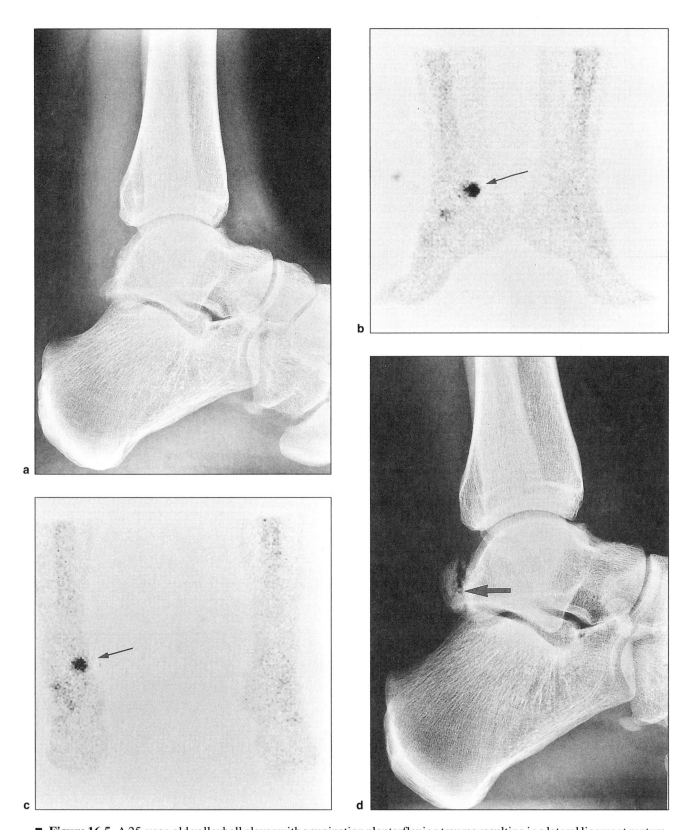

■ **Figure 16.5** A 25-year-old volleyball player with a supination plantarflexion trauma resulting in a lateral ligament rupture. After functional tape treatment, the patient developed a posterior impingement syndrome with painful, restricted plantarflexion. *(a)* The radiograph three months after trauma, apart from a small calcification, does not show an abnormality. Because of persisting symptoms 1 year postoperative, *(b and c)* a bone scan was made. *(c)* This bone scan shows a posteromedial hot spot. *(d)* A new radiograph was made, which showed posterior calcifications. Through a posteromedial approach, the calcifications were removed.

■ Diagnosis

A diagnosis or differential diagnosis can be made on the basis of the patient's history, physical examination, and radiographs.

History

Posterior ankle impingement syndrome is a pain syndrome. The patient experiences pain on the posterior aspect of the ankle joint. This pain is mainly present on forced plantarflexion. In some patients, forced dorsiflexion is also painful. In this dorsiflexed position, traction is applied to the posterior joint capsule and posterior talofibular ligament, which both attach to the posterior talar process.

Physical Examination

On examination, there is pain on palpation of the posterior aspect of the talus. This posterior talar process can best be palpated posterolaterally in between the peroneal tendons and the Achilles tendon (figure 16.1). Posteromedially, the neurovascular bundle and flexotendons are covering the talus (figure 16.6). Posteromedial pain on palpation therefore does not automatically mean impingement pain. The passive forced plantarflexion test is the most important test (figure 16.7). The test should be performed with repetitive quick and passive hyperplantarflexion move-ments in a neutral position. The test can be repeated in slight exorotation or slight endorotation of the foot relative to the tibia. The investigator can apply this rotation movement on the point of maximal plantarflexion, thereby "grinding" the posterior talar process/os trigonum between tibia and calcaneus. A negative test rules out a posterior impingement syndrome. A positive test in combination with pain on posterolateral palpation should be followed by a diagnostic infiltration. The infiltration is performed from the posterolateral side, so that the capsule between prominent posterior talar process and posterior edge of the tibia is infiltrated with Xylocaine. If the pain on forced plantarflexion disappears, the diagnosis is confirmed.

Radiograph

The anteroposterior (AP) ankle view typically does not show abnormalities. On the lateral view, often a prominent posterior talar process or os trigonum can be recognized. In post-traumatic cases, we look for signs of nonunion in this region. The posterior talar process or os trigonum is located posterolaterally. On the lateral view this posterolateral part is often superpositioned onto the medial talar tubercle (figure 16.8, a-c). Detection of a nonunion on a standard lateral view, therefore, is often difficult. Calcifications, for the same reason, sometimes cannot be detected by this standard lateral view. In post-traumatic

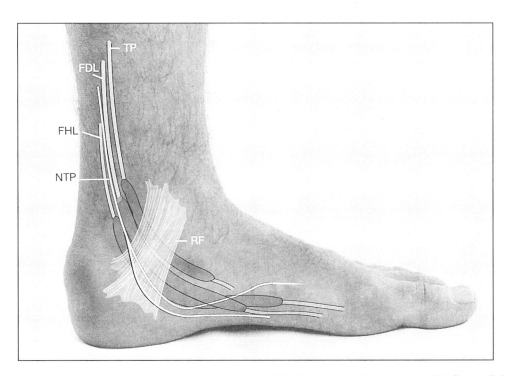

■ **Figure 16.6** Posteromedial structures: neurovascular bundle (NVB), posterior tibial tendon (TP), flexor digitorum longus tendon (FDL), and flexor hallucis longus tendon (FHL) are covering the talus. Together with the retinaculum (RF), it is not possible to exclusively palpate the posterior aspect of the talus from the medial side.

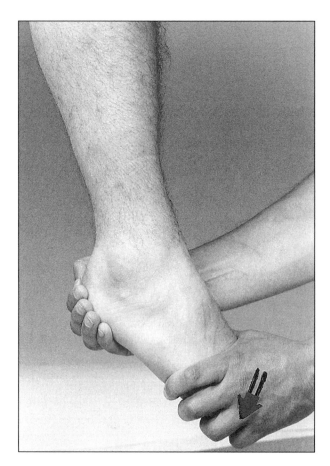

■ **Figure 16.7** The passive forced plantarflexion test. The test should be performed with repetitive quick and passive short hyperplantarflexion movements. In relation to the lower leg, the foot can be in relative endorotation, neutral position, or slight exorotation. At the point of maximal plantarflexion the investigator can apply a rotation movement, thereby "grinding" the posterior talar process/os trigonum between tibia and calcaneus.

cases, therefore, a bone scan must be performed if the radiograph does not show abnormalities (figure 16.9, a-d). A positive bone scan can be followed by CT scan. Especially in post-traumatic cases, a CT scan is important in order to determine the extent of injury and the exact location of calcification or fragments.

Differential Diagnosis

In the differential diagnosis, the following diagnoses must be considered:

1. Tendinitis flexor hallucis longus
2. Tarsal tunnel syndrome
3. Subtalar pathology

Conditions such as posterior tibial tendinitis, chronic synovitis of the ankle joint, posterior osteochondral effect, or osteoid osteoma usually have a different clinical presentation (van Dijk et al. 1990; van Dijk

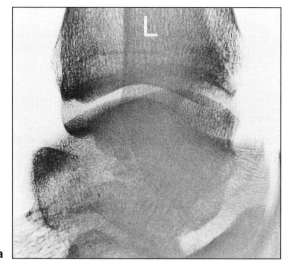

a

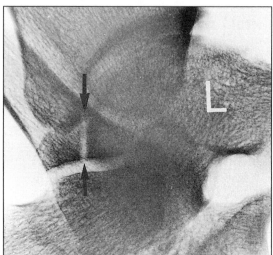

b

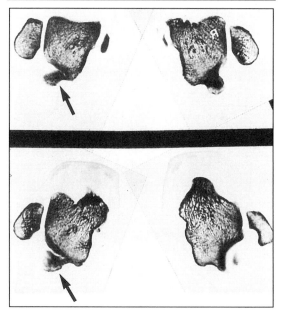

c

■ **Figure 16.8** A 24-year-old professional soccer player with persisting complaints 6 months after hyperplantarflexion trauma. (a) On the lateral radiograph, no pathology was recognized. (b) The 45° angle view however, shows a pseudarthrotic posterior talar process. (c) On the CT scan we see a big pseudarthrotic posterolateral fragment.

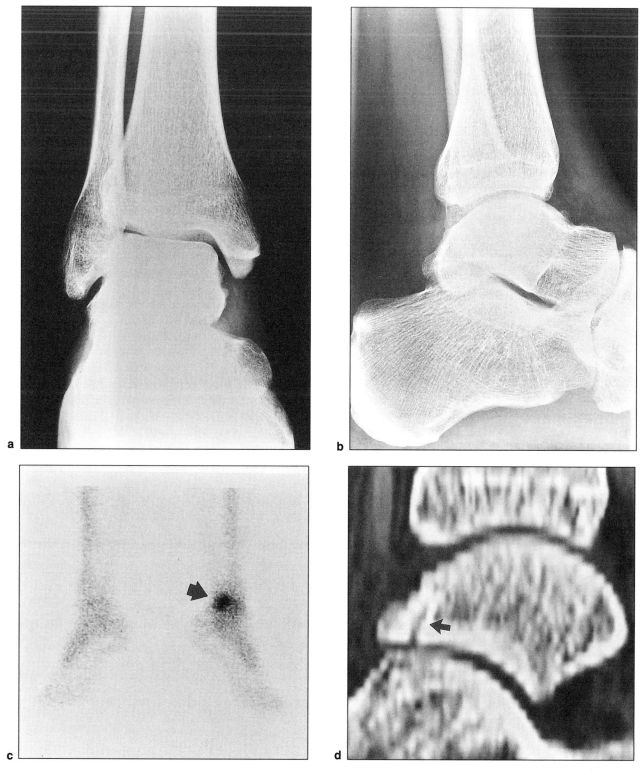

■ **Figure 16.9** *(a)* AP and *(b)* lateral view of a 28-year-old man who developed a posterior ankle impingement syndrome after a hyperplantarflexion trauma. *(b)* The radiographs do not show any abnormality. *(c)* The technetium scan shows a hot spot in the posterior aspect of the ankle joint. *(d)* The CT scan shows a slightly displaced pseudarthrotic posterior located fragment.

& Scholte 1997). A loose body in the posterior ankle joint can mimic a posterior ankle impingement. Flexor hallucis longus tendinitis in ballet dancers is most important in the differential diagnosis. The pain is located posteromedially. It is present in plié,

and especially in grand plié. The flexor hallucis longus tendon can be palpated behind the medial malleolus. By asking the patient to repetitively flex the toes with the ankle in 10-20° of plantarflexion, the flexor hallucis longus tendon can be palpated in its gliding channel behind the medial malleolus. The tendon glides up and down under the palpating finger of the examiner. In case of stenosing tendinitis or chronic inflammation, we feel for crepitus and pain, while sometimes a nodule in the tendon can be felt to move up and down under the palpating finger. Subtalar pathology of the posteromedial compartment is called "dancers' heel" (Marti & Besselaar 1983). The movement in the subtalar joint is a "gliding" and rotating movement. Even though there is little movement of the subtalar joint surfaces in relation to each other, a statistically significant increase in degenerative subtalar joint disease in retired professional female ballet dancers compared with a matched paired control group was found (van Dijk et al. 1995). The "dancers' heel" can be subdivided into three stages.

- Stage 1: Chondropathy without radiographic changes
- Stage 2: Subchondral changes, sometimes fragmentation
- Stage 3: Arthrosis (Marti & Besselaar 1983).

Because of the close relationship between the structures located in the tarsal tunnel and the posteromedial aspect of the subtalar joint, the dancers' heel can give rise to secondary tendon pathology.

■ Therapy

Nonoperative treatment involves modification of activities, physical therapy (massage, stretching, and muscle strengthening), icing, use of nonsteroidal anti-inflammatory medication, and injection of steroids. The steroids are injected posterolaterally into the posterior joint capsule between the prominent posterior tibial talar process and the posterior tibial edge. Physicians who are not familiar with this type of lesion are advised to perform the infiltration under fluoroscopic control. Analysis and correction of the patient's dance technique involves correction of sickling. Sickling in valgus is the result of hypertonic peroneal tendons and relative weakness of the posterior tibial tendon. Sickling in varus can be the result of a weakness of the peroneal tendons. Operative treatment involves the removal of a hypertrophic posterior joint capsule, an os trigonum, a hypertrophic posterior talar process, a pseudarthrotic fragment, or calcifications (figure 16.10, a and b).

In case of an isolated posterior impingement syndrome, a direct posterolateral approach is advised. The patient is placed in the lateral decubitus position or in the prone position. The posterior joint capsule is approached in between peroneal tendons and sural nerve. The capsulotomy is made with the ankle in a slight plantarflexed position. After

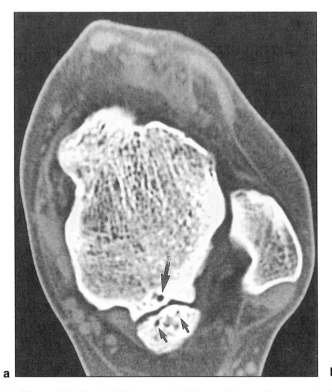
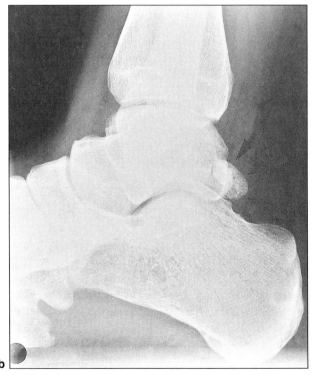

■ **Figure 16.10** *(a)* CT scan and *(b)* lateral view of a posterior impingement syndrome. A big os trigonum is present, which shows subchondral cysts in the "joint" between os trigonum and talus.

capsulotomy, the ankle is brought in dorsiflexion. Only in this position can the posterolateral aspect of the talus be seen and palpated. The os trigonum, or prominent posterior talar process, is located between the peroneal tendons and the flexor hallucis longus tendon. After removal of the prominence, by chisel or small bone elevator, the rest of the posterior aspect of the talus should be palpated with the ankle in a slight plantarflexed position to detect any remaining fragments or sharp edges.

Post-traumatic calcifications most often are located posteromedially. A posteromedial approach thus should be used. The neurovascular bundle, together with the tendons, is retracted posteriorly. The posterior part of the deltoid ligament and posterior capsule then can be excised. Subtalar joint pathology, in combination with secondary tendinopathy, needs the same approach. The tendon sheaths are opened and debridement of the subtalar joint is performed.

In case of combined posterior impingement and flexor hallucis longus tenosynovitis, a more posterior posteromedial incision can be used. The tendon sheath of the flexor hallucis longus is opened and the flexor retinaculum is divided. Lateral from the flexor hallucis longus, the posterolateral capsule of the ankle joint—with the ankle in slight plantarflexion—can be identified and excised. The os trigonum, or prominent talar process, then can be taken away.

Postoperatively, we apply a plaster cast for 5 days to prevent equinus deformation. After removal of the cast, functional treatment is started. Active range of motion is then stimulated. The patient is cautioned to expect up to 6 months until full recovery.

A new approach has been developed by means of minimal invasive surgery. The endoscopic approach offers an obvious advantage. Arthroscopic evaluation of posterior ankle problems by means of routine ankle arthroscopy using an anteromedial, anterolateral, and posterolateral portal is difficult because of the shape of the ankle joint. Pericapsular and extracapsular ankle pathology, such as a posterior ankle impingement syndrome, cannot be treated by means of routine ankle arthroscopy. We developed a two-portal endoscopic hindfoot approach, with the patient in the prone position, which offers excellent access to the posterior ankle compartment (van Dijk et al. 2000). When performing routine ankle arthroscopy, most surgeons feel that the posteromedial portal is contraindicated because of the potential vascular complications. The posterolateral portal is advocated as a routine portal by most authors. With the arthroscope shaft in place through the posterolateral portal, the trick is to angle the instruments (mosquito clamp, shaver) introduced through the posteromedial portal at 90° to the arthroscope shaft. The arthroscope shaft subsequently is used as a guide for the instruments to travel into the direction of the joint (van Dijk et al. 2000). The introduced instrument must be felt to touch the arthroscope shaft the whole way. In this manner, the neurovascular bundle is passed without a problem. Since 1995, we have performed over 100 consecutive endoscopic hindfoot procedures. Apart from one patient with a numbness of part of the heel skin, there were no complications. Removal of symptomatic os trigonum, or a nonunion of a fracture of the posterior talar process, involves partial detachment of the posterior talar ligament and release of the flexor retinaculum, both of which attached to the posterior talofibular prominence. Subsequently, by use of a 4-mm chisel, osteotome, or small rasp, the pathologic bone fragment can be removed. Release of the flexor hallucis longus involves endoscopic detachment of the flexor retinaculum from the posterior talar process. Adhesions surrounding the flexor tendon can be removed. The procedure is performed in an outpatient setting, with functional follow-up treatment.

■ Methods and Results

From 1976 till 1991, we analyzed the results of 27 surgical interventions for a posterior ankle impingement syndrome. All patients failed a period of conservative treatment for at least 6 months. The average follow-up is 4 years (between 1 year and 16 years). In 13 patients, the posterior impingement syndrome was caused by overuse, while 14 patients experienced trauma. Fifteen patients were operated on for an isolated posterior impingement, while 14 patients had additional pathology such as tenosynovitis of the flexor hallucis longus, a tarsal tunnel syndrome, or subtalar joint pathology.

There were no infections. One patient developed a sympathetic reflex dystrophy. One patient preoperatively had mild symptoms of a sympathetic reflex dystrophy, which did not resolve after the operation. Of the 13 patients with a posterior ankle impingement syndrome through overuse, there were 9 excellent results, 3 good results, and 1 fair result. Of the 16 patients with a post-traumatic posterior ankle impingement, there were 5 excellent results, 6 good results, 4 fair results, and 1 poor result. The 12 professional ballet dancers all resumed their work activity.

■ Conclusion

Posterior ankle impingement is a pain syndrome that is produced by forced plantarflexion. A distinction must be made between overuse injuries and traumatic injuries. Posterior ankle impingement as an overuse injury often occurs in ballet dancers.

The impediment is a prominent posterior talar process or an os trigonum. In ballet dancers tendinitis of the flexor hallucis longus and chondropathy of the posterior subtalar joint (dancers' heel) are important in the differential diagnosis. The distinction can be made through physical diagnostic means. In case of a posterior ankle impingement, the passive forced plantarflexion test is positive (a positive test means pain with recognition). A flexor hallucis longus tendinitis is detected by palpating the flexor hallucis longus behind the medial malleolus with the ankle in 10-20° of plantarflexion while the patient actively moves the toes from a neutral position to the grasping (plantarflexion) position. Crepitus, triggering, and pain (with recognition) can be appreciated.

Conservative measures include corticosteroid infiltration. In case of operative treatment for isolated posterior ankle impingement as an overuse injury, the posterolateral approach is advised. In combined injuries in which the flexor hallucis longus or tarsal tunnel are involved, resection should be performed by a posteromedial approach. Good and excellent results can be expected in over 90% of cases. Hyperplantarflexion trauma can result in fracture/pseudarthrosis, displacement of an os trigonum, or calcifications. These calcifications often are located posteromedially. Diagnosis can be difficult, since a pseudarthrotic fragment, an os trigonum, or calcifications can be invisible on the lateral radiograph. Bone scan and CT scan should be performed. Because of concomitant injuries in post-traumatic cases, the prognosis after surgical treatment is less favorable than in cases resulting from overuse.

Since 1995, we have used a two-portal hindfoot approach, with the patient in the prone position, for treatment of posterior impingement and flexor hallucis longus tendinitis, and flexor hallucis tendinitis (van Dijk 1997b, 2000). The approach offers not only excellent access to the flexor hallucis longus, but by means of this approach, the posterior ankle compartment, os trigonum, and subtalar joint can be visualized and treated. The removal of a symptomatic os trigonum, post-traumatic calcifications in the posterior capsule, posterior synovectomy, and capsulectomy all can be performed by means of this two-portal posterior hindfoot approach. Surgeons, used to the arthroscope, will find this endoscopic technique a more rewarding procedure.

■ References

Hamilton WG, Geppert MJ, Thompson FM. Pain in the posterior aspect of the ankle in dancers. J Bone Joint Surg 87A-10:1491-1500, 1996.

Hedrick MR, McBryde AM. Posterior ankle impingement. Foot Ankle Int 15:2-8, 1994.

Ludolph E, Hierholzer G. Anatomie des Bandapparates am oberen Sprunggelenk. Orthopäde 15(6):410-414, 1986.

Marti RK, Besselaar PP. Chronische Verletzungen des hinteren subtalar Gelenkes. In Chapchal G, editor. Sportverletzungen und Sportschäden, pp 250-252, Springer Verlag: Berlin, 1983.

Salyers SG, Fu FH. Posterior ankle impingement syndrome in a ballet dancer. Orthop Cons 10:9-12, 1989.

Stibbe AB, van Dijk CN, Marti RK. The os trigonum syndrome. In: Acta Orthop Scand (Suppl 262) 59-60, 1994.

van Dijk CN. Arthroscopie van het bovenste spronggewricht. In van Mourik JB, Patka P, editors. Letsels van de enkel en voet, pp. 69-86. Haren, the Netherlands: CSN, 1990.

van Dijk CN. On diagnostic strategies in patients with severe ankle sprain. University of Amsterdam, master's thesis, 1994.

van Dijk CN, Lim LSL, Poortman A, Strubbe EH, Marti RK. Degenerative joint disease in female ballet dancers. Am J Sports Med 23(3):295-300, 1995.

van Dijk CN, Scholte D. Arthroscopy of the ankle joint. J Arthroscopy 13:90-96, 1997a.

van Dijk CN, Scholte D, Kort N. Tendoscopy for overuse tendon injuries. In Srez and de Lee, editors. Operative techniques in sports medicine, 5(3): 170-178, 1997b.

van Dijk CN, Scholten PE, Krips R. A two-portal endoscopic approach for diagnosis and treatment of posterior ankle pathology. Arthroscopy 16(8):871-876, 2000.

Chapter 17

Fractures of the Fifth Metatarsal

Frank Spaas, MD, and Marc Martens, PhD

The fifth metatarsal is by far the most commonly fractured metatarsal. Metatarsal fractures are frequently overlooked or unsuccessfully treated and, thus, frequently the cause of prolonged disability. They are frequently the result of direct crushing injuries, and sometimes the associated soft tissue injury is of extreme importance. One can distinguish among three different groups of fractures of the fifth metatarsal: fractures involving the head and neck of the metatarsal, those involving the middle and distal diaphysis, and fractures of the base of the metatarsal. The first two groups can be treated like any other metatarsal fractures and will be discussed together. Fractures involving the base of the fifth metatarsal, however, have been a source of confusion in the literature with regard to classification and treatment, and will be discussed separately.

■ General Issues

Except for fractures of the neck of the metatarsal, displacement of simple fractures of the metatarsal is usually minimal, due to rigid ligamentous anchoring of the metatarsal bones to each other, particularly at the ends of the bones. Distally, there are the deep transverse ligaments, which pass horizontally between the metatarsal necks, and proximally, there are also strong ligaments connecting the bases of the metatarsals to each other.

In a fracture of the neck of the metatarsal, the head-neck fragment is commonly displaced beneath the distal metaphysis of the bone, because of the strong plantarflexing force of the lumbricals, interossei, and extrinsic flexors, which exert a strong plantar and proximal dislocating force on the distal fragment.

Different directions of displacement will produce different effects:

- Displacement of the distal fragment in a plantigrade direction results in increased loading of the metatarsal and may result in intractable keratosis under the metatarsal head.

- Dorsal displacement of the distal fragment decreases the load to the metatarsal and transfers greater pressure to the adjacent metatarsal heads.

- Persistent medial displacement of the fracture fragment can lead to mechanical impingement and interdigital neuroma formation.

- Lateral displacement of the distal fragment may lead to a bony prominence that can produce difficulties with shoe wear in the toe box.

Mechanism of Injury

Metatarsal fractures may result from direct or indirect forces. The fifth metatarsal in particular is often fractured by an indirect force, such as a twisting injury, in which the forepart of the foot is fixed as the patient turns, producing a mediolateral torque; it is more common in athletic endeavors and has been so commonly found in classical ballet dancers that the fracture has been referred to as the "dancer's fracture." These fractures are oblique and spiral, and displacement is unusual.

The direct injury with crushing is more common in industrial accidents, as a result of a direct blow on the dorsum of the foot, usually from some heavy object. Fractures of the metatarsal head may result from direct crush, or occasionally from bullet or shell fragment wounds.

Clinical Diagnosis

Fractures of the metatarsals in general are frequently overlooked, due to the fact that they often occur in motor vehicle accidents in which severe trauma to major bones or visceral organs is more apparent.

In the history, it is important to investigate the intensity of the original blow that produced the fracture. One has to caution against the practice of reducing a metatarsal fracture, placing the foot in a cast, and sending the patient home. Within 48 to 72 hours, the patient may return with skin slough, tendon damage, and intrinsic muscle damage. If there is soft tissue damage, it is therefore important to hospitalize the patient, irrespective of how minimal the underlying fracture appears to be.

The patient usually will complain of pain over the lateral side of the foot, with the inability to bear weight. The foot is swollen on the dorsolateral side. After the first 12 hours, ecchymosis over the fracture area will be present. If the patient is seen early, point tenderness may be present over the fracture site. With gross displacement, palpation of the fracture site may be possible. Grasping the distal fragment with the thumb and the forefinger and flexing and extending the fragment will produce motion, potential crepitus, and pain at the fracture site.

Radiology

Metatarsal fractures are visualized on routine anteroposterior, oblique, and lateral roentgenographs of the foot. The anteroposterior and oblique views are more useful due to the fact that the shafts of the metatarsals are superimposed on the lateral view. The fracture may be transverse, oblique, or segmental. The fracture may be angulated dorsally at the fracture site, due to the pull of the intrinsic muscles and the overpull of strong toe flexors. Axial or sesamoid views are particularly helpful in detecting this plantar displacement.

Fractures of the base of the metatarsal may require polytomograpy to delineate fracture fragment size and the occasional subluxation of the tarsometatarsal joint.

Treatment

As in any other fracture, treatment of a metatarsal fracture must take care of the soft tissue injury and the displacement of the fracture.

Open Fractures

Just as for other open long bone fractures, initial irrigation and debridement with appropriate antibiotic coverage are indicated. The wound is left open for delayed primary closure or skin grafting. The management of the fracture of the metatarsal is similar to that for closed fractures. However, axial Kirschner wire fixation is performed more routinely in open fractures to hasten bony union and to allow adequate treatment of the soft tissue injury.

Closed Fractures

If soft tissue damage is significant, placing the foot in a bulky dressing is considered. The foot is elevated

and ice applied until subsidence of the swelling permits more aggressive treatment of the fracture. Early weight bearing is important in the treatment of a metatarsal fracture, in order to help minimize long-term disability.

Undisplaced Fractures

Undisplaced (nondisplaced) fractures can be treated in a short leg walking cast or by taping the foot with adhesive tape and using a bunion-type shoe (figure 17.1). The choice is dependent on the patient's employment requirements. When comfort allows, the patient is transferred to a stiff-soled walking shoe or boot with a good arch support.

Displaced Fractures

A displaced fracture may produce residual morbidity unless it is accurately reduced. Healing with plantar angulation or displacement will result in an abnormal load on the metatarsal, with a buildup of callus under the metatarsal head and pain. Healing with dorsal angulation or shortening will result in transfer of weight to the fourth metatarsal head, with callus build-up and localized metatarsalgia. A displacement in the frontal plane may result in a callus formation on the lateral side of the foot.

Closed reduction is attempted by using a Chinese finger trap on the fifth digit under general anesthesia or regional ankle block, with a gentle manipulation at the fracture site. If reduction is obtained, consideration is given to percutaneous Kirschner wire fixation to the fourth metatarsal. Following reduction, patients are placed in a well-padded short leg cast with the foot held in traction. Weight bearing is allowed after the second week of immobilization.

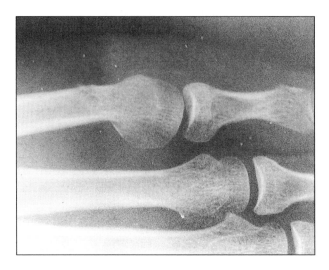

■ **Figure 17.1** A nondisplaced fracture of the neck of the fifth metatarsal.

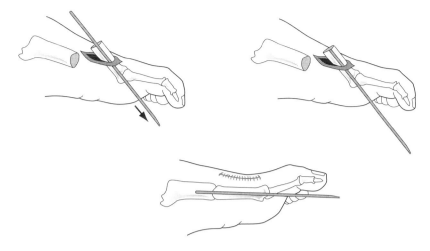

■ **Figure 17.2** Internal fixation with longitudinal intramedullary Kirschner wire. A Kirschner wire is inserted anterograde into the distal fragment first with the metatarsophalangeal joint in neutral dorsiflexion, and then advanced proximally into the fracture site.

If dorsoplantar angulation persists following closed reduction, open reduction and internal fixation with either longitudinal intramedullary or crossed Kirschner wires are utilized. A limited dorsal incision is made over the fracture site and a Kirschner wire is inserted anterograde into the distal fragment first with the metatarsophalangeal joint in neutral dorsiflexion, and then advanced proximally into the fracture site. The wire is bent at its tip and left protruding from the skin (figure 17.2).

If there is more than one displaced metatarsal fracture, internal fixation, either by percutaneous methods or by open reduction, may be necessary because of the loss of the splinting effect of adjacent metatarsals. Following open reduction and internal fixation, patients are kept nonweightbearing in a short leg cast for 2 weeks. Weight bearing is then initiated for an additional 6 weeks. The Kirschner wires are removed between 4 and 6 weeks.

■ Metatarsal Neck Fractures

If the metatarsal head and neck fragment is displaced, an attempt is made at closed reduction with Chinese fingertraps for traction and direct pressure beneath the metatarsal head to reduce the displacement. A short leg cast is applied, with a toe plate, with the traction in place. If the reduction is maintained, the patient is treated with weight bearing in the cast for 4 to 6 weeks, followed by the use of a stiff-soled shoe.

If the reduction is not acceptable, is unstable, or redisplaces in the cast, percutaneous Kirschner wire fixation of the fracture while in the Chinese finger traps is attempted. If this fails, open reduction through a dorsal incision and intramedullary Kirschner wire fixation as described previously is utilized. This Kirschner wire is left in place only 3 weeks and then

removed. Weight bearing in the cast is begun when swelling subsides. After removal of the wires, the patients are managed for an additional 2 weeks in a cast and then transferred to a stiff-soled shoe.

■ Metatarsal Head Fractures

Metatarsal head fractures are uncommon. If the metatarsal head fragment is small and the displacement does not affect the stability of the metatarsophalangeal joint, the fracture is treated by closed reduction under digital block anesthesia by applying longitudinal traction on the toe. If reduction is unsuccessful, and if the intra-articular fragment results in limiting the range of motion of the joint, open reduction with internal fixation is performed. Otherwise, the toe is treated as if the reduction were successful.

If the fragment is large enough that its displacement results in instability of the metatarsophalangeal joint, anatomic reduction and stable fixation is indicated. The fracture is treated by closed reduction under digital anesthesia, and if a stable acceptable reduction is obtained, a buddy taping to the fourth toe can be applied and the foot placed in a short leg cast.

If the reduction is not anatomic or displacement reoccurs, open reduction-internal fixation with smooth Kirschner wires is undertaken.

■ Metatarsal Base Fractures

Fractures of the base of the fifth metatarsal are the most common type of metatarsal fractures. Classically, they have been termed **Jones fractures** since Sir Robert Jones described the injury, which he sustained in his own foot in 1902. Jones described an acute transverse diaphyseal fracture of the fifth metatarsal, three-fourths of an inch from the base, at the junction of the diaphysis and the metaphysis, without extension distal to the intermetatarsal (4-5) articulation, involving the fourth and fifth intermetatarsal articular facet.

Other proximal fifth metatarsal fractures have indiscriminately also been called Jones fractures, which has created confusion. Laurence and Botte (1983) have stated that at least three fracture types have to be distinguished (figure 17.3): Besides the Jones fracture, there are the diaphyseal stress fracture and the tuberosity, or styloid process avulsion fracture.

The **diaphyseal stress fracture** is a pathological fracture of the proximal 1.5 cm of the fifth metatarsal shaft, the end result of the summation of repetitive, cyclic distraction forces, that causes prodromal symptoms and may herald an acute episode, resulting in a complete fracture. Stress fractures of the proximal shaft of the fifth metatarsal are different in their behavior than other metatarsal stress fractures. They are slow to heal, predisposed to reinjury, and often cause prolonged disability, particularly in the young athlete. Up to 50% of patients with stress fractures of the fifth metatarsal may give a history of discomfort over the lateral aspect of the foot several weeks prior to the roentgenographic evidence of the fracture, and show evidence of a lucent fracture line with periosteal reaction on the radiograph. Torg (Torg 1980; Torg et al. 1984) has divided fifth metatarsal diaphyseal stress fractures into three categories:

- In acute type 1 fractures, there is a periosteal reaction that demonstrates a previous attempt to heal an incomplete fracture.

- A type 2 fracture shows a widened fracture line and intramedullary sclerosis.

- Type 3 fractures demonstrate complete intramedullary obliteration (i.e., an established nonunion).

The third and most common fracture of the proximal fifth metatarsal is the **tuberosity** or **styloid process avulsion fracture**, which has also been called "tennis fracture." It is commonly extra-articular, although propagation of the fracture into the cubometatarsal joint is not infrequent. It may occur in association with a fracture of the lateral malleolus,

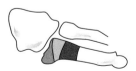

- ☐ Tuberosity fractures
- ☐ Jones fracture
- ☐ Diaphyseal stress fracture

■ **Figure 17.3** Fractures of the base of the fifth metatarsal.

which should be recognized and treated (figures 17.4 and 17.5).

Anatomy

The base of the fifth metatarsal is closely bound to the cuboid and to the fourth metatarsal by strong ligaments. Jones noted: "So powerful are these ligaments that dislocation of the base is the rarest of incidents." This was later confirmed by Kavanaugh in anatomic dissections. There are three articulations between these bones: the cuboid-fourth metatarsal, the cuboid-fifth metatarsal and the fourth-fifth intermetatarsal articulations.

The proximity of either a Jones fracture or a diaphyseal stress fracture to the extra-osseous plexus

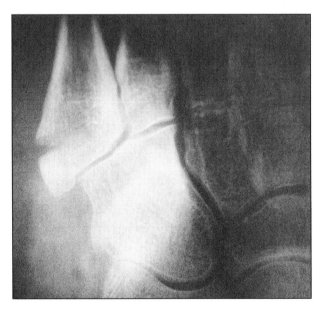

■ **Figure 17.4** Avulsion fracture of the tuberositas of the fifth metatarsal, also called "tennis fracture."

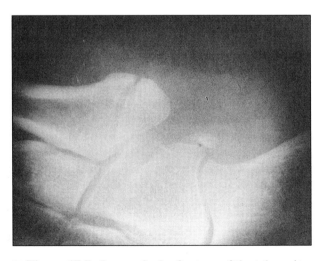

■ **Figure 17.5** Intra-articular fracture of the tuberositas of the fifth metatarsal.

and the nutrient foramen, located in the medial cortex at the junction of the proximal and middle one-third of the shaft, may play a role in the tendency of these fractures to heal slowly (Sheriff et al. 1991; Smith et al. 1992).

The tuberosity of the fifth metatarsal varies in size. It projects proximally (downward and laterally) beyond the surface of the adjacent cuboid, and has a certain potential for fracture because of this over-hang.

The lateral band of the plantar aponeurosis inserts onto the tip of the tuberosity, and is the most likely structure to cause a tuberosity avulsion fracture, contrary to the peroneus brevis tendon, which attaches broadly to the tuberosity and base.

Mechanism of Injury

Jones's original description of his own injury is classic: "I trod on the outer side of my foot, my heel at the moment being off the ground." Other authors also described a plantarflexion of the ankle while a large adduction force is applied to the forefoot, such as when one missteps on the lateral border of the foot, as the mechanism of injury.

A transverse or short oblique fracture results at the junction of the metaphysis and diaphysis, entering the 4-5-intermetatarsal joint, commonly with medial comminution, because motion of the base of the metatarsal in the adduction-abduction plane is severely limited.

Increased stress on the foot, secondary to increased activity, prolonged running, or participation in certain sports, may produce stress fractures of the proximal diaphysis, of the distraction type. It has been shown that the fifth metatarsal endures tremendous forces during vigorous propulsive activities, such as running, sprinting, or jumping. Angular deformities, such as genu varum, ankle varus, hindfoot varus, or forefoot supination, compound the stresses of the lateral forefoot. Also, dynamic muscle forces are concentrated on the proximal fifth metatarsal, which may play a role in creating a stress fracture.

Although the prominence of the tuberosity of the fifth metatarsal makes it at risk for direct trauma, fractures of the tuberosity by indirect violence are more common, secondary to the structures that attach to it. The structure most likely to cause an avulsion fracture is the lateral band of the plantar aponeurosis. Plantarflexion and inversion stress placed on the forefoot may avulse the styloid at the base of the metatarsal.

Diagnosis

The clinical diagnosis of a metatarsal base fracture is confirmed by radiographic examination.

Clinical Diagnosis

For the clinical diagnosis, the history as well as the physical examination are important.

■ **History.** Careful evaluation of the patient's history is essential to distinguish between fractures of acute onset and stress fractures, as the treatment differs for the two groups. An aching sensation on the lateral side of the foot may be the initial symptom of a fracture, which is then diagnosed by radiograph. Several weeks before the acute injury occurs, there may be prodromal symptoms of pain at the fracture site. In an acute fracture, there is usually a history of a twisting injury of the ankle. The patient will complain of pain when he or she puts pressure on the toes or the inner side of the foot, or with inversion of the foot.

■ **Physical examination.** There is local tenderness at the base of the lateral fifth metatarsal, and accentuation of the pain by inversion of the foot. Initially, swelling may be minimal, but increases especially when the foot is left dependent. After 24 hours there will be ecchymosis and edema. Generally there is no crepitus, no deformity, and no mobility at the fracture site.

Radiography

Anteroposterior and oblique views demonstrate the fracture best. An oblique radiograph is essential to evaluate the location of the fracture in relation to the fourth-fifth intermetatarsal articular facet, and to discover intra-articular involvement in the metatarso-cuboid joint and displacement.

Congenital anomalies at the base of the fifth metatarsal must be kept in mind: A secondary center of ossification is found in 25% of all children, and the apophysis unites to the shaft before the age of 12 years in girls and before the age of 15 years in boys. This ossification center may be distinguished from a fracture because of certain characteristics: The apophyseal line traverses the tubercle in a direction parallel to the long axis of the shaft and does not extend proximally into the joint, nor medially into the joint between the fourth and fifth metatarsal.

Two accessory bones must be distinguished from a fracture at the base of the fifth metatarsal:

■ The os peroneum, which is a sesamoid bone located in the tendon of the peroneus longus, as it curves under the cuboid.

■ The os vesalanium, a secondary ossicle in the peroneus brevis, on the proximal tip of the metatarsal. It has a smooth sclerotic surface, opposing the proximal portion of the fifth metatarsal, which differentiates it from a fracture.

One should look for the presence of the radiologic signs of a pre-existing stress reaction: a radiolucent line, periosteal reaction, callus, or intramedullary sclerosis.

Treatment

Treatment of fifth metatarsal base fractures depends on the fracture type.

Jones Fracture

The treatment of a patient with an **acute nondisplaced Jones fracture** consists of immobilization in a cast for 4 to 6 weeks, with partial weight bearing. It may take 8 to 12 weeks to get roentgenographic and clinical evidence of healing (figure 17.6). An exception may be the high-performance athlete, for whom operative treatment may be undertaken.

If clinical healing is present, a supervised rehabilitation program before returning to vigorous sports is recommended. In case of lack of healing after 6

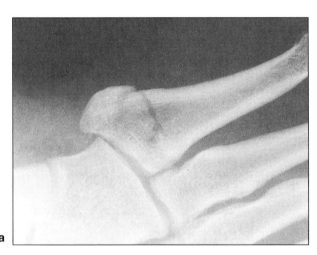

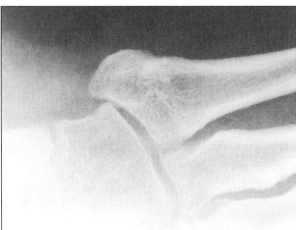

■ **Figure 17.6** (*a*) Acute Jones fracture of the fifth metatarsal; (*b*) radiographic healing in 7 months.

weeks of immobilization, treatment has to be individualized, according to the patient's needs. Continued immobilization or surgical intervention by intramedullary screw fixation or bone graft technique may be undertaken, although the deleterious effects of prolonged immobilization, including joint stiffness and muscle atrophy, need to be considered.

Displaced fractures may require open reduction and internal fixation by cross-pinning with Kirschner wires, tension band wiring, or an intramedullary screw. In elderly patients, a nonweightbearing cast for 4 to 6 weeks is recommended, followed by a stiff shoe.

Diaphyseal Stress Fractures

Diaphyseal stress fractures may take considerably longer to unite and frequently lead to delayed union or nonunion. In Dameron's series, 5 of 20 patients needed bone grafting for symptomatic nonunion (Dameron 1975). Arangio reported 38% delayed union and 14% nonunion with acute fractures (Arangio 1992a). Kavanaugh found that in 41% of so-called acute fractures, a stress reaction was evident, and in athletes not one of these united. Treatment must be individualized and based on the needs and desires of the patient (Dameron 1975; Kavanaugh et al. 1978; Zelko et al. 1979).

Acute type 1 fractures are treated as acute Jones fractures. In a high-performance athlete with a preexisting stress reaction, but without intramedullary sclerosis, a nonweightbearing cast is recommended until pain subsides, followed by a weightbearing cast until evidence of bone healing, when a molded arch support may be the most appropriate treatment (Zogby and Baker 1987). In the case of recurrent pain after the resumption of sport activities, operative treatment is recommended. In a high-performance athlete with a preexisting stress reaction, with intramedullary sclerosis, or for whom a loss of time from athletic activities is not acceptable, direct intramedullary screw fixation (De Lee et al. 1983; Kavanaugh et al. 1978) or bone graft procedure is recommended.

One must be careful with the approach and technique in intramedullary screw fixation, as surgical complications are common unless attention to detail is followed. Peroneus brevis tendon disruption or sural nerve injury may be avoided with isolation and protection of these structures. An incorrectly sized screw may fracture with insertion or may penetrate the cortex, because of the common plantar and lateral curvature of the metatarsal. If too long a screw is used, the gentle curvature of the metatarsal may ultimately straighten, leading to transfer of stress to the fourth metatarsal. Screw head prominence may irritate the soft tissues if the screw is not countersunk properly, and screw removal may be necessary after bony union. A cannulated screw system simplifies the intramedullary screw placement. The internal fixation is followed by a nonweightbearing cast for 2 weeks, followed by a short leg weightbearing cast and then a hard-soled shoe and progressive weight bearing. When pain is gone, patients are allowed to return to competitive sport, with a soft-soled shoe insert with protective padding over the lateral metatarsal base.

A reversed graft, by an asymmetrical trapezoid autograft, offers a simple and effective surgical solution: Through a dorsolateral incision, a trapezoid section of bone, measuring 0.7 × 2.0 cm and taken asymmetrically on the fracture, is outlined and removed. The canal is curetted and sclerotic bone removed. Next, the autograft is jammed back into its base as a reversed graft (figure 17.7) (Hens and Martens 1990).

After either intramedullary screw fixation or reversed grafting, a short leg cast is applied for 6 to 8 weeks and weight bearing is permitted after 2 weeks. Normal sporting activity may be regained in a mean of 3 months (figure 17.8).

In patients with low activity level, immobilization in a short leg walking cast is given, and according to progression towards union, eventually intramedullary screw fixation or bone grafting is carried out.

Avulsion Fractures

In nondisplaced **avulsion fractures**, only symptomatic treatment is necessary: strapping the foot until pain subsides, or a short leg cast until pain allows strapping of the foot. Weight bearing is also started, when the pain allows it, in a stiff-soled shoe. Almost all these fractures eventually unite, and even those that heal by fibrous union are rarely symptomatic (Dameron 1975).

In case of an intra-articular fragment, involvement of greater than 30% of the articular surface, or an articular stepoff exceeding 2 mm in a highly competitive athlete, open reduction and internal fixation with a small screw or tension band wiring is recommended. In the majority of cases, however, little disability results from allowing these fractures to heal in the displaced position. If a malunion or nonunion causes symptoms, the fragment can be excised.

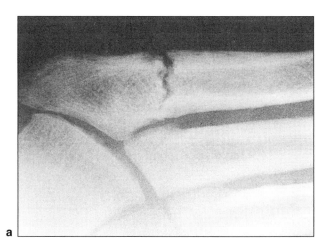

a

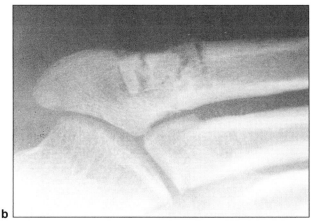

b

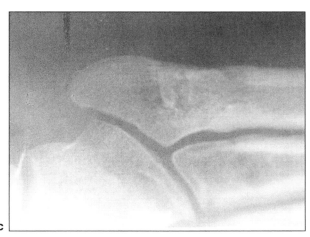

c

■ **Figure 17.8** *(a)* Diaphyseal stress fracture of the fifth metatarsal. *(b)* Treatment by reversed asymmetrical autograft. *(c)* Healing after 2 months.

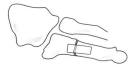 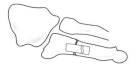

■ **Figure 17.7** Diaphyseal stress fracture of the fifth metatarsal. Treatment by reversed asymmetrical trapezoid autograft: A trapezoid section of bone, measuring 0.7 × 2.0 cm and taken asymmetrically on the fracture, is removed, and after curetting, all sclerotic bone is placed back into its base as a reversed graft.

■ References

Arangio GA. 1992a. The Jones fracture—transverse proximal diaphyseal fractures of the fifth metatarsal: frequency by radiology. Foot 1:201-204.

Arangio GA. 1992b. Transverse proximal diaphyseal fracture of the fifth metatarsal: a review of 12 cases. Foot Ankle 13(9):547.

Dameron TB Jr. 1975. Fractures and anatomical variations of the proximal portion of the fifth metatarsal. J Bone Joint Surg Am 57:788.

Hens J, Martens M. 1990. Surgical treatment of Jones fractures. Arch Orthop Trauma Surg 109(5):277-279.

Jones R. 1902. Fracture of the base of the fifth metatarsal by indirect violence. Ann Surg 35:679.

Kavanaugh JH, Brower TD, Mann RV. 1978. The Jones fracture revisited. J Bone Joint Surg Am 60:776.

Laurence S, Botte M. 1993. Foot Fellow's Review: Jones' fractures and related fractures of the proximal fifth metatarsal. Foot Ankle 14(6):358-365.

Sheriff MJ, Young GM, Kummer FJ, Frey CC, Greenridge N. 1991. Vascular anatomy of the fifth metatarsal. Foot Ankle 11(6):350-353.

Smith JW, Arnoczky SP, Hersik A. 1992. The intraosseous blood supply of the fifth metatarsal: implications for proximal fracture healing. Foot Ankle 13(3):143.

Stone HM. 1968. Avulsion fracture of the base of the fifth metatarsal. Am J Orthop Surg 10:190-193.

Torg JS. 1980. Fractures of the base of the fifth metatarsal distal to the tuberosity. Orthopaedics 13(7):731-737.

Torg JS, Balduini FC, Zelko RR, Pavlov H, Peff TC, Das M. 1984. Fracture of the base of the fifth metatarsal distal to the tuberosity. Classification and guidelines for non-surgical and surgical management. J Bone Joint Surg Am 66(2):209-214.

Zelko RR, Torg JS, Rachun A. 1979. Proximal diaphyseal fractures of the fifth metatarsal—treatment of the fractures and their complications in athletes. Am J Sports Med 7(2):95-101.

Zogby RB, Baker B. 1987. A review of nonoperative treatment of Jones fracture. Am J Sports Med 15:304-307.

Chapter 18

The Subtalar Joint: Instability

Elisha Freund, MD; Meir Nyska, MD; and Gideon Mann, MD

The subtalar joint plays a crucial role in the overall function of the foot. Injuries to this complex joint are often misdiagnosed and hence incorrectly treated. This chapter presents a review of the anatomy and traumatic pathology of the subtalar joint.

■ Anatomy

In order to understand the complexity of injuries of the subtalar joint, one must be familiar with its anatomy. Please refer to chapter 2, in which a full anatomical description is given.

■ Motion

The subtalar joint is a single inclined axis joint, which acts like a mitered hinge between the talus and the calcaneus. With the anterior talocalcaneal articulation lying further medially and having a higher center of rotation than the posterior one, the axis of the subtalar joint passes from medial to lateral at an angle of 16-23° and approximately 42° from the horizontal plane. Individual variations account for the ample variety observed in ambulating behavior.

At the time of heel strike, with the point of contact between the heel and the floor lying laterally to the ankle joint, there is an eversion of the subtalar joint, which reaches its maximum at foot flat. This eversion tends to unlock the midtarsal joints in order to permit plantigrade support of the forefoot, after which progressive inversion occurs until the time of toe-off. During walking, an inward rotation of the leg occurs at heel strike, reaching its peak at foot flat. Because of the inclined axis of the subtalar joint, which collapses into valgus when the foot is initially loaded, further rotation of the proximal limb over the fixed foot is possible. The overall rotation of the joint in a normal foot is about 24°, although during normal gait, only 6° are used. The importance of the subtalar movement lies in its capacity to allow the foot to adapt to uneven terrain during ambulation.

■ Assessment

Examination of the subtalar joint is an essential part of the clinical assessment of the foot. The clinical examination should include both the dynamic and the static motion of the joint.

Clinical Examination

Loading the foot with the body weight during the first half of stance phase, the foot should normally pronate, followed by an inversion of the heel and supination of the foot toward heel rise. The amount of pronation is subject to individual variation. It is important to note this sequence in order to assess, among other things, the integrity of the subtalar joint.

While standing, the weightbearing line of the body normally falls medial to the axis of the subtalar joint. Because of the linkage between the leg and the foot provided by the subtalar articulation, when the examiner rotates the leg externally, the heel will invert and the weight bearing will shift laterally (and vice versa). This will normally occur within the range of 10-15°. If the amount of rotation of the leg that is necessary to create a supination or pronation of the foot exceeds this range, it may indicate instability of the subtalar articulation. If a rotation of the leg of more than 15° would be needed to create supination or pronation, this would probably indicate instability of the subtalar joint. It should be remembered that subtalar instability is usually more an excessive gliding than excessive separation of the talus from the calcaneus (Clanton 1999; Kjaersgaard-Anderson et al. 1988; Astrom & Arvidson 1995).

When the patient is asked to rise onto his or her toes, the heel—under normal conditions—will promptly invert and the longitudinal arch will rise. Failure of these motions to occur should lead the examiner to suspect a malfunction of the subtalar joint (e.g., tarsal coalition) or other conditions, such as muscular weakness, tendon insufficiency, and arthritic changes of the hindfoot.

To accomplish the examination, the patient's feet are examined with the patient sitting on the examining table. The calcaneus is held in one hand of the examiner and placed in line with the long axis of the leg. With the other hand, the examiner inverts and everts the forefoot (including the transverse tarsal joint) to asses the subtalar motion. Usually there is twice as much inversion as eversion (2:1 ratio). The same examination can be done with the patient prone, the knee flexed to about 135° (in this position, the axis of the subtalar joint is close to horizontal), and the heel passively inverted and everted (Mann and Coughlin 1993).

Wernick and Langer (1972) and James et al. (1978) instruct the examiner to palpate the medial and lateral sides of the head of the talus as the foot is passively supinated and pronated in order to assess the subtalar congruency (with or without dorsiflexion of the ankle joint). The subtalar neutral position is reached when the head is felt to extend equally on both sides of the foot.

Radiological Examination

Imaging assessment of the subtalar joint is essential in achieving a correct diagnosis. Because the joint is complex, the imaging modalities include specific views and techniques.

Radiograph

Standard anterioposterior (AP) and standing lateral views are essential to rule out any bony abnormality. Subtalar instability will rarely have any significant findings in these studies.

Lateral stress radiographs of the ankle and subtalar joint may demonstrate lateral ligamentous instability of both the tibiotalar and the subtalar joints. The laterally viewed anterior drawer stress radiographs may reveal a separation of the articular surfaces of the talus and calcaneus (which are normally closely congruent). Mann and Coughlin (1993) wrote that a separation of 3 mm or more is indicative of an unstable subtalar joint. Both ankles should always be compared to each other.

Kato (1995) suggests dorsoplantar views of the subtalar joint with and without a positive anterior drawer stress. The amount of calcaneal anterior displacement is an indicator of the subtalar instability.

Broden's View

A more specific radiograph view of the subtalar joint is achieved by the Broden projection (with or without stress). This method visualizes the posterior facets of the subtalar joint, which are parallel under normal circumstances.

The patient is supine with the knee slightly flexed and supported by a sandbag. The foot rests on the film cassette with neutral dorsiflexion. The entire lower leg and foot is internally rotated 30-45°. The central beam is directed toward the lateral malleolus. Films are obtained at 10, 20, 30, and 40° of cephalic tilt (40° showing anterior, and 10° showing posterior facets).

A 40° Broden view with inversion stress applied to the foot may demonstrate divergence of the posterior facets (normally parallel), indicating instability (Clanton 1989).

Variations of these views include the lateral oblique axial, the lateral oblique, and the medial oblique axial.

■ **Lateral oblique axial view.** This view demonstrates the posterior subtalar facet. The foot is passively everted, dorsiflexed, and externally rotated 60°. The central beam is centered 1 inch below the tip of the medial malleolus with 10° cephalic tilt.

■ **Lateral oblique view.** This view demonstrates the anterior process of the calcaneus and the anterior facet of the subtalar joint. The patient is supine, with the inner border of the foot placed on the cassette and the sole inclined at 45°. The central beam is directed vertically and centered 1 inch below and 1 inch anterior to the tip of the lateral malleolus.

■ **Medial oblique axial view.** With the patient supine, the limb is internally rotated 30° to 45° with the ankle in neutral flexion. The beam is centered over the lateral malleolus.

Harris Beath View

The Harris Beath view demonstrates the body of the calcaneus, middle facet of the subtalar joint, and the sustenaculum tali.

The patient is erect. The sole of the foot is flat on the cassette. The central beam is angled at 45° toward the midline of the heel, caudally directed, on the cornal plane. A 35° or 55° angle is used to better visualize other facets of the subtalar joint.

Because the posterior and middle facets are in parallel planes at approximately 45° to the sole of the foot, these two areas are identified on axial view (Harris, or ski jump view). The effectiveness of Harris view for visualizing the subtalar joint is enhanced by measuring the angle of the posterior facet on the lateral radiograph and then adjusting Harris view to this inclination.

Arthrography

Arthrography of the posterior subtalar joint is an objective parameter, identifying peri- or intra-articular pathology as the cause of symptoms (Goossens et al. 1989). It is ideally combined with routine anterior drawer and talar tilt roentgenograms. The main value of this procedure, which is both invasive and expensive, is in diagnosing acute injuries rather than chronic ones.

Technique: With the patient supine, under fluoroscopic or radiographic control, a needle is inserted just lateral to the Achilles tendon and directed 15° caudal to the plantar surface of the foot and directed into the posterior subtalar joint. Two to four milliliters of radiographic contrast medium is injected.

A normal subtalar joint demonstrates free movement of the contrast dye with different foot position and well-defined medial and lateral joint recesses. In acute cases of injury, the dye may leak to the ankle joint, the sinus tarsi, or the surrounding soft tissue. In chronic lesions, the contrast medium will not fill the lateral recess normally, and the dye assumes a flat appearance along the anterior margin of the posterior subtalar joint (Clanton 1989).

Computed Tomography

Computed tomography (CT) is an essential tool in evaluating the subtalar pathology. It can be used to assess a variety of conditions, including fractures, neoplasms, infections, foreign bodies, osteochondral injuries, tendons, arthritis, and various abnormalities.

Choosing the correct planes of imaging (e.g., coronal, axial, or sagittal) is crucial for obtaining the desired view in order to evaluate the specific pathology (figure 18.1).

It is most important to use thin sections (5 mm or less) to avoid misdiagnosis. Axial images (on a plane perpendicular to the cephalocaudal line of an erect individual) are obtained with the patient supine, knees flexed, and the feet in neutral position. The angle of the gantry should be aimed to the estimated axial plane of the osseous structures rather than to that of the soft tissue. The coronal view (a plane perpendicular to the anteroposterior line of an erect individual) is obtained with the feet flat on the table and knees bent.

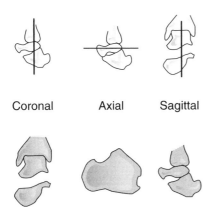

Coronal   Axial   Sagittal

■ **Figure 18.1** The coronal, axial, and sagittal planes of CT imaging.

The gantry is oriented perpendicular to the desired subtalar section to be examined.

Van Hellemondt et al. (1997) suggested a stress computerized tomography of the ankle joint. His work was further enhanced by Pearce and Buckley (1999), who emphasized the importance of CT in the evaluation of the subtalar joint as a means to assess its stability.

Magnetic Resonance Imaging

Magnetic resonance imaging (MRI) is considered to be the imaging modality of choice not only in the evaluation of soft tissue structures (such as the sinus and canalis tarsi, which are inaccessible by other methods), but also in diagnosing avascular necrosis and other bony lesions. The disadvantages of this method include the facts that it is not a dynamic investigation, the patient is not weight bearing during the investigation, and some patients may tolerate it poorly due to claustrophobia.

Axial, coronal (or oblique coronal), and sagittal views permit visualization of both superficial and deep ligamentous structures. In most instances, two planes are sufficient. The usual layer of adipose tissue surrounding tendons provides excellent contrast background (Ferkel 1996). In view of the complexity of the region, special scanning techniques have been developed, including three-dimensional reconstruction and inframillimetric slices (Shahabpour et al. 1992).

In an MRI study of the subtalar components, Klein and Spreitzer (1993) categorized the abnormalities of the tarsal sinus and canal by the type and amount of infiltration of the fatty tissue (synovitis or fibrosis). They also assessed the integrity of the ligaments by their appearance (either thickened or thin when the ligament was partially torn, and a complete absence if the ligament was disrupted). The occasional presence of fluid in the sinus was due to synovial cysts, although excessive fluid could represent an injured or ill joint, affected by trauma or by specific or nonspecific inflammatory changes. The amount of fluid collection in the tarsal sinus and canal and anterior microrecesses was more consistent with synovitis and nonspecific inflammatory changes, mainly in chronic cases.

Arthroscopy

Arthroscopy of the subtalar joint is not a routinely used method for the evaluation of the joint. The complexity of the vascular, tendinous, and neural elements surrounding the joint, as well as its convex shape and its small size, create difficulties regarding both the entry portals and the effective joint space visualization. Only the posterior facet may be viewed via an arthroscope, because the anterior and lateral facets are hidden by the interosseous ligament.

With the introduction of small instruments and precise techniques, the use of arthroscopy of the subtalar joint has expanded in the last decade. The indications for such a procedure are as follows:

- Diagnostic (inability to diagnose subtalar persisting symptoms with routine radiological methods).
- Therapeutic (removal of loose bodies, excision of adhesions, possible arthrodesis).

In their "Arthroscopic evaluation of the subtalar joint", Frey et al. (1999) stated that the term "sinus tarsi syndrome" as a cause for subtalar pain is a vague diagnosis and has to be replaced by a more specific one.

In their series, the preoperative diagnosis of sinus tarsi syndrome was made upon subjective complaints of pain and instability and objective findings of tenderness over the sinus and pain relief after an injection of local anesthetic, while their postoperative diagnosis was a torn interosseous ligament, fibrosis, or degenerative joint disease.

They have found that the previously diagnosed "sinus tarsi syndrome" as a cause for subtalar pain had a more specific diagnosis, which was determined by arthroscopy. Edema, infections, poor vascular flow, and advanced degenerative disease are contraindications for arthroscopy.

■ Causes of Instability

The so-called "subtalar instability syndrome" may be divided into three main categories according to etiology:

- **Active instability.** Active instability is a result of a malfunction of the nervous system (central or peripheral), a malfunction of the proprioceptive system, or a muscular-tendinous pathology.
- **Passive instability (laxity).** Some patients who might have been thought to have subtalar joint instability could have laxity of the interosseous talocalcaneal ligament, simply as a result of joint laxity.
- **Structural instability.** Structural instability is due to trauma that causes elongation or insufficiency of the ligaments. This is mainly caused by a great degree of stress to the foot.

Ligamentous Injury

In 1997, Karlsson et al. divided subtalar injuries into four groups according to the manner in which the injury occurred and the ligaments damaged in that injury:

- **Type I injury.** A type I injury is caused by a forceful supination of the hindfoot associated with a plantarflexion of the ankle. With the plantarflexed ankle, the anterior talofibular ligament, and possibly the cervical ligament, are torn first, followed by disruption of the calcaneofibular ligament and the lateral capsule.
- **Type II injury.** In a type II injury rupture of the interosseous talocalcaneal ligament also occurs.
- **Type III injury.** A type III injury occurs when the calcaneofibular ligament, cervical ligament, and the interosseous talocalcaneal ligament are ruptured with the ankle in dorsiflexion. The anterior talofibular ligament remains intact as it is without tension in this position.
- **Type IV injury.** A type IV injury is a combination of severe talotibial and subtalar ligament injury, and it is caused by a forceful supination of the hindfoot while the ankle is in dorsiflexion but subsequently rotating into plantarflexion.

When inversion stress is applied to a foot of a cadaver, rupture of the interosseous talocalcaneal ligament occurs only after rupture of the anterior talofibular ligament, followed by rupture of the calcaneofibular ligament. Total rupture of the cervical ligament and the interosseus ligament result in dislocation of the subtalar joint. In most cases, a severe lateral ankle sprain results only in a partial rupture or elongation of these ligaments. Elongation of the interosseous ligament may lead to an anterior displacement of the calcaneus. A rupture will cause a talar tilt (Kato 1995).

Sequential sectioning of the ligaments in vitro demonstrates the role of each ligament in stabilizing the subtalar joint:

- When the inferior extensor retinaculum lateral root (IERL) was divided, the stability of the ankle joint was not altered, but the subtalar joint gained 30% of movement, which only occurred in neutral and dorsiflexion. The other roots—inferior extensor retinaculum intermediate (IERI) and medial (IERM)—did not influence the stability of the subtalar or ankle joints.
- The division of the anterior talofibular ligament (ATFL) allowed some talar tilt within the ankle joint when the foot was plantarflexed, but otherwise, it did not contribute to stability.
- The lateral talocalcaneal ligament (LTC) did not demonstrate any stabilizing role.

■ After dividing the calcaneofibular ligament (CFL), in the absence of the ATFL, the ankle became unstable in all positions, but to a greater extent in plantarflexion.

■ Dividing the CFL also destabilized the subtalar joint, but to a lesser extent.

■ Sectioning of the posterior talofibular ligament (PTFL) did not alter subtalar stability.

■ The ligament of the anterior capsule of the posterior talocalcaneal joint (CPTC), and interosseous ligaments demonstrated a major role in subtalar stability

The cervical ligaments assist the CFL in promoting lateral subtalar stability, and tend to elongate with injury of the CFL. Not only could this lead to subtalar instability, but it could also lead to lingering subtalar instability even after the ankle regains its stability (with healing of the ATFL) (Martin et al. 1998).

■ Treatment

Nonoperative treatment, such as muscle strengthening, Achilles stretching, and proprioceptive re-education, may be sufficient to alleviate symptoms. Commercial or custom-made supports and braces can be useful in maintaining stability.

If these methods are ineffective or not tolerated by the patient, surgical intervention may be considered. Because subtalar instability is often associated with ankle ligamentous injury, most of the surgical procedures are aimed at resolving both.

Thermann et al. (1997) suggest an algorithm of surgical treatment of ankle/subtalar instability. The choice of the procedure is based on four prerequisites:

1. Ligament structure intact or scarred onto the osseous insertion = reconstruction or reinsertion.

2. Ligament elongation or scar remnants = periosteal flap repair.

3. Double ligament lesions = reconstruction of both ligaments or reconstruction of one ligament and a periosteal flap (modified Evans procedure).

4. Isolated subtalar instability = tenodesis (Chrisman-Snook procedure).

Cases of severe subtalar degenerative joint disease (DJD) may require an arthrodesis. The surgical procedures are described in chapter 31.

■ References

Astrom M, Arvidson T. 1995. Alignment and joint motion in the normal foot. J Orthop Sports Phys Ther 22:216-222.

Clanton TO. 1989. Instability of the subtalar joint. Orthop Clin N Am 20(4):583-592.

Clanton TO. 1999. Athletic injuries to the soft tissues of the foot and ankle. In Coughlin MJ, Mann RA, editors. Surgery of the foot and ankle. St Louis, MO: Mosby, pp. 1146-1147.

Ferkel RD. Whipple TL (Editor) Burst SE 1996. Arthroscopic surgery: The foot and ankle. Lippincott Williams & Wilkins, p. 2348.

Frey C, Feder KS, DiGiovanni C. 1999. Arthroscopic evaluation of the subtalar joint: does sinus tarsi syndrome exist? Foot Ankle Int 29(3):185-191.

Goossens M, De Stoop N, Claessens H, Van der Straeten C. 1989. Posterior subtalar joint arthrography. A useful tool in the diagnosis of hindfoot disorders. Clin Orthop Dec (249):248-255.

James SL, Bates BT, Ostering LR. 1978. Injuries to runners. Am J Sports Med 6(4):40-50.

Karlsson J, Eriksson BI, Renström PA. 1997. Subtalar ankle instability. Sports Med 24(5):337-345.

Kato T. 1995. The diagnosis and treatment of instability of the subtalar joint. J Bone Joint Surg Br 77(3):400-406.

Kjaersgaard-Anderson P, Wethelund J, Helmig P et al. 1988. The stabilizing effect of the ligamentous structures in the sinus and canalis tarsi on movements in the hindfoot: an experimental study. Am J Sports Med 16:512-516.

Klein MA, Spreitzer AM. 1993. MR imaging of the tarsal sinus and canal: Normal anatomy, pathologic findings and features of the sinus tarsi syndrome. Radiology 186 (1): 223-240

Mann RA, Coughlin MJ. 1993. Surgery of the foot and ankle. 6th ed. St. Louis, MO: Mosby.

Martin LP, Wayne JS, Monahan TJ, Adelaar RS. 1998. Elongation behavior of calcaneofibular and cervical ligaments during inversion loads applied in an open kinetic chain. Foot Ankle Int 19(4):232-239.

Pearce TJ, Buckley RE. 1999. Subtalar joint movement: clinical and computed tomography scan correlation. Foot Ankle Int 20(7):428-432.

Shahabpour M, Handelberg F, Opdecam M, Osteaux M, Spruyt D, Vaes P, Verhaven E, Zygas P. Magnetic resonance imaging (MRI) of the ankle and hindfoot. Acta Orthop Belg. 1992;58 Suppl 1:5-14.

Thermann et al. 1997. Treatment algorithm of chronic ankle and subtalar instability. Foot Ankle Int 18(3):163-169.

van Hellemondt FJ, Louwerens JW, Sijbrandij ES, van Gils AP. 1997. Stress radiography and stress examination of the talocrural and subtalar joint on helical computed tomography. Foot Ankle Int 18(8):482-488.

Wernick J, Langer S. 1972. A practical manual for a basic approach to biomechanics. Vol. 1. New York: Langer Acrylic Laboratory.

Chapter 19

Midfoot Sprain

Meir Nyska, MD, and Gideon Mann, MD

Acute inversion injury of the foot usually causes sprain or tear of the lateral ligaments of the ankle. The inversion forces acting on the foot may be transmitted forward to cause injury to the midfoot—the calcaneonavicular and talonavicular joint (Chopart) and the tarsometatarsal joint (Lisfranc). The accumulating force may cause a sprain of the ligaments of these joints and eventually fracture-dislocations. Sprains of ligaments may be graded as

- grade I: stretching,
- grade II: partial tear, or
- grade III: complete tear, which usually causes mechanical instability.

The stretching or tearing of ligaments might take place at the midsubstance or at the insertion to bone. If the tear is at the insertion, it may include a small avulsion fracture, which can be seen clearly on plain radiography.

■ Anatomy and Pathophysiology

In the following paragraphs, we will review in brief the anatomical structures previously discussed in chapter 2.

The posterior border of the midfoot is the talonavicular and the calcaneonavicular joint, which are known as the Chopart joint. The anterior border of the midfoot is the tarsometatarsal joint, which is known as the Lisfranc joint. The dorsal talonavicular ligament and the plantar talonavicular ligament stabilize the talonavicular joint and make up the spring ligament. On the lateral side there are dorsal and plantar calcaneonavicular ligaments and the bifurcate ligament. The bifurcate ligament is a major stabilizer of the calcaneonavicular joint. It runs from the anterior calcaneal tuberosity in two strong bands to the lateral side of the navicular and the dorsal surface of the cuboid. The second metatarsal is the keyhole bony stabilizer of the Lisfranc joint, because it sits firmly between the medial and lateral cuneiforms. The short and thick Lisfranc ligament runs from the medial base of the second metatarsal to the lateral side of the medial cuneiform, and locks the base of the metatarsals and cuneiforms tightly. The tight construction of the midfoot provides the insertion to the strong dorsiflexor and plantarflexor tendons of the foot. These include the peroneus longus and brevis, tibialis posterior, and tibialis anterior tendons.

Midfoot sprain may involve the lateral column, including calcaneocuboid ligamentous injuries and bifurcate ligament injury; or it may involve the medial column, including the talonavicular ligaments, the Lisfranc ligament, and the intercuneiform ligaments (Holmer et al. 1994, Sondergaard et al. 1996).

The motion of the midfoot is limited and includes adduction, abduction, supination, pronation, dorsiflexion, and plantarflexion. Most of these motions are passive, therefore excessive motion occurs only in trauma. The classification of injuries of the midtarsal joints is well known and is based on the nature of the deforming force: medial, longitudinal compression, lateral, plantar, and crush type (Main and Jowett 1975). Forced pronation (inversion) of the forefoot causes tension on the lateral column of the foot and compression of the medial column. Forced supination (eversion) of the forefoot causes dorsal translation of the medial column and plantar translation of the lateral column. During inversion injury, both of the forces acting on the foot are usually also accompanied by axial compression, leading to tears and avulsion injuries of the lateral column and compression injuries of the medial column.

■ Incidence

There are few reports in the literature on midfoot sprain, and most of those that do exist relate to sport injuries. Meyer et al. (1994) found an occurrence of 4% per year in football players, with offensive linemen incurring 29.2% of the injuries. In another retrospective review concerning foot injuries in athletes, midfoot injuries made up 12.7% of the total (Clanton et al. 1986). In a survey of 766 patients having ankle inversion sprain, most of the injuries occurred during sport activity (Holmer et al. 1994). Sport was more dominant as the cause of injury in the lateral ankle ligaments than in the midfoot. In Holmer's study, there were two main locations of maximum tenderness. The first was around the lateral malleolus (in 61% of the patients), and the other was at the lateral midfoot (in 24% of the patients). The location pointed to injury of the transverse tarsal joint (Chopart's joint). The median age of patients with symptoms evolving from the midfoot was 29.7 years versus 23.1 years for patients with lesions around the lateral malleolus. Females experienced a larger percentage of midfoot lesions than males. In an epidemiological study of running injuries among 4,358 males, Marti et al. (1988) noted a 3.2% incidence of midfoot injuries. They did not, however, specify the exact nature of these injuries.

In another follow-up study of 162 patients having midtarsal injuries and 161 patients having lateral ankle sprain, Sondergaard et al. (1996) did not find differences between the groups in the persistence of residual symptoms after 1-year follow-up. The frequencies of both pain (48%) and swelling (36%) were significantly lower in the group of midfoot lesions when compared with the group of isolated lateral ligament lesions (61% and 36%, respectively) after 1 month. Similar observations were seen for swelling after 3 months (12% vs 39%).

Agnholt et al. (1988) found clinical signs of damage to the bifurcate ligament of the midfoot in 40.5% of 106 patients with history of acute ankle sprain. It seems that this injury is much more common than is reported in the literature.

■ Assessment

Clinical examination should raise suspicion of a midfoot sprain, as diagnostic measures as well as treatment are considered differently in midfoot sprains and in ankle sprains.

■ **Clinical evaluation.** Patients may complain of diffuse pain following a midfoot sprain, and they may find it difficult to locate the exact location of that pain. The pain may involve the hindfoot, or even the ankle, and may radiate to the whole leg. The pain will be increased by weight bearing or any other activity. Clinical examination will demonstrate the maximal point of tenderness and swelling to be located in the midfoot. Pain may be located at the lateral midfoot over the calcaneocuboid and the bifurcate ligament, on the medial side at the talonavicular ligament, or at

the Lisfranc ligament. It is not difficult to differentiate these locations of pain from the maximal point of tenderness occurring in lateral ankle ligament injury (Sondergaard et al. 1996). In order to locate the exact injury, stress the midfoot in all directions and determine the exact location of pain. It may be medial on the talonavicular joint, on the tarsometatarsal medial joint, or on the bifurcate ligament.

■ **Radiological evaluation.** Plain radiography, including standard anterioposterior and lateral oblique views, will demonstrate most of the fractures occurring in the midfoot. In complete tears of the tarsometatarsal ligaments, including the Lisfranc ligament, there might be instability of the midfoot. Even plain radiography can demonstrate subtle widening of the intercuneiform space or displacement of the second metatarsal from the intermediate cuneiform. It is important to note that the second metatarsal should be in line with the intermediate cuneiform in all radiographic projections. Stress radiographs with pronation-abduction and supination-adduction can assist in disclosing instability of the tarsometatarsal joint (Zwipp et al. 1986). If a patient experiences chronic pain after injury of the midfoot, but radiography is normal, increased uptake on a Technetium bone scan would raise the suspicion of midfoot injury. Groshar et al (1995) presented a patient with inversion injury of the foot. Radiography was inconclusive, whereas radionuclide bone scintigraphy showed marked increased uptake at the injured site. Hyperemia and local abnormalities of permeability associated with the injury process caused the increased uptake observed in the three-phase bone scintigraphy. This scintigraphic pattern associated with the clinical picture made a specific diagnosis of a Lisfranc joint sprain possible. The patient had a slow recovery under conservative treatment. If a bone scan demonstrates increased uptake, computerized tomography may demonstrate the exact nature of the injury. Magnetic resonance imaging could occasionally be used to exclude avascular necrosis or occult nondisplaced fractures.

■ Injury of the Lateral Midfoot

Although injury to the lateral midfoot (including the bifurcate ligament) is rarely reported in the literature, Nielsen et al (1987), in a prospective study, found that 40% of the patients who sustained an acute ankle sprain had clinical signs of a lesion of the bifurcate ligament, and 20% had radiological pathology indicating injury to the bifurcate ligament. The clinical presentation consists of localized pain and swelling just anterior to the lateral malleolus at middistance between the tip of the lateral malleolus and the base of the fifth metatarsal (Gellman 1951). The scope of injury includes avulsion fractures of the ligament insertions; fracture of the tip of the anterior tuberosity of the calcaneus; fracture of the lateral part of the navicularis; and fracture of the dorsal lateral part of the cuboid. A tear of the midsubstance of the ligament may lead to late sequelae, including calcification with painful limitation of the subtalar motion (Nyska et al. 1994). We reviewed four patients who demonstrated this injury.

■ The first patient sustained an inversion injury during a basketball game and developed painful limitation of the subtalar motion. This limitation lasted for 4 years and was accompanied by localized pain just over the bifurcate ligament. Injection of a local anesthetic to that area relieved the pain. Plain radiography was normal and a bone scan demonstrated increased activity of the lateral midfoot. Computerized tomography demonstrated calcification of the bifurcate ligament. Excision of the calcification alleviated the pain, and the patient regained painless subtalar motion (figure 19.1).

■ The second patient, a middle-aged skier in her early forties, sustained a rotation injury while skiing. Fracture of the lateral malleolus was diagnosed, and she underwent open reduction and internal fixation (figure 19.2a). Follow-up plain radiography 6 weeks later demonstrated an avulsion fracture of the lateral side of the navicularis (figure 19.2b). She was treated conservatively by physiotherapy. At 6 months, the patient still complained of some localized pain and swelling over the lateral midfoot.

■ The third patient, in his mid-twenties, sustained an inversion injury. Plain radiography demonstrated a fracture of the anterior process of the calcaneum. Conservative treatment by immobilization in a cast for 4 weeks, followed by physiotherapy for 2 months, led to complete recovery (figure 19.3).

■ A fourth patient who sustained an avulsion injury of the dorsolateral part of the cuboid had chronic localized pain but refused excision of the fragment.

Recently, we encountered three patients, each of whom sustained an inversion injury of the foot and presented with chronic pain that was increased by physical activity and that continued 3 to 6 months after injury. The patients had localized pain over the lateral midfoot. The pain was increased by supination of the midfoot. Plain radiography was interpreted as normal, but a bone scan showed increased uptake in the midfoot. Computerized tomography of the midfoot demonstrated an avulsion fracture of the anterior tip of the calcaneum in one patient, and an avulsion chip fracture of the lateral dorsal area of the cuboid in the other two patients. At 1-year follow-up, the patient

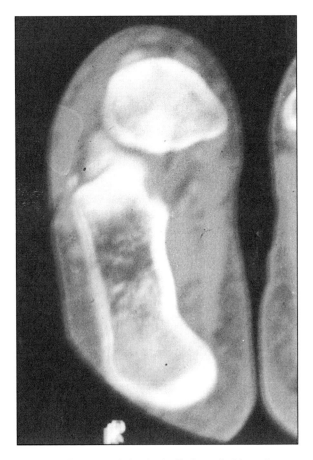

■ **Figure 19.1** A male basketball player in his early twenties sprained his right ankle and continued to experience persistent lateral midfoot pain. A computerized tomogram in the transverse plain identified a large calcification on the anterior aspect of the calcaneum, indicating damage to the bifurcate ligament.

with the fracture of the anterior tuberosity of the calcaneum recovered completely, but the other two still had some pain, mainly during sport activity. They refused any further treatment.

Howie et al.(1986) presented seven patients with damage to the anterior process of the calcaneum at the calcaneocuboid joint. All seven patients had prolonged symptoms. Three had persistent but not disabling pain 3 years after injury, and four patients developed calcaneocuboid joint arthritis.

Sondergaard et al (1996) followed 172 patients with isolated sprains to the midfoot. Of these, 7% (17 patients) had a total of 19 avulsions: 7 to the cuboid bone, 7 to the calcaneum, 2 to the navicular bone, and 3 to the talus. Thirteen of the patients with avulsions had sprains involving only the dorsal midfoot, and the duration of residual symptoms in this group was significantly higher (9 months) than for the group of patients with sprains located at the same joints but without a concomitant avulsion (6 months). Pain during activity was the main disability in all cases.

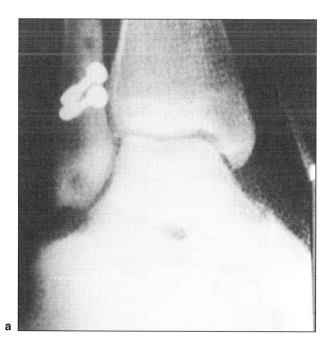
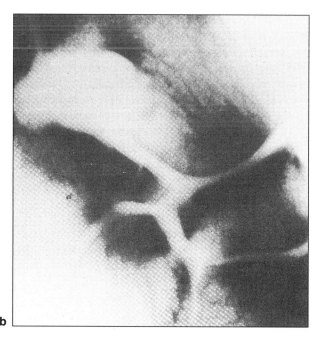

■ **Figure 19.2** A female middle-aged skier suffered a rotation injury of the foot and ankle while skiing. *(a)* A lateral malleolar fracture was diagnosed, and was surgically reduced and fixed. *(b)* Pain persisted, and 6 weeks later an oblique radiograph of the foot revealed an avulsion fracture of the lateral side of the navicular bone, indicating avulsion of the intact bifurcate ligament.

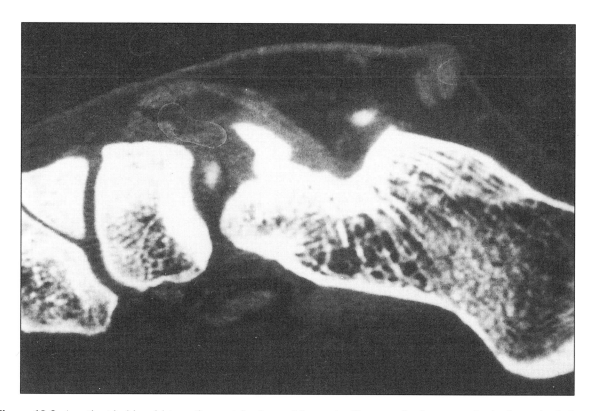

■ **Figure 19.3** A patient in his mid-twenties sustained an ankle sprain. Computerized tomography in the sagittal plane was performed because of persistent midfoot pain, and revealed an avulsion fracture of the anterior-superior calcaneum, indicating an avulsion by the intact bifurcate ligament. This later formed a bony union with the calcaneum, which was seen on a follow-up computerized tomogram. At this stage the patient was asymptomatic.

However, those patients who did not have avulsions recovered and had residual symptoms similar to those of patients who sustained a lateral ligament injury. The benign course of the injury in these patients is most probably attributed to patient selection, because the included cases of ankle sprain were not differentiated according to stages of severity. Patients having grade I injury of the midfoot or of the lateral ligaments of the ankle should usually be considered as having a minor injury that will ultimately fully recover.

■ Injury of the Medial Midfoot

Fracture-dislocations of the tarsometatarsal joints are well known and widely documented injuries that necessitate operative reduction and fixation (Main & Jowett 1975, Resch & Stenstrom1990). However, subtle injuries to these joints, which mainly involve the medial and intermediate cuneiform and the base of the medial metatarsal, are infrequently reported. Diastases of these joints may be easily overlooked. The interspace between the medial and intermediate cuneiform is about 1.3 mm. A space of 2 mm or more is pathological (Faciszewski et al. 1990). The authors demonstrated that the extent of the diastases did not correlate with patient's functional result. However, others could not confirm this conclusion (Clanton & Schon 1993, Resch & Stenstrom 1990, Howie 1986). Lateral weightbearing radiographs can demonstrate loss of the longitudinal arch by measuring the distance between the medial cuneiform and the fifth metatarsal. Normally, the medial cuneiform lies dorsal to the fifth metatarsal (Faciszewski 1990). A negative distance indicates flattening of the arch and is a reliable indicator of how much flattening of the longitudinal arch has occurred. The flattening of the arch is associated with a poor prognosis. Reduction and fixation of diastases of these joints is recommended (Zwipp et al. 1986). Three patients were evaluated 4 months after sustaining an inversion injury of the foot, with resulting localized pain in the medial midfoot that was increased by physical activity and by supination of the midfoot. Plain radiography of these patients was normal. A bone scan demonstrated increased uptake in the midfoot. The computerized tomography of the three patients was normal and two of them recovered within 9-12 months. One patient underwent exploration, and a chondral marginal distal navicular osteophyte was resected, leading to full recovery. It should be concluded that when imaging techniques demonstrate any pathology in the medial midfoot, a slow recovery should be expected and surgical treatment may eventually be needed.

■ Conclusions

Midfoot sprains are common injuries but are seldom reported. Recovery from these sprains, if they are simple, is rapid and faster than recovery from a lateral ankle ligament sprain. However, if the midfoot sprain is significant or includes an avulsion fracture or a tear of the bifurcate ligament, the recovery should be expected to be slow and, occasionally, operative treatment may be required.

■ References

Agnholt J, Nielsen S, Christensen H. Lesion of the ligamentum bifurcatum in ankle sprain. Arch Orthop Trauma Surg, 107(5):326-328, 1998.

Clanton TO, Butler JE, Eggert A. Injuries to metatarsophalangeal joints in athletes. Foot Ankle 7:162-176, 1986.

Clanton TO, Schon LC. Athletic injuries to the soft tissues of the foot and ankle—midfoot sprain. In Mann RA, Coughlin MJ, editors. Surgery of the foot and ankle. St. Louis, MO: Mosby, 1184-1191, 1993.

Faciszewski T, Burks RT, Manaster BJ. Subtle injuries of the Lisfranc joint. J Bone Joint Surg 72A:1519-1522, 1990.

Gellman M. Fracture of the anterior process of the calcaneus. J Bone Joint Surg 33A:382. 1951.

Groshar D, Alperson M, Mendes DJ, Barski V, Liberson A. Bone scintigraphy findings in Lisfranc joint injury. Foot Ankle Int. 16(11):710-711, 1995.

Holmer P, Sondergaard L, Konradsen L, Nielsen PT, Jorgensen LN. Epidemiology of sprains in the lateral ankle and foot. Foot Ankle Int 15(2):72-74, 1994.

Howie CR, Hooper G, Hughes SP.Occult midtarsal subluxation. Clin. Orthop. 209:206-209, 1986.

Main BJ, Jowett RL. Injuries of the midtarsal joints. J Bone Joint Surg 57B:89-97, 1975.

Marti B, Vader JP, Minder CE et al. On the epidemiology of running injuries. The 1984 Bern Grand-Prix Study. Am J Sports Med 16:285-294, 1988.

Meyer SA, Callaghan JJ, Albright JP, Crowley ET, Powell JW. Midfoot sprains in collegiate football players. Am J Sports Med 22(3):392-401, 1994.

Nielsen S, Agnholt J, Christensen H. Radiologic findings in lesions of the ligamentum bifurcatum of the midfoot. Skelet Radiol 16:114-116, 1987.

Nyska M, Mann G, Finsterbush A, Matan Y, Elishuv O, Bar-Ziv Y. Injuries of the ligamentum bifurcatum. Medicina Sportiva 3(3):100, 1994.

Resch S, Stenstrom A. The treatment of tarsometatarsal injuries. Foot Ankle 11:117-123, 1990.

Sondergaard L, Konradsen L, Holmer P, Jorgensen LN, Nielsen PT. Acute midtarsal sprains: frequency and course of recovery. Foot Ankle Int 17(4):195-199, 1996.

Zwipp H, Krettek C. Diagnostic und therapy der akuten und chronischen bandistabilitat des unteren sprunggelenkes. Orthopade 15:472-478, 1986.

Part V

Conservative Treatment

Generally speaking, there is very little role, if any, for surgical treatment in acute ankle sprains. The mainstay of appropriate treatment is conservative. Late surgical ankle reconstruction is at least as good as any attempt at acute ankle ligament repair. There are few fields in orthopedics where the physiotherapist has such a major role as in ankle sprain rehabilitation. This role includes the basic management of the acute injury; the rehabilitation program aimed at regaining motion, force, balance, and proprioceptive abilities; and, of course, rehabilitation after any surgical intervention. As Michael Freeman of London pointed out in 1965, rehabilitation by a physiotherapist could probably drop the rate of recurrent sprain by two or three times.

Chapter 20

Management of Acute Ankle Sprains

Per Renström, MD, PhD, and Scott A. Lynch, MD

Ankle injuries are underestimated and, unfortunately, very common. Each day, approximately 23,000 ankle ligament injuries occur in the United States (Makhani 1962; McCulloch et al. 1985).

Seven percent to 10% of those who are examined at emergency departments of the hospitals in Scandinavia have sprained ankles (Viljakka & Rokkanen 1983). In a prospective study in Sweden, 18% of the patients who were treated at a surgical emergency ward of a major hospital had an acute sprain of the ankle (Axelsson et al. 1980).

These injuries tend to occur primarily in young people (Broström 1965), perhaps because many of these injuries result from sport. In fact, ankle injuries are the most common injuries in sport and recreational activity (Balduini et al. 1987; Brand et al. 1977; Fiore & Leard 1980; Garrick 1977; Garrick & Requa 1988; Glick et al. 1976; Hardaker et al. 1985; Lassiter et al. 1989; McConkey 1987). In 1973, Garrick and Requa studied 1,650 high school students in several sports. Ankle injuries occurred frequently in most sports. The percentage was highest for basketball, where 53% of the injuries involved the ankle. In a study of 19 sports over a 7.5-year period, approximately one-quarter of all the injuries occurred to the foot and ankle, with about 21% occurring in basketball and figure skating (Garrick & Requa 1973). In 1990, Ekstrand and Tropp reviewed 41 soccer teams and found ankle sprains to account for 17% to 21% of all injuries. In 1982, Ekstrand noted that 46% of soccer players had a history of ankle sprains. Sandelin et al. (1988) observed that 29% of all injuries of the lower extremities in soccer were in the ankle, and of the ankle injuries, 75% involved the lateral ligament structures. Mack (1982) found ankle ligament injuries to constitute about 25% of injuries occurring in running and jumping sports. Ankle ligament injuries are the most common trauma in modern dance and classical ballet (Hardaker et al. 1985). At the United States Military Academy at West Point, one-third of the cadets can be expected to sprain an ankle during their 4-year term (Balduini et al. 1987).

In spite of the high frequency of ankle injuries, there is great variation in clinical diagnostic techniques and methods of treatment. The biomechanics of the ankle joint, and the function of its ligaments and their evaluation, are not yet well understood, which could be an explanation for these variations.

■ Grades of Injury

The damage after an ankle ligament injury can be classified a number of ways. There is no standardized system for grading ankle sprain severity, but the most frequently used terms are **mild, moderate,** and **severe**. By Hamilton's (1982) description, these would be defined as follows: A grade I, or mild, sprain involves a ligament stretch without macroscopic tearing, little swelling or tenderness, minimal or no functional loss, and no mechanical joint instability. A grade II, or moderate, sprain consists of a torn anterior talofibular ligament (ATFL) with an intact calcaneofibular ligament (CFL), involving a partial macroscopic ligament tear with moderate pain, swelling and tenderness, some loss of joint motion, and mild joint instability. A grade III, or severe, sprain consists of a tear of the entire lateral ligament complex, involving a complete ligament rupture with marked swelling, hemorrhage, and tenderness. Lindenfeld (1988) finds these terms quite subjective. Others (Black et al. 1978; Cox 1985) prefer to classify lateral ligament injuries as single or double ligament tears rather than first-, second-, or third-degree sprains. A "single" would involve only the ATFL, and a "double" would involve both the ATFL and the CFL (figures 20.1-20.4).

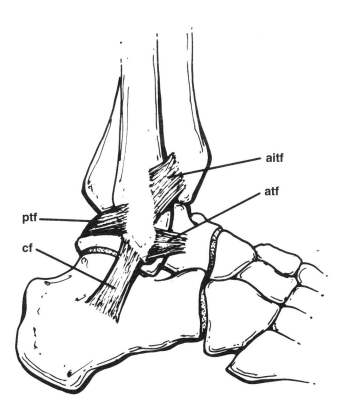

■ **Figure 20.1** The lateral ligamentous complex of the ankle consists of the anterior talofibular (ATF), calcaneofibular (CF), and posterior talofibular (PTF) ligaments. AITF = anterior inferior tibiofibular ligament.

■ **Figure 20.2** Ankle ligaments viewed from the posterior. PITF = posterior inferior tibiofibular ligament, PTF = posterior talofibular ligament, CF = calcaneofibular ligament, and D = deltoid ligament.

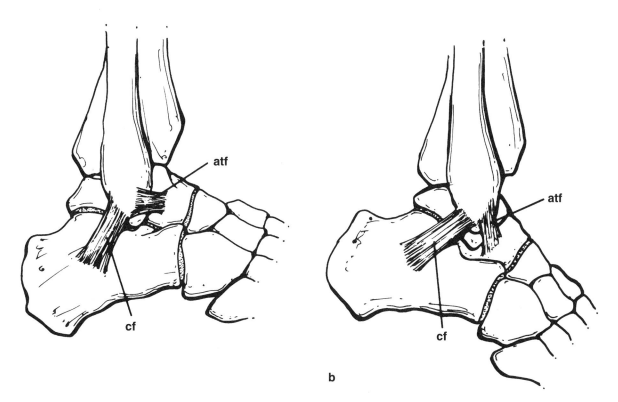

a

b

■ **Figure 20.3** *(a)* The anterior talofibular (ATF) ligament runs parallel to the axis of the foot when the foot is in neutral position. CF = calcaneofibular ligament. *(b)* When the foot is in plantarflexion, the ATF ligament assumes a course parallel to the axis of the tibia and fibula.

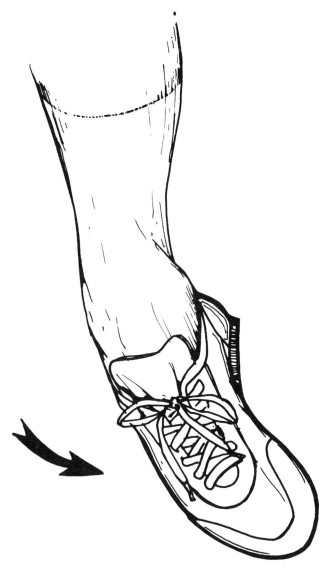

■ **Figure 20.4** A typical injury mechanism of an ankle sprain: plantarflexion, inversion, and adduction.

■ Conservative Versus Surgical Treatment

Once the diagnosis has been made, a treatment regimen must be decided on. Almost all authors have agreed that patients who have grade I or grade II injuries recover quickly with nonoperative management (Balduini et al. 1987; Brand et al. 1977; Diamond 1989; Lassiter et al. 1989) and that the prognosis is, almost without exception, excellent or good (Balduini & Tetzlaff 1982; Balduini et al. 1987; Brooks et al. 1981; Derscheid & Brown 1985; Hamilton 1988; Jackson et al. 1974; Lassiter et al. 1989; McCulloch et al. 1985; Prins 1978; Ryan et al. 1989). The treatment program, usually called functional treatment, includes four phases. Immediately

after the injury, rest, ice (cold), compression, and elevation (RICE) are used. Then there is a short period of immobilization and protection with supportive bandaging, taping, or bracing to control pain and swelling. After this, early active range-of-motion exercises are started, followed by weight bearing, proprioceptive training with a tilt board, strengthening exercises for the peroneal muscle, and finally gradual return to work and sport. These stages are further detailed in the following pages. Jackson et al. (1974) found that in cadets who followed this type of regimen, the duration of disability was 8 days for a grade I injury and 15 days for a grade II injury.

The treatment of grade III sprains of the lateral ligament complex is more controversial. Many uncontrolled, nonrandomized studies have suggested that primary repair is the method of choice, since most patients who had operative treatment seem to have a mechanically stable ankle and satisfactory subjective results (Anderson et al. 1962; Brand et al. 1981; Jaskulka et al. 1988; Korkala et al. 1982; Niethard 1974; Redler et al. 1977; Reichen & Marti 1974; Ruth 1961; Staples 1975). However, similar results have been reported after conservative treatment (Adler 1976; Chirls 1973; Drez et al. 1982; Hansen et al. 1979; Henning & Egge 1977; Jakob et al. 1986; Leonard 1949; McMaster 1943).

Kannus and Renström Review

A review by Kannus and Renström in 1991 includes an extensive evaluation of all the prospectively randomized studies (n =12) available in the literature at that time that compared cast immobilization, strapping with early mobilization, and surgery followed by casting. In general, according to the 12 studies, the results after treatment of an acute grade III sprain of the lateral ligaments of the ankle were excellent. In most patients (75% to 100%), irrespective of the therapy (repair and cast, cast alone, or early controlled mobilization), the 1-year prognosis was excellent or good and fully acceptable, and only a few patients had residual symptoms. Interestingly, these overall results were better than those reported in earlier studies (Bosien et al. 1955; Hansen et al. 1979; Leonard 1949; Staples 1975; Termansen et al. 1979). Furthermore, the 12 studies could not identify any difference between the patients who had an isolated rupture of the anterior talofibular ligament and those who had a combined injury of the anterior talofibular and calcaneofibular ligaments. These findings may partially explain why in all retrospective, uncontrolled studies, the treatment that is presented has led to fine results, and why such a controversy about proper treatment can persist for years.

In each study, the authors reached a final conclusion about the proper treatment of acute grade III sprains of the lateral ligaments of the ankle. Of the five studies in which treatment with an operation and a cast was compared with treatment with a cast alone, the authors of three (Garrick 1977; Jozsa, Reffy et al. 1988; Jozsa, Thoring et al. 1988) concluded that conservative treatment (cast alone) is the method of choice, even though they indicated that early mobilization might give better results. Clark et al. (1965) also recommended conservative treatment, with one exception, a young athlete who had a severe tear and a talar tilt of more than 15°, for whom they recommended operative treatment. Prins (1978) recommended operative repair as the best method of treatment. In all seven studies that had three treatment groups, the authors recommended functional treatment as the primary choice. Four (Freeman et al. 1965; Moller-Larsen et al. 1988; Sommer & Arza 1989; van Moppens et al. 1992) recommended functional treatment without any reservations, and three (Broström 1966; Gromnark et al. 1980; Korkala et al. 1982) cited one reservation: the young, active athlete, for whom primary operative repair should be considered.

In their review, Kannus and Renström (1991) concluded that functional treatment should be the first method of choice for complete lateral ankle ligament rupture. This type of treatment includes a short period of ankle protection by tape, bandage, or brace, and allows early mobility and weight bearing.

Additional Studies

The study by Kannus and Renström (1991) has been repeated by Shrier (1995). His data analysis also shows that the concept of early mobilization with the proper rehabilitation program should be the treatment of choice. Kaikkonen et al. (1996) also evaluated surgical treatment with early mobilization versus functional rehabilitation for grade II ankle sprains in a prospectively randomized trial. At 9-month follow-up, 87% of the rehabilitation group and 60% of the surgical group had good or excellent results. This further supports functional rehabilitation.

Konradsen et al. (1992) published the results of treatment of grade III ankle ligament injuries as defined by talar tilt of more than 9° and anterior talar translation of more than 10° by stress radiographs. Eighty patients with a mean age of 23 years were randomized to either cast immobilization or treatment with an Aircast functional brace for 6 weeks. Results at 1 week showed that 22% of the early mobilization patients could walk normally. At several weeks, 100% of the patients treated with early mobilization could walk normally and resumed work. This was compared to 81% of the cast immobilization group that were able to walk normally and return to work. By 3 months, both groups had reached 100% for these categories, but 86% of the early mobilization group had returned to sport as compared with only 49% of the casted patients. Ten percent of all patients complained of residual disability at 1 year; the complaints included functional instability, occasional pain with sport, and/or secondary sprains.

Sommer and Schreiber (1993) found functional treatment to be superior to immobilization in a cast both in terms of recurrent ankle instability and the cost of treatment. Leanderson and Wredmark (1995) compared the use of a semirigid brace with a compression bandage in 73 patients. They found that the group treated with a semirigid air stirrup brace was more mobile, showed a larger range of motion in the initial phase of rehabilitation, and had the shortest sick leave.

Although initial protective treatment of severe ankle sprains is necessary to prevent further injury of the damaged joint and ligaments, rehabilitation exercises are considered by some to be the most important step in the treatment process (Cox 1985; Lindenfeld 1988). The goal of rehabilitation is to return the injured ankle to its pre-injury condition by reestablishing ankle range of motion, muscle strength, and neuromuscular control. If functional treatment fails, late surgery is as successful as early surgery (Kitaoka et al. 1997).

■ Four Basic Phases of Treatment and Rehabilitation

In the postinjury phase, an ideal treatment and rehabilitation program fulfills four requirements: (Kannus & Renström 1991)

1. Immediately after the injury, the ankle should be treated with the RICE principle: rest, ice (cold), compression, and elevation. The aim is to minimize hemorrhage, swelling, inflammation, cellular metabolism, and pain in order to offer the best possible conditions for the healing process (Burry 1975; Järvinen & Lehto 1993).

2. The second requirement is protection of the injured ligaments during the first 1 to 3 weeks. In this phase of healing (the proliferation phase), immobilization is followed by undisturbed fibroblast invasion of the injured area, which leads to undisturbed proliferation and production of collagen fibers. In this phase, mobilization too early leads to more prolonged type III collagen formation with weaker healing tissue than during optimal immobilization (Järvinen 1976; Järvinen & Lehto 1993; Lehto 1983). Protection is

needed to prevent secondary injuries and early disruption and lengthening of the injured ligaments.

3. Approximately 3 weeks after the injury, the maturation phase of the collagen and the formation of final scar tissue begins (Järvinen 1976; Lehto 1983; Montgomery & Steadman 1985). In this phase the injured ligaments need controlled mobilization, and perhaps even more importantly, the ankle itself must avoid the deleterious effects of immobilization on joint cartilage, bone, muscles, tendons and ligaments (Akeson et al. 1980; Haggmark & Eriksson 1979; Jozsa et al. 1987; Jozsa et al. 1988; Montgomery & Steadman 1985; Noyes 1977; Ogata et al. 1980). Controlled stretching of muscles and movement of the joint enhance the orientation of collagen fibers parallel with the stress lines (i.e., the normal collagen fibers of the ligaments), and they can prevent the atrophy caused by immobilization (Järvinen & Lehto 1993; Lehto 1983). Repeated exercises will also increase the mechanical and structural properties of the ligaments (Woo et al. 1987).

4. Approximately 4 to 8 weeks after the injury, the new collagen fibers begin to withstand almost normal stress, and the goal for rehabilitation is rapid recovery and full return to work and sport. If treated according to the guidelines mentioned above, there is no pathophysiological reason to continue the protection any longer. In other words, each component of the ankle is ready for a gradually increasing mobilization and rehabilitation program, keeping in mind that final maturation and remodeling of the injured ligaments takes a long time, from 6 to 12 months.

■ Functional Treatment Protocol

The exact treatment protocol varies from clinic to clinic (Balduini & Tezlaff 1982; Drez et al. 1982; Hamilton 1988; Lassiter et al. 1989; Ryan et al. 1989), but its principles are the same at most centers. All agree that RICE therapy should start immediately after the injury:

- ■ R = rest, which means rest until a diagnosis is secured and, thereafter, gradually increasing motion exercises.
- ■ I = ice, which has its greatest effect on pain. Ice may also have some effects on cell metabolism, and thereby on swelling.
- ■ C = compression, which is very important initially in an ankle injury.
- ■ E = elevation, which means that the ankle should be kept clearly elevated in order to decrease the swelling.

Protection should be used for the ankle for 1 to 3 weeks followed by early controlled mobilization with some kind of ankle support.

Protection

The protection can be given by tape, Ace wrap, brace (orthosis), or cast.

Tape and Strapping

Traditionally, ankle ligament injuries have been treated with strapping and/or with taping, or with immobilization. Adhesive tape offers protection against ankle sprains during sport activity.

The primary purpose of taping is to provide a semirigid and sometimes rigid splint around the ankle. There are studies indicating that taping of the ankle is of value in the prevention of ankle injuries. Garrick and Requa (1973) found that the combination of taping prophylactically and the use of high-top shoes in basketball reduced the amount of ankle sprains. Lindenberger et al. (1990) found that tape had a significant prophylactic effect against injuries to the lateral ligaments of the ankle. In their study, players in team handball were studied prospectively during two full seasons. Six top-level teams participated in the first year. In three teams the players were taped, and in three teams the players were not taped. During the first season, 13 ankle sprains occurred; all of these occurred in the non-taped group. In the second season nine teams participated. Twenty-one ankle sprains occurred. Twenty of these were in the non-taped group, and only one occurred in the taped group. Taping of the ankle was, in other words, shown to have a significant effect in preventing injuries to the lateral ligaments of the ankle in this prospective study.

There has been a question regarding whether tape would influence performance and technique during sport activity. Taping of an injured ankle will decrease the range of motion for up to 2 to 3 hours of physical activity (Fiore & Leard 1980). Thomas and Cotton (1971) found no change in agility drills during taping, while Coffman and Mize (1989) found a decrease in sprint speed and vertical jump. Tape, applied incorrectly, might not only lead to decreased performance, but may also predispose for and add to injury of either the joint immobilized or to other joints along the kinetic chain. The mechanism behind the effect of ankle taping is not well known. Tape not only restricts excess joint motion, but also enhances the proprioceptive feedback mechanism and shortens the recruitment time of the dynamic ankle stabilizers.

Tape may give many athletes skin reactions; therefore skin protections may be used. Delacerda (1975) found no difference in support between tape directly on the skin and tape with skin protections. Because of these skin problems and its high cost, tape is used mostly by elite athletes and not by recreational athletes. It has, therefore, become common clinical practice to use conventional strapping with an Ace wrap or an ankle brace for treatment of grade I or II ankle sprains. Strapping with an Ace wrap produces some compression and is, thereby, helpful in controlling the swelling after an ankle sprain. It also allows early motion and can be part of an early functional treatment program.

The supportive function of strapping with an Ace wrap is not as high as that with a cast or brace. This kind of treatment should be combined with crutches if needed. Weight bearing starts as tolerated. Strapping with the Ace wrap has been used by Broström (1966) in his classic PhD thesis, in which he showed that patients using an Ace wrap were doing well, and had medical end results after 1 year that could be compared with those for patients with 6 weeks immobilization in a cast. There was, however, a sequelae frequency after ankle sprains of about 20%, which can be compared with the literature as a whole, which reports 10% to 20% sequelae, such as chronic instability and/or pain, after ankle sprains.

Plaster Cast Immobilization

Fifty years ago, ligaments were believed to require immobilization in order to heal. Based on this philosophy, cast immobilization became a very common treatment. In Shrier's review, there is no difference in the static stability of ankles treated with early mobilization as compared with cast immobilization (Glasgow et al. 1980; Ozeki et al. 1990; Sandelin et al. 1988; Shrier 1995). Most articles at that time stressed objective findings, such as static stability, instead of subjective findings, such as pain or functional instability. Broström (1966) noted that static mechanical stability did not correlate with symptoms.

Immobilization with a plaster cast is used extensively around the world and is very common in many emergency rooms in the United States for ankle sprains. Application of a plaster cast has the advantage of immobilizing the joint, allowing healing, and at the same time decreasing swelling and pain. It also allows the patient to be weight bearing within a few days. Cast immobilization has not, however, been shown to reduce time off work for mild (Brand et al. 1977) or severe sprains (Dias 1979). The disadvantages are that the joint is immobilized, with all of the secondary effects of immobilization. The effects of immobilization on the histology of the ligaments are not well documented in the literature, but there are grounds to believe that the effects are very much the same as those described in tendons. Immobilization seems to cause a decrease in total collagen mass of ligaments (Amiel et al. 1984; Klein et al. 1988), although this has not been uniformly found.

Broström (1966) and Lindstrand (1976) included plaster cast immobilization as a treatment group in their studies. They showed that after 1 year, the results were similar to those of surgery and functional treatment, although surgery resulted in less residual problems. Other studies that have used immobilization have demonstrated similar results (Korkala et al. 1987; Milford & Dunleavy 1990; Sommer & Arza 1989; van Moppens & van den Hoogenband 1992). The conventional risks of immobilization are well known, and they should be balanced with the benefits of good protection and decreased joint pain.

Ankle Braces

The use of ankle orthoses has increased over the past decade. Ankle taping has been extensively used for ankle sprains, but it is expensive and, as noted above, creates skin problems. Therefore, ankle orthoses have been developed. One of these types, the Aircast Air-Stirrup Ankle Brace, has been used extensively since the 1970s because it provides good support in inversion and eversion. At the same time, this device allows some motion in plantarflexion and dorsiflexion.

When a patient walks with an Aircast, the pressure pulsates, rising with the muscular contraction and flexion of each step. Tests show the pulsation is significantly stronger under the distal air cell. This massaging compression is believed to contribute to a reduction in swelling and an increase in comfort and mobility (Alves et al. 1992; Bergfeld et al. 1986). The effectiveness of the Aircast is shown in several clinical studies (Fritschy & Bonvin 1987; Konradsen et al. 1992; Raemy & Jacob 1993; Stover 1986). Milford & Dunleavy (1990) compared 60 patients with treatment using an Aircast versus daily strapping with elastoplast bandages. They found that the return to function was shorter with the Aircast. In a prospective, randomized study of 80 patients with grade III lateral sprains, Konradsen et al. (1992) found that early immobilization with the air stirrup brace provided earlier return to work and sport than cast immobilization.

Although other ankle braces have been developed and used—in particular the lace-on braces—they have not yet been substantially evaluated scientifically. One study comparing prophylactic ankle taping and wrapping with laced braces (Bunch et al. 1985) found that initially adhesive tape provided the best support, but it quickly lost its effect. Rovere et al. (1988) studied retrospectively the effectiveness of taping and laced ankle braces on ankle sprains of college football players. They found that the most effective prophylactic device was a combination of low-top shoes and laced ankle stabilizers. Ankle taping was less effective in injury prevention then laced ankle braces. Both tape and braces seem to work well for the athletes, although scientific evidence for this effect is limited.

There have been discussions about the effect on performance by braces. Coffman and Mize (1989) evaluated the effects of tape and Aircast's Sport Stirrup on sprinting and vertical jump. They found decreased speed in the sprint as well as a decrease in vertical jump with the tape but not with the brace. Burks (Burks et al. 1991) compared tape with two different lace-on braces (Kallassy and Swede-O-Universal) in terms of performance in a broad jump, vertical jump, 10-yard shuttle run, and 40-yard sprint. Overall, the Kallassy restricted performance the least, with significant differences found only in vertical jumping. Greene and Wight (1990) compared the effect of Swede-O-Universal, Aircast Air Stirrup, and DonJoy ALP on the athletes' ability to run around the bases on a softball field. The Aircast significantly slowed base running, but neither the DonJoy or Swede-O-Universal had a significant effect on base running completion time. Gross et al. (1994) compared the DonJoy ALP with Aircast Sport Stirrup during a 40-m sprint, figure-of-eight run, and vertical jump, and found no significant difference in performance between braced and unbraced condition. The Aircast brace was rated as more comfortable. Studies on performance changes are thus somewhat confusing, but appear to indicate that orthoses tend to restrict performance less than tape. The measured studies are, however, carried out with normal subjects. In the only study of bracing and performance on functionally unstable ankles, Jerosch et al. (1997) found that both bracing and taping significantly enhanced performance in special single-leg jumping and side stepping tests.

Shoes

Studies support the use of high-top shoes for ankle sprain prevention because of their ability to limit extreme range of motion, provide additional proprioceptive input, and decrease external joint stress (Barrett & Bilisko 1995). Few clinical studies, however, have been carried out to examine the effect shoes have on the incidence of ankle sprains. The biomechanical support has not been shown through clinical trials to translate into a lower rate of ankle sprains when using high-top shoes. Further studies are needed.

Ankle Mobilization

Ankle mobilization is started as soon as possible with limited plantarflexion and dorsiflexion. The patient should be more careful with starting inversion/eversion activities, as these activities usually cause pain and may stretch the healing ligaments. Weight bearing should usually start as early as tolerated. If the patient cannot bear weight within 7 to 10 days, a more serious injury should be suspected.

An active rehabilitation program must include stretching, strengthening, and proprioceptive exercises. All muscle groups around the ankle, especially the evertors of the foot, should be exercised. Assisted eversion exercises should be performed in dorsiflexion for peroneus brevis and tertius, and in plantarflexion for peroneus longus. Some recent studies have implicated an imbalance of the invertor/evertor muscle strength ratio as a cause of ankle sprains (Wilkerson et al. 1997). Thus, we must not neglect the training of the other muscle groups. For conditioning, the patient can start stationary cycling or swimming immediately.

Proprioception training with a tilt board is allowed and should start as early as possible; however, in practice, for grade III sprains the patient cannot start these kinds of exercises until after about 4 weeks. The aim of this training is to improve balance and neuromuscular control. Tropp et al. (1985) have shown that it should be carried out for a minimum of 10 weeks, the time when the effect usually reaches a maximal plateau. Wester et al. (1996) have confirmed the positive effects of tilt board training. See chapters 5, 22, 23, and 24 for details on proprioceptive training.

■ Supportive Treatment Modalities

Passive physical therapy modalities are often recommended to promote healing in the early rehabilitation phase. The most frequently used are ultrasound, temperature contrast baths, short waves, and various current therapies including dynamic or interference current therapy, or electrogalvanic stimulation. The effect of these modalities is under question, as no randomized controlled studies have verified their efficacy. Of the different types of passive physical therapy, only cryotherapy has been proven to be effective (Cote et al. 1988).

Nonsteroidal anti-inflammatory drugs (NSAIDs) have been studied in prospectively randomized double-blind trials and found to be more effective than placebo concerning ankle function, tenderness, swelling, and pain. However, the differences were not striking and seemed to disappear during an extended follow-up (Dupont et al. 1987; Viljakka & Rokkanen 1983).

In cases with chronic postinjury swelling, moist heat packs, warm whirlpool baths, contrast baths, electrogalvanic stimulation, and intermittent pneumatic compression (IPC) have been tried (Balduini et al. 1987). Only IPC has been shown in prospectively randomized studies to have an independent capacity to reduce the amount of swelling (Airaksinen 1989; Airaksinen et al. 1988). The IPC device consists of a compressor and a compressive stocking, which is placed over the lower extremity. A compressive wave begins from the distal part of the stocking and continues proximally, and, thereby, reduces the ankle edema and increases the mobility of the joint.

■ Surgery

Although primary repair has long been considered the treatment of choice by many authors, more recent studies have found little difference in long-term results in patients treated conservatively with functional treatment and those treated surgically. Therefore, the treatment of choice in acute cases is functional treatment. However, some authors have recommended operative repair of acute grade III ankle sprains in young athletes (Arms et al. 1988; Jackson & Hutson 1986; Ozeki et al. 1990). Indications for acute repair in athletes as listed by Leach and Schepsis (1990) are

- a history of momentary talocrural dislocation with complete ligamentous disruption,

- a clinical anterior drawer sign,

- 10° more tilt on the affected side with stress inversion testing,

- clinical or radiographic suspicion of tears in both the ATFL and CFL, and

- osteochondral fracture.

Technique

Most techniques described for repair of acute ligament injuries are similar. The incision begins above the level of the tibial plafond, approximately 1 cm in front of and parallel to the anterior border of the fibula, and is carried distally approximately 2 cm past the tip of the fibula. The intermediate dorsal and lateral dorsal cutaneous nerves must be protected during subcutaneous dissection. Extensive capsular disruption usually makes arthrotomy unnecessary. The ATFL is identified, and thereafter the peroneal sheath is opened distally, and the CFL is identified. Application of anterior drawer stress makes identification of the posterior talofibular ligament (PTFL) easier. After irrigation and appropriate debridement, absorbable sutures are placed in the ends of the ATFL and CFL, but they are not tied. Repair of the PTFL is desirable but is not critical if the other two ligaments are appropriately repaired. Once the ATFL and CFL sutures are in place, sutures are placed in the antero-

lateral capsule. The sutures are tied from posterior to anterior, with the ankle held in neutral dorsiflexion and eversion. The peroneal sheath is repaired with absorbable sutures, the wound is closed, and a posterior plaster splint is applied with the foot in neutral dorsiflexion and slight eversion.

Postoperative Management

No weight bearing is allowed for the first week, but isometric calf contractions may be performed in the splint. The splint is removed at 1 week. A removable walking boot is worn for another 3 weeks, during which weight bearing to tolerance is allowed, and dorsiflexion and eversion exercises are begun. At 4 weeks the boot is removed, and an ankle stirrup brace is fitted. Active dorsiflexion and plantarflexion, peroneal strengthening, gentle active inversion, and Achilles stretching exercises are begun. Proprioceptive training and resistive exercises with Theraband (Hygienic Co., Akron, OH) or isokinetic equipment also are started. Gradual progression from walking to straight line running is encouraged, progressing to figure-of-eight running, and eventually cutting maneuvers, if ankle pain and swelling are absent.

If the patient participates in sport on any level, a general program including strengthening of all the lower leg muscles and stretching of the peroneal and calf muscles, in combination with ankle exercises, should be prescribed. Heel and toe raises; walking; exercises with rubber Therabands; rope-skipping; climbing up and down stairs; straight ahead jogging or running; backward running; running in circles and figure-of-eights clockwise and counterclockwise; 90° cuts when running; and running zigzags at 45° should start gradually as part of the rehabilitation for return to sport (Balduini et al. 1987; Lassiter et al. 1989). Sport-specific activities may be gradually resumed, and return to play is allowed when all the exercises listed here can be accomplished without pain or swelling. A protective ankle brace or taping is used to protect the repair for 6 months.

■ Conclusions

The treatment of acute grade III tears of the lateral ligaments of the ankle has generated much controversy, but a critical review of the literature shows that functional treatment should be the method of choice. This functional treatment includes a short period of protection with tape, bandage, or brace, and allows early weight bearing. Range-of-motion exercises, as well as neuromuscular training of the ankle, should begin early. This program provides the quickest recovery to full range of motion and return to work and physical activity. This treatment does not produce an increasing number of residual problems (not even increased mechanical instability). If residual problems are present, secondary surgical reconstruction or delayed anatomic repair of the ruptured ligaments can be performed even years after the injury with good results. These results seem to be comparable with those of primary repair.

■ References

Adler H: Therapie and prognose der frischen aussenknochelbandlasion (Treatment and prognosis of the fresh ankle ligament ruptures). Unfallheikunde 79:101-104, 1976.

Airaksinen O: Changes in posttraumatic ankle joint mobility, pain, and edema following intermittent pneumatic compression therapy. Arch Phys Med Rehabil 70:341-344, 1989.

Airaksinen O, Kolari P, Herve R, et al: Treatment of post-traumatic edema in lower legs using intermittent pneumatic compression. Scand J Rehab Med 20:25-28, 1988.

Akeson WU, Amiel D, Woo S L-Y: Immobility effects on synovial joints: the pathomechanics of joint contracture. Biorheology 17:95-100, 1980.

Alves J, Alday R, Ketcham D, Lentell G: A comparison of the passive support provided by various ankle braces. J Ortho Sports Phys Ther, Jan 1992.

Amiel D, Frank L, Harwood P, et al: Tendon and ligaments: A morphological and biochemical comparison. J Orthop Res 1:257-265, 1984.

Anderson KJ, LeCocq JF, Clayton ML: Athletic injury to the fibular collateral ligament of the ankle. Clin Orthop 23:146-160, 1962.

Arms SW, Renström P, Incavo S, et al: A-P laxity of the human ankle and the effect of ATFL resection. 34th annual meeting of the Orthopaedic Research Society, Atlanta, Georgia, February 1-4, 1988 (abstr).

Axelsson R, Renström P, Svenson H-O: Acute sports injuries in a central hospital (in Swedish). Lakartidningen 77:3615-3617, 1980.

Balduini FC, Tetzlaff J: Historical perspectives on injuries of the ligaments of the ankle. Am J Sports Med 1:3-12,1982.

Balduini FC, Vegso JJ, Torg JS, et al: Management and rehabilitation of ligamentous injuries to the ankle. Am J Sports Med 4:364-380, 1987.

Barrett J, Bilisko T: The role of shoes in the prevention of ankle sprains. Sports Med 20(4):227-280, 1995.

Bergfeld J, Cox J, Drez D, Raemy H, Weiker G: Symposium: Management of acute ankle sprains. Contemp Ortho 13(3):83-116, 1986.

Black HM, Brand RL, Eichelberger MR: An improved technique for the evaluation of ligamentous injury in severe ankle sprains. Am J Sports Med 6(5):276-282, 1978.

Bosien WR, Staples OS, Russell SW: Residual disability following acute ankle sprains. J Bone Joint Surg 37A:1237-1243, 1955.

Brand RL, Black HM, Cox JS: The natural history of inadequately treated ankle sprain. Am J Sports Med 5(6):248-249, 1977.

Brand RL, Collins MDF, Templeton T: Surgical repair of ruptured lateral ankle ligaments. Am J Sports Med 9:40-44, 1981.

Brooks SC, Potter BT, Rainey JB: Treatment for partial tears of the lateral ligament of the ankle: A prospective trial. Brit Med J 282:606-607, 1981.

Broström L: Sprained ankles III—clinical observations in recent ligament ruptures. Acta Chir Scand 130:560-569, 1965.

Broström L: Sprained ankles V—treatment and prognosis in recent ligament ruptures. Acta Chir Scand 135:537-550, 1966.

Bunch RP, Bednarski K, Holland D, et al: Ankle joint support: a comparison of reusable lace-on braces with taping and wrapping. Phys Sportsmed 13:59-62, 1985.

Burks RT, Bean BG, Marcus R, et al: Analysis of athletic performance with prophylactic ankle devices. Am J Sports Med 19(2):104-106, 1991.

Burry HC: Soft tissue injury. Sport Exerc Sports Sci Rev 3:275-301, 1975.

Chirls M: Inversion injuries of the ankle. J Med Soc 70:751-753,1973.

Clark BL, Derby AC, Power GRI: Injuries of the lateral ligament of the ankle. Conservative vs. operative repair. Canadian J Surg 8:358-363, 1965.

Coffman JL, Mize NL: A comparison of ankle taping and the Aircast Sport-Stirrup on athletic performance. Athl Train 24(2):123, 1989.

Cote DJ, Prentice VVE, Hooker DN, et al: Comparison of three treatment procedures for minimizing ankle sprain swelling. Phys Ther 68:1072-1076, 1988.

Cox JS: Surgical and nonsurgical treatment of acute ankle sprains. Clin Orthop Rel Res 198:118-126, 1985.

Delacerda F: Ankle taping. Athletic Journal 56, October 2, 1975.

Derscheid GL, Brown WC: Rehabilitation of the ankle. Clin Sports Med 4:527-544, 1985.

Diamond JE: Rehabilitation of ankle sprains. Clin Sports Med 8:877-891, 1989.

Dias LS: The lateral ankle sprain: An experimental study. J Trauma 19(4):266-269, 1979.

Drez D, Young JC, Waldmar D, et al: Nonoperative treatment of double lateral ligament tears of the ankle. Am J Sports Med 10: 197-200, 1982.

Dupont M, Beliveau P, Theriault G: The efficacy of anti-inflammatory medication in the treatment of the acutely sprained ankle. Am J Sports Med 15:41-45, 1987.

Ekstrand J: Soccer injuries and their prevention. (medical dissertation No. 130), Linköping University, Linköping, Sweden 1982.

Ekstrand J, Tropp H: The incidence of ankle sprains in soccer. Foot Ankle Int 11(1):41-4, 1990.

Fiore RD, Leard JS: A functional approach in the rehabilitation of the ankle and rear foot. Athl Train 15:231-235, 1980.

Freeman MAR, Dean MRE, Hanham IWF: The etiology and prevention of functional instability of the foot. J Bone Joint Surg 47B:678-685, 1965.

Fritschy D, Bonvin J: Functional treatment of severe ankle sprain. J Traumatol Sport 4:131-136, 1987.

Garrick JG: The frequency of injury, mechanism of injury and epidemiology of ankle sprains. Am J Sports Med 5:241-242, 1977.

Garrick JG, Requa RK: Role of external support in the prevention of ankle sprains. Med Sci Sports 5(3):200-203, 1973.

Garrick JG, Requa RK: The epidemiology of foot and ankle injuries in sports. Clin Sports Med 7(1):29-36, 1988.

Glasgow M, Jackson A, Jamieson AM: Instability of the ankle after injury to the lateral ligament. J Bone Joint Surg 62B(2):196-200, 1980.

Glick JM, Gordon RB, Nashimoto D: The prevention and treatment of ankle injuries. Am J Sports Med 4:136-141, 1976.

Greene TA, Wight CR: A comparative support evaluation of three ankle orthosis before, during and after exercise. J Ortho Sports Phys Ther 11(10):453-466, 1990.

Gromnark T, Johnsen O, Kogstad O: Rupture of the lateral ligaments of the ankle: A controlled clinical trial. Injury 11:215-218, 1980.

Gross MT, Everts JR, Roberson SE, et al: Effect of DonJoy ankle ligament protector and Aircast Sport-Stirrup orthoses on functional performance. J Orthop Sports Phys Ther 19(3):150-156, 1994.

Haggmark T, Eriksson E: Cylinder or mobile cast brace after knee ligament surgery. Am J Sports Med 7:48-56, 1979.

Hamilton WG: Sprained ankles in ballet dancers. Foot & Ankle 3(2):99-102, 1982.

Hamilton WG: Foot and ankle injuries in dancers. Clin Sports Med 7:143-173, 1988.

Hansen H, Damholt V, Termansen NB: Clinical and social status following injury to the lateral ligaments of the ankle. Follow-up of 144 patients treated conservatively. Acta Orthop Scand 50:699-704, 1979.

Hardaker WT, Margello S, Goldner JL: Foot and ankle injuries in theatrical dancers. Foot Ankle 6(2):59-69, 1985.

Henning CE, Egge LN: Cast brace treatment of acute unstable ankle sprain. A preliminary report. Am J Sports Med 5:252-255, 1977.

Jackson DW, Ashley RL, Powell JW: Ankle sprains in young athletes. Relation of severity and disability. Clin Orthop 101:201-215, 1974.

Jackson JP, Hutson MA: Cast-brace treatment of ankle sprains. Injury 17(4):251-255, 1986.

Jakob RP, Raemy H, Steffen R, et al: Zur funktionellen Behandlung des frischen Aussenbandrrisses mit der Aircast-Shiene (Functional treatment of the fresh lateral ligament ruptures by Aircast Brace). Orthopade 15:434-440, 1986.

Järvinen M: Healing of a crush injury in rat striated muscle with special reference to treatment of early mobilization and immobilization. Academic dissertation (thesis), University of Turku, Turku, Finland, 1976.

Järvinen M, Lehto M: The effects of early mobilization and immobilization on the healing process following muscle injuries. Sports Med 15:78-89, 1993.

Jaskulka R, Fischer G, Schedl R: Injuries of the lateral ligaments of the ankle joint. Operative treatment and long-term results. Arch Orthop Traumat Surg 107:217-221, 1988.

Jerosch J, Thorwesten L, Frebel T, Linnenbecker S: Influence of external stabilizing devices of the ankle on sport specific capabilities. Knee Surg, Sports Traumatol, Arthroscopy 5(1):50-57, 1997.

Jozsa L, Järvinen M, Kannus P, et al: Fine structural changes in the articular cartilage of the rat's knee following short-term immobilization in various positions: A scanning electron microscopical study. Int Orthop 11:137-140, 1987.

Jozsa L, Reffy A, Järvinen M, et al: Cortical and trabecular osteopenia after immobilization. A quantitative histological study of the rat knee. Int Orthop 12:169-172, 1988.

Jozsa L, Thoring J, Järvinen M, et al: Quantitative alterations in intramuscular connective tissue following immobilization: An experimental study in the rat calf muscles. Exp Mol Path 49:267-278, 1988.

Kaikkonen A, Kannus P, Järvinen M: Surgery versus functional treatment in ankle ligament tears. Clin Orthop 326:194-202, 1996.

Kannus P, Renström P: Current concepts review: Treatment for acute tears of the lateral ligaments of the ankle. J Bone Joint Surg 73A(2):305-312, 1991.

Kitaoka HB, Lee MD, Morrey BF, Cass JR: Acute repair and delayed reconstruction for lateral ankle instability: twenty-year follow-up study. J Orthop Trauma 11(7):530-535, 1997.

Klein J, Schreckenberger C, Roddecker K, et al: Operative oder konservative behandlung der frischen aussenbandruptur am oberen sprunggelenk. Radnomisierte klinische studie (Operative or conservative treatment of recent rupture of the fibular ligament in the ankle. A randomized clinical trial). Unfallchirurg 91:154-160, 1988.

Konradsen L, Holmer P, Sondergaard L: Early mobilizing treatment for Grade III ankle ligament injuries. Foot Ankle 12(2):69-73, 1992.

Korkala O, Lauttamus L, Tanskanen P: Lateral ligament injuries of the ankle. Results of primary surgical treatment. Ann Chir Gynaec 71:161-163, 1982.

Korkala O, Rusanen M, Jokipii P, et al: A prospective study of the treatment of severe tears of the lateral ligament of the ankle. Int Ortho 11:13-17, 1987.

Lassiter TE, Malone TR, Garrett WE: Injury to the lateral ligaments of the ankle. Orthop Clin North Am 20:629-640, 1989.

Leach RE, Schepsis AA: Acute injury to ligaments of the ankle. In Evarts CM, ed. Surgery of the Musculoskeletal System. Vol 4. New York: Churchill Livingstone, 1990, 3887-3913.

Leanderson J, Wredmark T: Treatment of acute ankle sprain. Acta Orthop Scand 66(6):529-531, 1995.

Lehto M: Collagen and fibronectin in a healing skeletal muscle injury: An experimental study in rats under variable conditions of physical exercise. Academic dissertation (thesis), The University of Turku. Annales Universitatis Turkuensis, Medica Odontological Series D, vol. 14, 1983.

Leonard NM: Injuries of the lateral ligaments of the ankle. A clinical and experimental study. J Bone Joint Surg 31A:373-377, 1949.

Lindenberger U, Reese D, Anfreasson G, Renström P, Peterson L: The effect of prophylactic taping of ankles. FIMS World Congress, Amsterdam, 1990.

Lindenfeld TN: The differentiation and treatment of ankle sprains. Orthopedics 11(1):203-206, 1988.

Lindstrand A: Lateral lesions in sprained ankles, Medical dissertation, Lund University, 1976.

Mack RP: Ankle injuries in athletes. Clin Sports Med 1:71-84, 1982.

Makhani JS: Diagnosis and treatment of acute rupture of the various components of the lateral ligaments of the ankle, Am J Orthop 4:224-230, 1962.

McConkey JP: Ankle sprains, consequences and mimics, Med Sport Sci 23:39-55, 1987.

McCulloch PG, Holden P, Robson DJ, et al.: The value of mobilization and non-steroidal anti-inflammatory analgesia in the management of inversion injuries of the ankle. Brit J Clin Pract 39:69-72, 1985.

McMaster PE: Treatment of the ankle sprain. Observations in more than five hundred cases. J Am Med Assn 122:659-600, 1943.

Milford PI, Dunleavy PJ: A pilot trial of treatment of acute inversion sprains to the ankle by ankle supports. J Roy Nav Med Serv 76:97-100, 1990.

Moller-Larsen F, Wethelund JO, Jurik AG, et al: Comparison of three different treatments for ruptured lateral ankle ligaments. Acta Orthop Scand 59(5):564-566, 1988.

Montgomery JB, Steadman JR: Rehabilitation of the injured knee. Clin Sports Med 4:333-343, 1985.

Niethard FU: Die stabilitat des sprunggelenkes nach ruptur des lateralen bandapparates (The mechanical stability of the ankle joint after rupture for the lateral ligament). Arch Orthop Unfallchir 80:53-61, 1974.

Noyes FR: Functional properties of knee ligaments and alterations induced by immobilization. Clin Orthop 123:210-242, 1977.

Ogata K, Whiteside LA, Andersen DA: The intra-articular effect of various postoperative managements following knee ligament repair: an experimental study on dogs. Clin Orthop 150:271-276, 1980.

Ozeki S, Yasuda K, Kaneda K, et al: Simultaneous measurement of strain changes and determination of zero strain in the collateral ligaments of the human ankle. 36th Annual Orthopedic Research Society, New Orleans, LA, 1990 (abstr).

Prins JG: Diagnosis and treatment of injury to the lateral ligament of the ankle. A comparative clinical study. Acta Chir Scand (Suppl) 486, 1978.

Raemy H, Jacob R: Functional treatment of fresh fibular lesions using the Aircast splint. Swiss J Sports Med 31, 1993.

Redler I, Brown GG Jr, Williams JT: Operative treatment of the acutely ruptured lateral ligament of the ankle. Southern Med J 70:1168-1171, 1977.

Reichen A, Marti R: Die frische fibulare bandruptur—Diagnose, therapies resultate (Rupture of the fibular collateral ligaments—Diagnosis, surgical treatment, results). Arch Orthop Unfallchir 80:211-222, 1974.

Rovere GD, Clarke TJ, Yates CS, et al: Retrospective comparison of taping and ankle stabilizers in preventing ankle injuries. Am J Sports Med 16:228-233, 1988.

Ruth CJ: The surgical treatment of injuries of the fibular collateral ligaments of the ankle. J Bone Joint Surg 43A:229-239, 1961.

Ryan JB, Hopkinson WJ, Wheeler JH, et al: Office management of the acute ankle sprain. Clin Sports Med 8:477-495, 1989.

Sandelin J, Santavirta S, Lattila R, et al: Sports injuries in a large urban population: occurrence and epidemiological aspects. Int J Sports Med 9(1):61-66, 1988.

Shrier I: Treatment of lateral collateral ligament sprains of the ankle: A critical appraisal of the literature. Clin J Sports Med 5:187-195, 1995.

Sommer HM, Arza D: Functional treatment of recent ruptures of the fibular ligament of the ankle. Int Orthop 13:157-160, 1989.

Sommer HM, Schreiber T: Early functional conservative therapy of a fresh fibular rupture of the capsular ligament from a socioecomonic point of view. Sportverletz Sportschaden 7:40-46, 1993.

Staples OS: Ruptures of the fibular collateral ligaments of the ankle. Results of immediate surgical treatment. J Bone Joint Surg 57A: 101-107, 1975.

Stover C: Functional sprain management of the ankle. Ambulatory Care 6(11):211, 1986.

Termansen NB, Hansen H, Damholt V: Radiological and muscular status following injury to the lateral ligaments of the ankle. Follow-up of 144 patients treated conservatively. Acta Orthop Scand 50:705-708, 1979.

Thomas JR, Cotton DJ: Does ankle taping slow down athletes? Coach Athlete 34(4):20, 1971.

Tropp H, Askling C, Gillquist J: Prevention of ankle sprains. Am J Sports Med 13(4):259-262, 1985.

van Moppens Fl, van den Hoogenband CR: Diagnostic and therapeutic aspects of inversion trauma of the ankle joint. Thesis, University of Maastricht. Utrecht/Antwerpen: Bohn, Scheltema & Holkema, 1992.

Viljakka T, Rokkanen P: The treatment of ankle sprain by bandaging and antiphlogistic drugs. Ann Chir Gynaecol 72:66-70, 1983.

Wester JU, Jespersen SM, Nielsen KD, Neumann L: Wobble board training after partial sprains of the lateral ligaments of the ankle. J Orthop Sports Phys Ther 23(5):332-336, 1996.

Wilkerson GB, Pinerola JJ, Caturano RW: Invertor vs. evertor peak torque and power deficiencies associated with lateral ankle ligament injury. J Orthop Sports Phys Ther 26(2):78-86, 1997.

Woo SLY, Inoue M, McGurk-Burleson E, et al: Treatment of the medial collateral ligament injury. II: Structure and function of canine knees in response to different treatment regimens. Am J Sports Med 15:22-29, 1987.

Chapter 21

Rehabilitation of the Acute Lateral Ankle Sprain

Deborah Mandis Cozen, PT, and Richard D. Ferkel, MD

The goal of conservative treatment is early rehabilitation and prevention of chronic functional instability, such as mechanical instability, peroneal weakness, and traction neuritis.

Conservative treatment consists of strengthening and flexibility exercises, balance and proprioceptive agility drills, and bracing and/or taping. Functional treatment is broken down into four general phases (Ferkel 1996):

■ In the first phase, modalities of ice and compression are initiated, along with rest and elevation, in order to control acute symptoms (RICE principle).

■ The second phase encourages early range of motion to within normal limits and progression to full weightbearing status, with supportive taping or bracing as indicated.

■ In phase three, proprioception training begins with emphasis on peroneal strengthening.

■ After the patient progresses through phase three, he or she begins phase four, which consists of specific sport or activity training and testing to evaluate the patient's capacity to return to prior level of function.

Conservative treatment is indicated for all grade I and II ankle sprain injuries. Grade III sprains are more controversial. Recent studies have shown that in first-time grade III lateral ankle sprains, early mobilization allowed earlier return to work than in those patients who were casted. Other studies have recently shown that early mobilization gave better results in grade III ankle sprain than surgery.

Indications for surgery in grade III ankle sprains include large avulsion fractures of the fibula, prior symptomatic chronic instability, displaced osteochondral fractures, and significant peroneal tendon tears or dislocation. In addition, some ankle experts feel that surgery should be considered in grade III ankle sprains for professional ballet dancers, but this needs to be determined on a case-by-case basis.

Five principles are basic to successful ankle rehabilitation:

1. The effects of mobilization must be minimized.
2. Never overstress healing tissue.
3. There is more to ankle rehabilitation than strengthening.
4. Each rehabilitation program must be uniquely adapted to the patient.
5. The physician, physical therapist, and patient must work together as a team to formulate an adequate treatment plan to successfully achieve goals.

The ultimate goal of rehabilitation is to safely return each individual to his or her prior level of function and to prevent reinjury in the future.

■ The Four-Phase Rehabilitation Program

The following protocol is a four-phase rehabilitation program for acute lateral ankle sprains. Each phase can be modified, if necessary, to accommodate the needs of each patient.

Phase I: Acute

The goals of treatment during the acute phase are to

1. decrease inflammation/pain,
2. provide controlled forces that will have a positive effect on healing collagen tissue, and
3. initiate safe cardiovascular training to promote overall conditioning.

During the acute phase, the rehabilitation program employs a wide array of techniques to achieve these goals. Most of these techniques will be discussed at greater length later in this chapter.

1. Control of inflammation and pain can be achieved through the use of

   - compression,
   - elevation,
   - cryotherapy, and
   - high voltage galvanic stimulation.

2. Applying controlled forces that will positively affect healing collagen tissue may require most of the following techniques:

   - Control the forces that act on the injured structures to stimulate collagen alignment by
     - limiting eversion and inversion,
     - promoting dorsiflexion and plantarflexion, and
     - bracing with an Aircast.
   - Restore flexibility, emphasizing the
     - gastrocnemius and
     - soleus.
   - Minimize soft tissue dysfunction by initiating range of motion in the acutely injured joint through
     - gentle passive motion exercises and
     - nonweightbearing activities in the pool (figure 21.1).

- Prevent kinesthesia shutdown by initiating balance activities in nondependent position.
- Initiate neuromuscular control through gentle manual isometric strengthening exercises as tolerated.

3. Initiate cardiovascular training using

   - Upper body ergometer (UBE) for safe cardiovascular training without involving the lower extremity (figure 21.2) or
   - deep water pool exercises (avoiding active ankle involvement).

Phase II: Subacute

The goals of treatment during the subacute phase are to

1. continue to control forces to facilitate the healing process,
2. control and diminish swelling,
3. improve proprioception,
4. increase joint range of motion and flexibility, and
5. increase strength.

During the subacute phase, passive modalities should be decreased to promote more active patient participation. Cardiovascular endurance training is continued using a stationary bike. The rehabilitation program utilized in this phase is as follows:

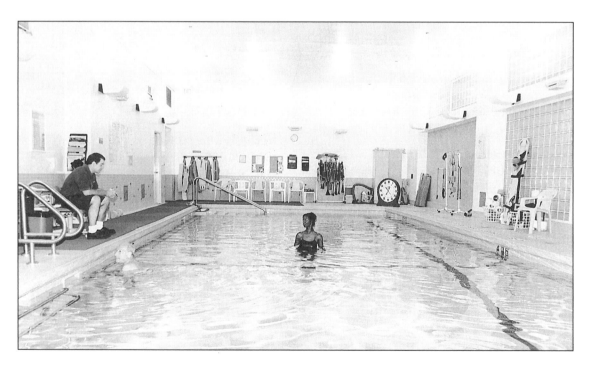

■ **Figure 21.1** Pool treatment for early phases of rehabilitation. Also used for cardiovascular conditioning with athletes.

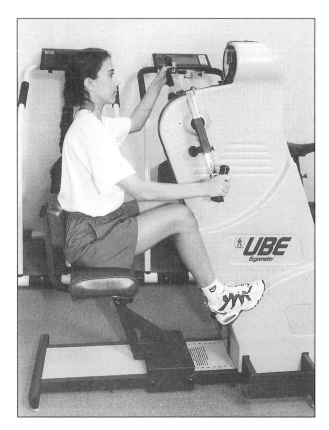

■ **Figure 21.2** Upper body ergometer (UBE) for cardiovascular conditioning.

1. Control forces using the following measures:
   - Bracing and taping
   - Evaluating limb alignment
   - Assessing for orthotics
2. Control/diminish swelling with the following:
   - Ice
   - Electrical stimulation
   - Soft tissue massage
3. Improve proprioception with exercises in a dependent position.
   - Patient should perform one-legged balance drills on floor, progressing to trampoline.
   - Initiate dynamic training by progressing patient from sitting BAPS to standing, as appropriate.
4. Increase joint range of motion and flexibility with the following methods:
   - Normalized arthrokinematics
     - Joint mobilization to the talocrural and subtalar joints (grade I and II joint mobiliza-

tion may also be used to control pain symptoms)
     - Physiological glides
   - Continuing flexibility exercises
5. Increase strength with the following techniques:
   - Strengthening exercises
     - Dynamic strengthening with tubing supination and plantarflexion with an emphasis on eversion and dorsiflexion concentric/eccentric strengthening
     - Intrinsic muscle strengthening
     - Strengthening entire lower kinetic chain from pelvis to foot, with emphasis on hip abduction
   - Pool rehabilitation
     - Gait training in shallow water
     - Deep water running

Phase III: Advanced

A patient qualifies for this phase only if all of the following conditions are met:

- The patient has full nonpainful range of motion.
- The patient has good "manual" muscle testing for eversion/dorsiflexors.
- The patient's improvement in proprioception is a minimum of 50% to 70%.
- The patient passes a clinical exam satisfactorily.

The goals of treatment during the advanced phase are to

1. increase active strengthening;
2. continue progressive proprioception and coordination training, especially in weightbearing positions;
3. continue weightbearing cardiovascular training; and
4. increase flexibility.

The rehabilitation program in this advanced phase uses a wide variety of techniques, as follows:

1. Increase active strengthening with strengthening exercises:
   - Dynamic strengthening exercises with an emphasis on eccentrics
   - Power and endurance intervals
   - Plyometric training for balance and power training

2. Continue progressive proprioception and coordination training with the following:

- Proprioceptive training

  - Advanced balance drills (e.g., balance on trampoline while throwing plyoball)

  - Advanced dynamic balance activities (e.g., sports cord activities, retro stair stepper without support, Fitter or Skiers Edge)

- Initiation of agility drills and functional return to sport

3. Continue weightbearing cardiovascular training with the following:

- Weightbearing activities

  - Treadmill

  - Stair stepper

  - Skiing machines

  - Slide board

  - Running front, back, and sideways with sports cord

- Patient should be instructed to monitor his or her target heart rate and working intensity

4. Increase flexibility with the following:

- Flexibility exercises

- Evaluate the entire lower kinetic chain, including the pelvis, for soft tissue restrictions

Phase IV: Return to Activity

The patient qualifies to return to his or her competitive sport or job only if all of the following conditions are met:

- The patient has full nonpainful range of motion with good accessory joint motion.

- The patient exhibits normal "manual" muscle testing of the ankle, especially in stabilizing muscles that support the medial arch and subtalar joint.

- The patient's proprioceptive tests are 95% or higher on the contralateral side.

- The patient passes a clinical exam satisfactorily.

- The patient exhibits normal flexibility in the lower extremity, especially the gastrocnemius, hamstring, hip flexor, and hip abductor.

- The patient exhibits good subtalar joint positioning.

The goal of treatment during this phase is to return the patient to his or her preinjury level of function. The rehabilitation program used in this phase is as follows:

1. Establish a maintenance program.

- Strengthening exercises

- Balance/proprioception/agility drills

- Flexibility exercises

- Continued external support (i.e., brace or taping)

2. Use sport-specific training.

3. Work hardening and conditioning to safely return patient to previous job or activities.

■ Keys to Successful Return to Activity

Phase IV involves a creative use of rehabilitation techniques to duplicate the athlete's or worker's environment in order to efficiently and effectively train the individual. However, no matter how creative at duplicating environments they are, and no matter how skillful at applying specific techniques specialists may be, if they fail to take all four of the following factors into account, the success of their rehabilitation efforts will remain in doubt.

- The interdependence of the entire kinetic chain

- Teamwork

- Technical elements of the program

- Proper diagnosis

■ **The interdependence of the entire kinetic chain.** A common error in rehabilitation is that the trainer, physical therapist, and physician tend to focus solely on the injured joint, the area where the patient complains of pain and other symptoms. Most importantly, once the ankle symptoms have decreased, the source of the problem, possibly higher up in the chain, needs to be identified and treated appropriately in order to effectively correct the problem that may have originally predisposed the patient to injury. Thus, whatever techniques you are using, it is vital to keep in mind that the body functions as a unit. Each joint depends on the proper functioning of the proximal segment. If there is a dysfunction higher up in the chain, the distal segments will compensate as necessary for this dysfunction. Evaluating and assessing the patient's upper body and back while she performs a particular activity is important in order to identify associated weaknesses and/or soft tissue dysfunction. Analysis of posture, especially in specific work-related or sport positions, may need attention. These problems should be addressed as part of the patient's rehabilitation program.

■ **Teamwork.** Never forget the importance of the team concept. Both the patient and the physical therapist are vital members of the rehabilitation team. Proper patient education and instruction in a thorough home exercise program is key to success. Patient education is critical in the rehabilitation process for avoiding reinjury. It should begin early and should be emphasized throughout the entire rehabilitation program. The physical therapist spends much more time with the patient than the physician does. It is the physical therapist's responsibility to adequately document significant subjective and measurable objective information after each patient visit. Over a period of 3 to 4 weeks, data is collected to formulate a progress note for the physician at the time of the patient's return visit. The purpose of the progress note is to inform the physician of the patient's current status, which includes present problems, goals achieved or not achieved, treatment plan, and the physical therapist's recommendation regarding continuation of physical therapy or discharge plans. The physical therapist's feedback on the patient's recovery is vital for the physician to direct further rehabilitation plans.

■ **Technical elements of the program.** Key points of acute lateral ankle sprain rehabilitation include early control of the inflammatory process and protected mobilization of the ankle joint. Once this has been achieved, this is followed by proper rehabilitation to decrease the acute symptoms, emphasizing restoring normal range of motion, strengthening of muscle groups, retraining proprioceptive awareness of the ankle joint to prevent chronic lateral ankle joint instability, and identification and correction of the source of the problem.

■ **Proper diagnosis.** The best rehabilitation techniques in the world will prove useless unless the source of the problem is identified and corrected. If rehabilitation is not successful, remember to look for other diagnoses. Diagnoses commonly overlooked include fractures (talar lateral process fracture), bony disorders (OCD), or other soft tissue problems, inflammatory conditions, and neurological injuries.

■ Closed Kinetic Chain Rehabilitation Exercises

Closed kinetic chain exercises are used to increase strength, endurance, power, and proprioception in the lower extremity. Closed chain exercises should also be used whenever possible to assess function (Appenzeller 1988). There are many different exercises you can use in the patient's rehabilitation program after an acute lateral ankle sprain. The exercises discussed in this section are very specific to strengthening the ankle and foot stabilizing muscles (intrinsic and extrinsic muscle groups) and also increasing proprioception. The base of movement must be strong and stable in order for efficient, controlled movement to occur. After an acute lateral ankle sprain, stability in the ankle and foot is significantly weak, especially laterally, and proprioception is diminished. Thus, the following exercises are of utmost importance.

Windshield Wipers

The patient sits with both feet flat on the ground, shoulder width apart. Both fists are placed between the knees to stabilize them. While keeping the feet completely flat on the ground, the patient pivots on both heels and touches his big toes together. It is very important to keep the first metatarsal as close as possible to the ground. For normal range of motion, the great toes should touch one another. Internal rotation should go past midline. External rotation and internal rotation should be equal. If the patient has full pronation and supination range of motion, he can use a Theraband for added resistance. Normal strength would be 40 repetitions easily with a green Theraband.

This test evaluates the following:

■ The strength of and functional relationship between the posterior tibialis and the peroneus longus

■ The functional range of motion between pronation and supination

■ Rotation of the tibia on the femur

Internal rotation strengthens the posterior tibialis and external rotation strengthens the peroneus longus. Rotation of the tibia connects functionally between the foot and the SI joint. There must be proper tibial rotation for efficient movement of the SI joint. Decrease in internal tibial rotation may indicate soft tissue tightness superior to the tibiofemoral joint and/or tight medial hamstrings. The popliteus, hamstrings, and calf muscles should be assessed for soft tissue tightness. Remember that tissues tighten adaptively in the direction of the dysfunction. A decrease in external tibial rotation indicates tight lateral structures (lateral hamstrings and/or iliotibial band).

Intrinsic Muscle Strengthening

Sufficient foot and ankle stability is extremely important in the rehabilitation process. The following exercises increase strength in the intrinsic muscles of the foot.

Towel Curling

When the knees are placed at 90°, the long toe flexors are emphasized. When the knees are at less than 90° of flexion, the short toe flexors are emphasized. The patient sits with both feet flat on the ground. The feet should be on a towel spread over a smooth surface. Emphasize to the patient the necessity of maintaining the ankle in a neutral position. The toes are flexed repeatedly to curl the towel up underneath the arches (see figure 21.3). The motion of all toes should be symmetrical and the toes should flex enough that the proximal phalange of the toes is in flexion compared to the plane of the metatarsals. Normal strength is considered to be able to curl the towel under the arch several times without fatigue. Encourage the patient to also extend the toes, keeping the metatarsals flat on the ground.

Toe Raises With Toes Flexed

The patient tightens the toes against the floor and then raises the heels. This exercise is especially good for patients suffering from shin splints.

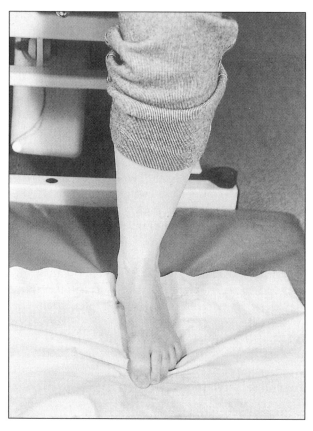

■ **Figure 21.3** Towel curls for intrinsic muscle strengthening.

Gastroc-Soleus Strengthening

Soleus: Seated Toe Raises

The patient sits with legs bent and feet flat on the ground. The patient raises the heel by plantarflexing the foot. A weight may be placed on the knee for added resistance. Assess whether the movement is smooth and controlled.

Gastrocnemius

The following two exercises are excellent for strengthening the gastrocnemius:

■ Toe raises with lower leg. The patient stands with her toes and midfoot on a step and her heels hanging off it, then rises onto her toes. Assess the strength throughout the entire range. Can the patient hold a position in various ranges?

■ Top one-half toe raises. This is a very important exercise for patients involved in leaping sports (e.g., basketball). The patient stands on both feet and rises as high as possible onto his toes. This is repeated as in the previous exercise, without letting the heels come back down to a level position. The greatest weakness in the gastrocnemius muscle is in the top one-half of the range. Make sure that the patient comes up over the first metatarsal, avoiding supination.

As strength increases, these exercises can be used with weight for added resistance.

Single-Leg Knee Bends

This exercise evaluates the ability of the patella to track properly through the femoral groove during closed chain knee flexion. The patient stands with both feet flat on the ground and flexes her knees to about 45°. The patella should track directly over the second toe. Weak hip abductors or tight hip internal rotators can be easily observed with this exercise. Tennis players between the ages of 35 and 55 tend to squat into this position with their knees going in. This is a problem that needs to be addressed in the clinic before the patient is allowed to go back on the court. The patient needs to be instructed to keep the knee directly over the second toe. To progress with this exercise, have her perform a squat against the wall, holding dumbbell weights in her hands. The patient can also use an elastic resistive band, performing mini-squats for timed intervals. Once she is efficient in performing this exercise, have the patient perform mini-squats with the sports cord unilaterally. Repetitions and time can be increased as appropriate.

Pronation-Supination

Twisting Hips

This exercise helps the patient to learn to initiate awareness of movement, and is also used for assessment. The patient stands still with both feet flat on the ground. Have the patient initiate a twisting motion with the hips to the right and to the left. His feet should be rotating through pronation and supination, with one foot pronating and the other supinating.

Active Inversion/Eversion: Standing

This exercise requires more muscular involvement than does the previous one. The patient stands with both feet on the ground. While using the feet and lower legs only, she initiates inversion/eversion motion. Both feet are moved through inversion than eversion cycle together. While the patient is moving her feet, use your index finger and thumb to palpate the head of the talus medially and laterally, to insure that her foot goes through a full range of motion.

Active Inversion/Eversion: Sitting

This exercise is more difficult than the previous one because rotation of the leg is not allowed. The patient sits with both feet on the floor. Have the patient invert and evert the feet without moving the knees. The medial and lateral edges of the foot rise up off the ground.

Sitting Subtalar Pronation/Supination

The patient sits, as in the previous exercise. This time, he pronates and supinates the subtalar joint without allowing the medial and lateral edges of the foot to come off of the floor. The pronation/supination motion must be made through the movement of the calcaneus and talus, not the metatarsals or the toes. Touch the patient on the medial side of the heel and then on the lateral side of the heel to increase his awareness of isolating talar movement.

Standing Subtalar Pronation/Supination

This exercise is performed exactly as the previous exercise, except the patient is standing. This exercise can be progressed to single limb.

Stork Exercises

The following exercises are referred to as "stork exercises." These exercises increase proprioception and control, as well as strength and endurance, spe-cifically in the lower extremity and foot- and ankle stabilizing muscles.

Basic

The patient stands on one leg, without using any supports. Have her stand in a doorway if you think balance may be a problem. The patient's knee is straight and her legs should not be touching one another. The arms are down to the sides. Normal is considered to be able to stand for 30 seconds while keeping the shoulders fairly level and having minimal movement of the nonweightbearing leg (the other body muscles should not have to assist to maintain balance). The basic stork exercise tests the function of the posterior tibialis and peroneal longus muscles. If the patient is not able to keep the subtalar joint in neutral and falls into pronation, this indicates dysfunction of the posterior tibialis. Peroneal dysfunction is indicated by supination.

Eyes Closed

This exercise is performed as described in the previous paragraph, except the eyes are closed. The patient should be able to maintain balance.

Functional Activities

This is the same as the basic stork exercise. However, throwing, batting, dance moves, and walking motion with the nonweightbearing leg are incorporated while standing on one leg and maintaining balance. Make sure that the patient is maintaining the subtalar joint in a neutral position throughout the entire activity.

Twisting Exercises While Balancing

The pelvis and femur should stay in alignment as the patient twists. The femur should be independent of pelvic movement. Adductor muscle dysfunction is indicated in patients who are unable to maintain this alignment. This dysfunction is a result of hip adductor weakness and/or lack of endurance in these muscles.

Stork Toe Raises

The standing position is the same as in the basic stork exercise. The patient rises as slowly as possible up onto her toes and lowers as slowly as possible down again. Have the patient rise up only as high on her toes as she is able to slowly lower herself and maintain her balance. The motion up and down should be so slow that you have to look closely to see it. Normal is considered to be able to do three repetitions. This exercise is a combination of proprioception and strength. Again, the movement needs to be very slow and controlled. The patient can perform this exercise with her eyes open, and then, as she progresses, with her eyes closed.

■ Therapeutic Modalities

The most commonly used modalities in the treatment of an acute lateral ankle sprain include the following: interferential electrical stimulation, medium frequency electrical stimulation, iontophoresis, phonophoresis, ice or ice massage, and contrast baths.

Interferential Electrical Stimulation

The primary application for interferential electrical stimulation is in pain management. Medium frequency currents are believed to be more penetrating, thus selectively treating the larger and deeper pain fibers instead of the smaller and more superficial fibers that are addressed with traditional TENS. The use of four electrodes in a crisscross pattern allows for the centralization of the perceived sensation, which makes interferential therapy effective for localized and deep-seated pain (see figure 21.4). Some units also have vacuum suction cups with which to apply the electrodes. This type of application adds an additional mode of pain reduction through the counterirritation to the skin, and may also promote superficial blood flow under the cups. Patients will experience a massage-like effect. Avoid using the vacuum electrodes on patients with sensitive skin or immediately after an injury.

Medium Frequency Electrical Stimulation

Medium frequency stimulation was developed in Russia in an attempt to provide high levels of stimulation while minimizing sensory nerve recruitment. This type of stimulation is capable of producing a strong enough contraction to result in muscle strengthening. To produce changes in the strength of a muscle, the electrical stimulus must produce a contraction capable of producing at least 60% of the torque of that individual's maximal voluntary contraction for that muscle. To avoid causing rapid muscle fatigue, the typical treatment guidelines of a 1:3 or 1:4 duty cycle are followed. The combination of medium frequency stimulation and voluntary contractions produces a better increase in muscle torque than either voluntary contractions or electrical stimulation alone. For example, have the patient isometrically contract the peroneal muscles in conjunction with the medium frequency stimulation. The goal of utilizing electrical stimulation for strengthening is to promote an independent exercise program for the patient. At lower intensities, this type of stimulation can be used for muscle re-education, keeping the level of stimulation in a comfortable range and merely providing feedback to the patient to aid in initiating a contraction. Lower intensities with shorter off times could be used for pain modulation, as with high voltage and interferential stimulation.

Iontophoresis

Iontophoresis (figure 21.5) is the process whereby ions in solution are transferred through the intact skin

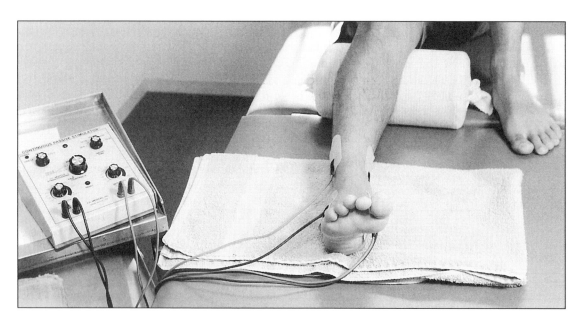

■ **Figure 21.4** Electrical stimulation for control of pain and swelling.

via electrical potential, using electrodes with positive or negative polarity. Positive ions are driven through the skin at the anode, and negative ions are driven through the skin at the cathode. The greatest concentrations of ions are driven into the skin along sweat glands and hair follicles. The velocity of ion movement is directly proportional to the voltage used. The quantity depends on the current flow and the duration of flow. Medication can penetrate up to 3 mm, depending on dosage, skin impedance, and underlying structures. Iontophoresis is indicated for areas of localized specific pain. It is very effective for lateral ankle pain after a lateral ankle sprain. Palpate to feel the most uncomfortable area to place the electrode. The effects of iontophoresis are seen from 24 to 48 hours after the first treatment. Some patients report pain relief within 2 to 4 hours. These treatments appear to have a cumulative effect, as relief is more apparent after the third to fourth treatment. On the day following treatment, there may be an area of redness. This is a normal response. If blistering or a deeper wound is present, the skin was burned. In either instance, repeat application should not be made at the same site. Ultrasound may be used after the iontophoresis, as this may promote deeper penetration of the medication.

Phonophoresis

Phonophoresis (figure 21.6) is very effective in the treatment of acute lateral ankle sprains for the reduction of pain and inflammation. Ten-percent hydrocortisone ointment is commonly used with phonophoresis. Post-ultrasound with a therapeutic intensity of .5 watts/cm^2 to 1.0 watts/cm^2 is recommended to avoid the thermal and, thus, pro-inflammatory effects of continuous mode ultrasound. In acute lateral ankle sprains, pain is usually located around the distribution of the peroneal tendons, the anterior inferior aspect of the lateral malleoli, and other soft tissues surrounding the ankle joint, and phonophoresis is used after treatment for the control of pain and inflammatory symptoms.

Cryotherapy

Soft tissue inflammation is a physiological response to stress of soft tissues. When traumatized (excessively stressed or irritated), the involved soft tissues produce inflammatories, which are designed to promote the healing process. These inflammatories include histamine, bradykinin, and prostaglandins. Soft tissue traumatized during a precipitating event for an inversion ankle sprain will, of course, experience such inflammation. Cryotherapy is of great value in the treatment of this inflammation because it

- slows, through tissue cooling, the reaction of destructive enzymes and toxins;
- desensitizes sensory nerves previously sensitized by histamine and bradykinin; and
- retards the production of prostaglandins by slowing the sensory nerve release of histamine.

The treatment of soft tissue inflammation by cooling is best performed by cryotherapeutic applications including ice packing, ice massage, and ice bath. Of these devices, which provide deep tissue cooling,

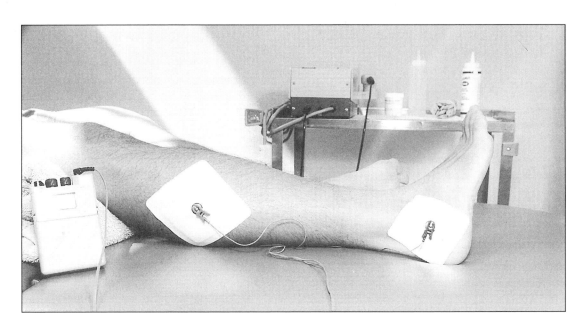

■ **Figure 21.5** Iontophoresis to decrease pain.

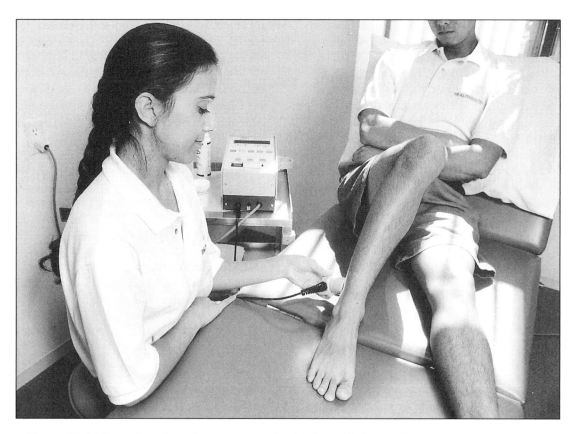

■ **Figure 21.6** Phonophoresis to decrease generalized pain and inflammation.

the most commonly applied and easiest to use is the ice pack.

Vasoconstriction may also be affected by cold applications to the skin via affected sympathetic afferent and efferent nerve fibers innervating the skin and blood vessels (capillary beds included). This reflexive behavior is used for control of acute edema by the direct application of ice to the affected area. Ice massage is very effective when treating areas of isolated inflammation and pain.

Contrast Baths

The penetration of cold and heat is superficial with deeper reflexive effects on circulation. Contrast baths may promote more vigorous circulatory effects than cold alone. They are an effective alternative for pain management, especially in the distal extremities such as the foot and ankle. Contrast baths serve as an excellent modality for subacute trauma, inflammatory conditions, sprains and strains, tendinitis, and chronic edema.

■ Case Studies

The following two case studies illustrate rehabilitation programs for inversion injuries of different severity.

Example 1

A 28-year-old female suffered an inversion injury to her right ankle while walking on the sidewalk. She noted immediate pain and swelling. Before this incident, she was running 40 miles per week with no problems in her ankle. She had no previous ankle injuries. Plantarflexion inversion stress test and anterior drawer test appear to be increased compared to the left ankle. MRI revealed soft tissue swelling only. Radiography was negative. Inversion stress test radiographs showed an increased talar tilt on the right (5° compared to 13°). Based on these findings, the patient was determined to have a grade III ankle sprain.

The goals of treatment during phase I are to

1. decrease acute symptoms of pain and swelling,

2. support lateral ankle structures,

3. increase range of motion,

4. introduce gentle strengthening, and

5. increase gait status to weight bearing as tolerated.

During phase I, the rehabilitation program consists of the following techniques to achieve the desired goals.

1. **Pain and swelling** can be decreased through the use of ice and elevation, electrical stimulation, soft tissue massage (figure 21.7), grade 1-2 gentle ankle and forefoot joint mobilization, active ankle pumps, and TED stockings.

2. **Lateral ankle support** is achieved with an ankle brace or a controlled action motion (CAM) walker.

3. **Range of motion** is increased by initiating gentle passive range of motion as well as ankle and forefoot mobilization, grades II and III.

4. **Gentle strengthening** can be initiated by performing gentle ankle isometrics and active range-of-motion exercises.

5. **Weight bearing as tolerated** is encouraged by emphasizing heel-toe gait training with strong push-off, progressing from weight bearing as tolerated to full and equal weight bearing.

The goals of treatment during phase II (1-3 weeks) are to

1. alleviate pain and swelling,

2. achieve full active range of motion,

3. strengthen ankle stabilizing muscles,

4. increase proprioception/control/coordination,

5. increase strength in the lower kinetic chain, and

6. maintain cardiovascular fitness.

During phase II, the rehabilitation program consists of the following modalities and exercises.

1. **Pain and swelling are alleviated** by applying ice with elevation for swelling/pain and applying iontophoresis for localized pain.

2. **Full range of motion** is achieved through manual ankle mobilization, gentle inversion and eversion stretches, and stretches of hamstring, gastrocnemius, and soleus.

3. **Increased strength in ankle stabilization muscles** is attained through the following exercises: standing heel raises, sitting heel raises, windshield wipers, stork exercises, towel curls, resistive band ankle exercises in all planes of motion, and toe push-ups.

4. **Increased proprioception/control and coordination** are accomplished by performing the following exercises: balancing and weight shifting exercises on a trampoline, various balancing and weight shifting exercises performed on a piece of equipment referred to as a biomechanical ankle platform system (BAPS board), stork exercises, and chain reaction exercises.

5. **Exercises for general lower extremity strengthening** include wall squats, step downs, agility drills, hamstring curls, leg press, and hip strengthening in multiple planes.

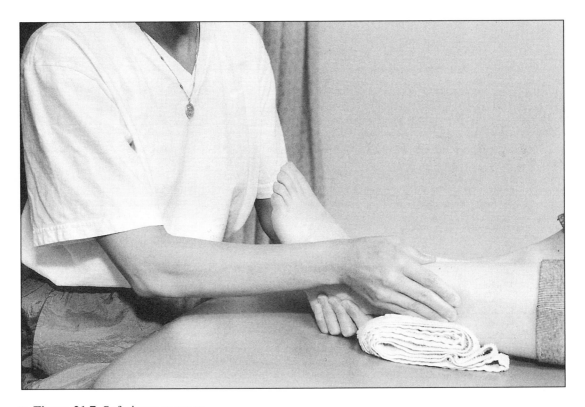

■ **Figure 21.7** Soft tissue massage.

6. **Cardiovascular fitness is maintained** by using the following pieces of exercise equipment: stationary bike, treadmill, stair stepper, and upper extremity ergometer (UBE).

Before initiating phase III of the rehabilitation program, the following criteria should be met:

- able to maintain subtalar joint neutral with all exercises
- no pain or swelling
- discharge modalities
- discharge passive range of motion/mobilization
- discharge external support

The goals of treatment during phase III are to

1. increase functional strength and proprioception,
2. initiate sport-specific training, and
3. increase sport-specific endurance.

During phase III, the rehabilitation program continues to emphasize strengthening and proprioception training while incorporating sport-specific techniques.

1. **Increase functional strength and proprioception.** Use single-leg balancing on a trampoline, throwing a weighted ball, and agility drills using an elastic band for resistance (running).

2. **Design a sport-specific training program.** At 4 weeks post-op, interval training on a treadmill (running) is initiated; the patient's running technique is assessed; the patient's upper body, back, pelvis, and other parts of the body are assessed for dysfunction or weakness; patient education on proper running form and technique is carried out; the patient is videotaped while running to further assess details of form and technique; the need for orthotics is assessed; and the patient's running shoes are assessed for proper fit and support. Areas of weakness or dysfunction are addressed by incorporating appropriate exercises and stretches.

3. **Increase sport-specific endurance.** Use the slide board (figure 21.8), fitter, pedal stepping on stair stepper, and deep water running (timed intervals).

During phase IV (5-6 weeks), the rehabilitation program is as follows:

1. Return to running with appropriate progression to previous training level.

2. Incorporate light hill training and plyometric training drills.

3. Develop a thorough home exercise program to avoid reinjury.

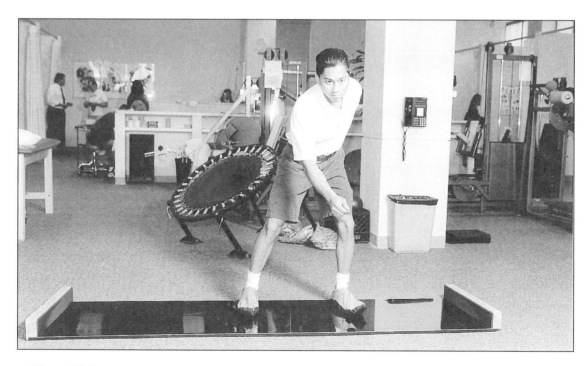

■ **Figure 21.8** Slide board for general lower extremity conditioning and cardiovascular training.

Example 2

A 55-year-old female suffered a severe inversion injury to her left ankle while jumping on a trampoline. Radiographs revealed an avulsion of the anterior talofibular ligament from the fibula. Surgical arthroscopy also revealed a partial tear of the deltoid ligament. The patient then underwent an open reduction internal fixation (ORIF) of the fracture, with a screw fixation.

In phase I (1-3 weeks), the patient is casted and nonweightbearing. In phase II (3-6 weeks), the patient remains in a cast and is partial weight bearing until 4 weeks post-op, and then is full weight bearing.

The goals of treatment in phase III (6-10 weeks) are to

1. decrease pain and swelling,
2. increase active range of motion in all directions,
3. increase strength in lower extremities, as well as ankle and foot stabilizing muscles,
4. increase proprioception, control, and coordination, and
5. maintain cardiovascular fitness.

In phase III, the cast is removed and the patient's foot is placed into a CAM walker. The subtalar joint must be maintained in a neutral position for all exercises. Physical therapy is initiated utilizing pool therapy one time per week and land therapy two times per week. Gait training is initiated in the pool without the CAM walker. Extreme plantarflexion must be avoided. The rehabilitation program during this phase is as follows:

1. **Decrease pain and swelling** with ice, elevation, phonophoresis, soft tissue massage, and active ankle pumps.

2. **Increase range of motion** with ankle and forefoot mobilization, gentle passive range of motion, and stretches of the hamstring and calf.

3. **Increase strength** using ankle stabilizing exercises, Theraband exercises in all planes including plantarflexion, manual resistance (proprioceptive neuromuscular facilitation [PNF] stretching), hamstring curls, leg press, and the multihip machine.

4. **Increase proprioception** by utilizing trampoline balancing, BAPS board sitting → standing, and stork exercises.

5. **Increase/maintain cardiovascular fitness** with Nitron and deep water pool exercises.

The goals of treatment in phase IV (10-12 weeks) are to

1. increase strength,
2. increase proprioception/control/coordination, and
3. increase cardiovascular fitness.

In this phase, the CAM walker is removed and the patient is progressed to a shoe. The pool, mobilizations, and modalities are all discharged, except for ice and iontophoresis (for local pain).

The exercises described in phase II for strength and proprioception are progressed in the rehabilitation program for this phase. Additionally, the following exercises are incorporated.

1. **Increase strength** by focusing on ankle stabilizing muscles, chain reaction (sports cord), fitter, slide board, lunges, stepdowns, subtalar joint neutral exercises, toe raises with weight, and agility drills with sports cord.

2. **Increase proprioception** (advanced exercises) with trampoline (throwing plyoball, etc.), retro stair stepper, and stork exercises with dynamic movement of uninvolved side.

3. **Increase cardiovascular fitness** by utilizing treadmill walking (with incline), retro stair stepper, slide board, and fitter.

The goals of treatment during phase V (3 months) are to

1. return the patient to sport-specific training,
2. return the patient to full duty on the job, and
3. develop a thorough home exercise program in preparation for discharge.

This is the final phase of the rehabilitation program. The patient must wait approximately 3 months post-op before returning to the previous sport.

The patient's rehabilitation program is progressed with the following exercises:

- Jumping activities
- Progression from jogging to running
- Plyometrics
- Sport-specific and job-specific training
- Patient education to avoid reinjury
- Overall assessment for associated dysfunction, similar to phase III of Example 1.

■ References

Appenzeller O, ed. 1988. Sports medicine. 3rd ed. Baltimore: Urban and Schwarzenberg.

Ferkel RD. 1996. Arthroscopic surgery: the foot and ankle. Philadelphia: Lippincott- Raven.

Suggested Readings

Corrigan B, Maitland GD. Practical Orthopaedic Medicine. Butterworth & Co., 1983.

DeMaio M, Paine R, Drez D Jr. Chronic lateral ankle instability—inversion sprains. Orthopedics 15:87-96, 1992.

DeMaio M, Paine R, Drez D Jr. Chronic lateral ankle instability—inversion sprains: Part II. Orthopedics 15:241-248, 1992.

Ferkel RD, Scranton PE. Current concepts review: Arthroscopy of the ankle and foot. J Bone Joint Surg 75A:1233-1242, 1993.

Ferkel RD. Differential diagnosis of chronic ankle sprain pain in the athlete. Sports Med Arthroscopy Rev 2:274-283, 1994.

Lehmkuhl LK. Clinical Kinesiology 4th ed. Philadelphia: F.A. Davis, 1983.

Payton OD. Manual of Physical Therapy. New York: Churchill Livingstone, 1989.

Pitman CA. Rehabilitative exercises following ankle injuries. Orthopedics 13:723-725, 1990.

Voss De, Ionta MK, Myers BJ. Proprioceptive Neuromuscular Facilitation. 3rd ed. Philadelphia: Harper and Row, 1985.

Wilkerson LA. Ankle injuries in athletes. Prim Care 19:377-392, 1992.

Chapter 22

Proprioceptive Retraining of Chronic Ankle Instability

David Mencher, DC, PhD

Chronic instability often follows seemingly moderate injury to the anatomical structures supporting the ankle. Many studies have linked these late symptoms of ankle injury to differentiation in the acute and subacute stages, with resultant loss of motor coordination, leading to what Freeman et al. (1965) termed "functional instability." In the years since Freeman first proposed the model of "functional" as well as anatomical instability in chronic ankle injury, the importance of proprioception and kinesthesia in the mechanism of development of recurrent injury and in the successful rehabilitation of ankle injury and prevention of chronic injury has been widely recognized (Lephart et al. 1997; Leanderson et al. 1996; Konradsen et al. 1993). In this chapter, the contribution of proprioceptive pathways to ankle injury, stability, and rehabilitation will be briefly reviewed, and the basic tenets of proprioceptive retraining, as developed by Janda (Janda & Va'Vrova 1996), will be presented along with current protocols for the application of these principles in the clinical setting.

■ Proprioception in Ankle Sprains

Lephart et al. (1997) defined proprioception as a specialized variation of the sensory modality of touch that encompasses the sensation of joint movement (kinesthesia) and joint position (joint position sense). Proprioception relies on sensory receptors in the skin, muscles, and joints, as well as ligaments, tendons, and visual and vestibular centers, for afferent input regarding tissue deformation, body position, and balance (Lephart et al. 1997). This neural stimulation travels to the central nervous system via cortical and reflex pathways. Damage to cutaneous, muscle, and articular sources of proprioceptive feedback in acute ankle sprain has been implicated in the development of chronic instability (Freeman 1965; Lofvenberg et al. 1995). In addition, it has been suggested that proprioceptive deficits may be a primary factor in the etiology of the acute ankle sprain (Leanderson et al. 1996; Lofvenberg et al. 1995).

By measuring changes in muscle contraction patterns, Sheth et al. (1997) were able to demonstrate an increased frequency of ankle inversion control in healthy subjects receiving 8 weeks of proprioceptive (ankle disk) training, as compared with untrained subjects. Similarly, Tropp et al. (1985) reported a decreased rate of ankle sprains in soccer players after 10 weeks of ankle disk training, also suggesting that the degree of afferent stimulation is critical to the mechanism of ankle injury.

In studies of postural sway, stabilometry, and muscle reaction times following ankle injury, it has been generally shown that postural stability is impaired in the injured ankle, regardless of the degree of mechanical stability retained (Leanderson et al. 1996; Lofvenberg et al. 1995; Lephart et al. 1998). Compared with immobilization, active rehabilitation of these injuries, including proprioceptive training, efficiently restores these components of dynamic stabilization (Regis et al. 1995). Although some controversy exists regarding the relative contribution of articular vs. musculotendinous mechanoreceptors (Robbins & Waked 1998) to joint position sense, it is clear that a program of exercises that challenges the components of balance can effectively improve the resistance of the ankle joint to chronic and acute inversion injury.

The section titled "Further Thoughts on Proprioceptive Training As a Therapeutic Measure" was written by Dr. Rüdiger Reer and Dr. Jörg Jorosch.

■ Principles of Proprioceptive Retraining

The goal of proprioceptive retraining is to restore and improve the unconscious motor responses to unexpected joint loading. This is achieved through a graded program of challenges to balance, progressing from simple two-legged sways, to one-legged stance, to rocker board, to special "wobble" balance sandals worn for a few minutes each day. Although not usually included under this heading, comprehensive exercise routines, such as Tai Chi, employ important components of postural training and have been proven valuable in the rehabilitation of elderly and challenged populations.

Because most proprioceptive information originates from mechanoreceptors located in the neck, sacroiliac joints, and the soles of the feet, the exercises that make up proprioceptive retraining are effective for a number of conditions involving chronic instability, including chronic ankle and knee sprain, faulty posture syndromes, and chronic low back pain. They are also effective training as compensation for decreased proprioception in the elderly.

In the "Sensory Motor Stimulation" program developed by Janda and Va'Vrova (1996), a general plan of proprioceptive retraining is implemented, directed toward improving motor activities involved with posture and gait. Although rehabilitation of the chronically unstable ankle focuses on the foot and lower limb exercises, the retraining of posture- and gait-related motor patterns at the knee, pelvis, and torso should be viewed as necessary components of any ankle rehabilitation program. The following protocol is adapted from Janda's Sensory Motor Stimulation, with specific emphasis on ankle-related exercises.

■ Protocol for Proprioceptive Retraining of Chronic Ankle Instability

Indications for the following protocol include posttraumatic ankle instability; chronic ankle instability associated with low back pain; and coordination and balance deficiencies associated with lower limb joint hypermobility.

Contraindications for the protocol include acute pain syndromes of the lower limb; mechanical instability; and extreme peripheral dysfunction. (Peripheral dysfunction should be normalized first to minimize pathological proprioceptive information during rehabilitation.)

The following principles underlie this protocol:

- To maximize correct proprioceptive input, the exercises are performed in bare feet.
- Integrity of the skin, joints, muscles, and related structures should be optimized (stretching and balancing) to improve balance.
- Exercises should not provoke pain or lead to physical fatigue.
- The program progresses from stable to more uncertain surfaces, from "predictable" to "less predictable" positions.

Janda has found that a supinated foot posture with relaxed toes ("short foot") improves afferent input from receptors on the soles (Janda & Va'Vrova 1996). The therapist should help the patient develop the short foot stance through the following measures:

1. The short foot is first achieved passively, while seated, through molding by the therapist.
2. Once attained, the short foot design is practiced actively, with aid from the therapist.
3. Finally, the patient actively forms the short foot (sitting), while the therapist loads the calf muscles with pressure through the knee.

The short foot should be taught at the beginning of therapy, but it is not necessary to achieve proficiency before proceeding to the balance regimen. With progress, the short foot will become automatic.

Standing Balance Exercises

1. Simple balance. Simple balance exercises may be necessary at first: feet parallel, shoulder-width apart, and swaying from front to back with heels and soles flat on the floor. This can also be done with knees slightly (20-30°) flexed. The therapist should lightly touch chest and buttocks to check the range of sway.

2. Balance minus visual cues. Once mastered, sway may be attempted without visual cues (blindfolded or eyes closed— this will be difficult, and should not be attempted for more than 5 seconds at a time), on one foot, etc. Sway exercises not only enhance position sense at the lower limb and feet, but also improve balance and body awareness.

Rocker Board Exercises

A rocker board is employed after progress and proficiency in the floor exercises (the exercises relating to simple balance and balance minus visual cues). Rocker boards should be wooden, approximately 35 cm × 25 cm × 15 cm high, and should have a nonslip surface appropriate for bare feet.

1. Simple balance. Simple balancing is practiced at first, with rocking in the anterioposterior plane, gradually increasing in frequency and amplitude with practice. Patients may practice this at home, with periodic monitoring by the therapist in the clinic.

2. Floor exercises. Balancing then progresses similarly to floor exercises: rocking at a 45° angle; one-legged stance; resisting challenges (taps, pushes, brushes) by the therapist; and, eventually, rocker board exercises without visual cues. Flexed knee postures should be encouraged while on the rocker board, as they strengthen the vastus medialis and enhance pelvic mobility.

3. Jumps. Finally, the patient may practice jumps, at first landing on both feet on the floor, then progressing to two-legged and one-legged jumps onto the rocker board. This advanced stage of proprioceptive training is valuable for strengthening the spinovestibulocerebellar response to sudden changes in terrain, lessening the likelihood of falls and chronic reinjury.

Balance Sandals

Balance sandals for proprioceptive retraining were recently introduced by Bullock-Saxton and Janda. Their value for therapy in chronic ankle instability derives from the ease of their use, the automatic, unconscious response to their challenge, and the rapid response in muscle coordination usually achieved with regular use (Bullock-Saxton et al. 1993; Janda & Va'Vrova 1996). Balance sandals have a firm, inflexible sole, with a solid rubber hemisphere 5-7 cm in diameter placed at the center of gravity. The fit is approximate, and the single strap should allow for heel movement.

Patients should be instructed to

- attempt to control posture (head, shoulder, and pelvis) rather than bending;
- take short, quick steps;
- hold feet parallel; and
- maintain natural movement of the pelvis while walking.

Initially, support may be necessary to prevent lack of coordination and falls. Patients may benefit from practicing gait in front of a mirror.

Balance sandals have been shown to be effective for postural control and dynamic muscle coordination after only a few weeks of indoor use at 5-10 minutes per day (Bullock-Saxton et al. 1993). Patient motivation and compliance with balance sandal exercise is very high, perhaps because of the simplicity of their use.

■ Conclusion

Failure of mechanisms of dynamic stabilization has been implicated in chronic ankle injury, as well in as low back pain, knee instability, and postural syndromes. Proprioceptive retraining, directed toward improving the speed and coordination of muscle contraction, should be an integral component of any program of ankle rehabilitation. The methods discussed here (short foot, floor exercises, rocker board, and balance sandals) are easily mastered, require little sophisticated equipment, and are easily adapted to patients' individual needs and capabilities.

■ Further Thoughts on Proprioceptive Training As a Therapeutic Measure

It has recently been determined that, as in other joints, the stability of the upper ankle joint can to a major extent be traced back to coordinative and proprioceptive abilities. Because of this, interest has increased regarding understanding neurophysiological relations, as well as regarding how that understanding should affect current practice in prophylaxis and therapy, particularly as applied to sport. As shown in several studies, proprioceptive perception can be positively influenced by coordinative training (Freeman et al. 1965). In contrast, Berenberg et al. (1987) could not prove any improvement of proprioception by a special coordinative training using special mirror tests.

Conservative-Functional Therapeutic Approaches

In several studies, good results of functional therapy after supination traumas of the ankle joint could be confirmed (Freeman et al. 1965). MRI controlled studies show a scarred restitution of the ligamentous continuity.

Sommer and Schreiber pointed to the socioeconomic advantages that have been documented over many years (1993). Three different treatment methods were compared: Method A (immobilization in a plaster cast for three weeks, followed by mobilization with a brace), method B (mobilization with a brace), and method C (Unna's paste dressing for 2 weeks with subsequent tape dressings and in each case immediate mobilization). Comparison of direct costs of the different methods revealed results in favor of method B (DM 175) compared to method C (DM 206) and method A (DM 340). The direct costs after early functional treatment are the lowest compared with surgical treatment in a hospital setting (in 1991, the cost of one day in a hospital in West Germany was DM

319). The indirect sequential costs resulting from loss of working hours are also lower when an early functional treatment approach is used. Aftercare with braces leads to a decrease in the rehabilitation time by several weeks. Renström et al. (1997) emphasized the substantial advantage of treatment with brace and bandage in comparison to plaster. The following principles are suggested for the treatment of ankle supination trauma:

- Analgesia, antiphlogistic therapy, structural adaptation
- Strain protection of the structural damage
- Securing of the periarticular trophic
- Mobilization and manipulative therapy before hypomobility
- Early axial strain and proprioceptive stimulation
- Muscle stretching
- Integrative muscular strength training
- Neuromuscular coordinative training
- Improvement of posture and body sense
- Aiding adaptation

From these considerations, the following treatment techniques can be derived:

- RICE (rest, ice, compression, elevation), with limited load and functional immobility
- Cryo-cuff
- Tape, lace-on brace, stirrup brace
- Iontophoresis, ultrasound, lymphatic drainage, two-cell bath
- Manual therapy, CPM, motion bath, aquajogging
- Walking exercises on treadmill
- Passive and active stretching and relaxation techniques
- Isometric exercises, PNF, ergometry, isokinetic exercises
- Proprioceptive training
- Spine rehabilitation and training, skill training
- Insole supports, footwear care, training, and sport consultation

Recent Changes in Therapeutic Techniques

Today, post-traumatic plaster immobilization is to a large extent obsolete. The plaster treatment leads to various unwelcome side effects: reduction of collagen synthesis and reduction in thickness of fibers, which results in insufficient scar tissue. The muscular deficit that results from immobilization, and the os-

teoporosis that is often generated by it, both complicate and lengthen rehabilitation. After these problems were discovered, different ankle braces were developed. The type of device to use was determined by its limitation of pronation and supination. The plantarflexion and dorsal extension of the foot should be less than 10°-0°-20°, and the rotation should also be substantially limited.

It has became obvious that, as with other joints, the stability of the injured upper ankle joint can to a great extent be improved through the restoration of coordinative and proprioceptive (sensomotory) abilities. According to several studies, the necessary sensomotory processing can be positively influenced by coordinative training. Gleitz et al. (1993) and Freeman et al. (1965) showed the improvement of post-traumatic proprioception by coordinative and reflex training. According to their suggestion, this training effect can be achieved by means of training the remaining intact receptors and by an improved central regulation. Tropp et al. (1985) showed a prophylactic effect of regular proprioceptive training among soccer players with unstable ankle joints. Janda and Bullock-Saxton (1994) pointed especially to the influence of proprioceptive abilities on the stability of complex movement patterns of the lower extremities. They came to the conclusion that this effect was due to an extreme instability of the movement control resulting from a central nervous system adaptation deficit, as well as an arthrogenic proprioception deficit.

As already described previously (see chapter 5), the work of Jerosch et al. demonstrated that the aim of stability testing should be to identify the individual sensomotory deficits of each patient with special tests in order to design a precise proprioceptive training program that will address the unique needs of that patient.

Recommendations for Sensomotory Training

In the future, change in rehabilitative therapy of joint injuries in general, and ankle joint traumas in particular, is likely. The therapy will be oriented to the individual deficits of each patient. Possible emphases of such custom-designed therapy include the following:

- Static and dynamic muscle balance
- Stability
- Gait rhythm
- Control of the axis of the leg
- Balance training
- Kinetic reflex facilitation

Simple aids for proprioceptive-coordinative training of the ankle joint include soft mat, trampoline, wobble board, sloping board, Pezzi ball, and the whole range of balance exercises—for example, one-leg stand test with eyes closed. By means of these exercises, proprioceptors are continuously activated with the constant change in positon and motion of the ankle joint and the entire body. This continuous activation of proprioceptors leads to a reaction that facilitates the maintenance of postural equilibrium. Thus, the afferent central and efferent parts of the proprioceptive-sensomotory system are continuously challenged.

The following sections describe recommended prophylactic and therapeutic exercises for increasing proprioceptive capabilities that are particularly important in sport.

Soft Mat

The unstable surface of the soft mat (figure 22.1) leads to increased requirements for the foot and the maintenance of equilibrium.

Possible exercises include the following:

- Standing on tiptoe
- Falling into the lunge position and trying to stop and stabilize the movement

- Keeping one leg stabilized and carrying out dynamic, gait-typical movements with the free leg (this leads to an improvement in muscle activity)
- Improving proprioceptive-sensomotory gait skills by exercising with the resistance of a Theraband (figure 22.1)
- Carrying out gait-typical crossover movements

Trampoline

The trampoline (figure 22.2) offers the advantage of a joint-sparing exercise. The fast movements make coordinative demands on the muscles of the entire body, and jumping strongly emphasizes upward movement.

The following exercises offer stimuli for the proprioceptive-sensomotory system:

- Straddle jumps and standing jumps with a strong emphasis on the process of elevation; rotation jumps with impulse intensification of the rotation pattern of the spine during walking; and jumping with dynamic arm movements.
- One-leg stand test, which leads to an increased strain on the standing leg. This leads to high demands on intra- and intermuscular coordination ability, because the free leg is unstable.

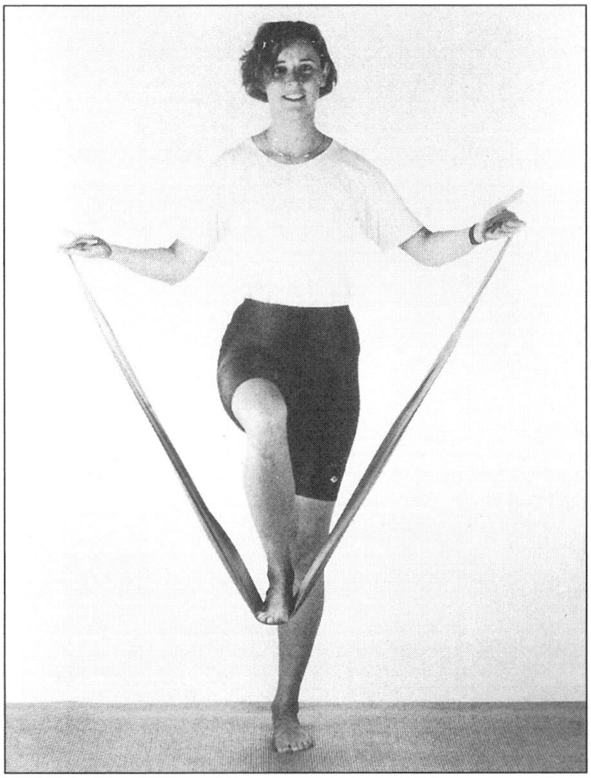

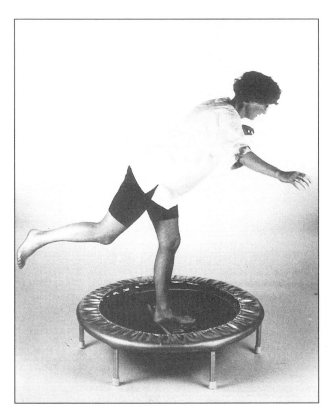

■ **Figure 22.1** Set-up of proprioceptive-coordinative training using the soft mat and the Theraband.

■ **Figure 22.2** Set-up of proprioceptive-coordinative training using the trampoline.

- Scale position, which leads to an increased strain on the standing leg and to increased demands on the equilibrium response due to the use of the extremities as levers (figure 22.2).

Wobble Board

Because of its unstable base, the wobble board (figure 22.3) offers ideal conditions for developing the proprioceptive capabilities of the ankle joint.

Possible exercises include the following:

- Two-leg or one-leg stand on the wobble board, which requires balancing of the entire body.

- Weight shift to the right/left side and to the front/back using two-leg and one-leg stands. respectively. This leads to continuous stimulation of the proprioceptive systems and, therefore, to tightening of the muscle links.

- Throwing and catching objects, which requires a controlled braking and steering of small movements (fine motor control) and therefore leads to a continuous alteration between concentric and excentric muscle activities.

- Lifting of objects on the wobble board, which, because of the shifting of the longitudinal axis of the body on an unstable base, presents a strong challenge for equilibrium conditions (figure 22.3)

Sloping Board

The sloping board (figure 22.4) leads to proprioceptive requirements and increments of the footwork by creating an oblique plane.

Possible exercises include the following:

- Loading on the outer edge of the foot in downhill position and on the inner edge of the foot in uphill position

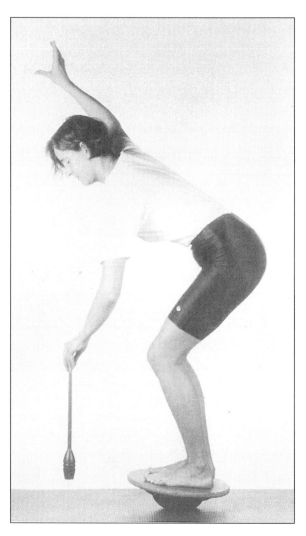

■ **Figure 22.3** Set-up of proprioceptive-coordinative training using the wobble board.

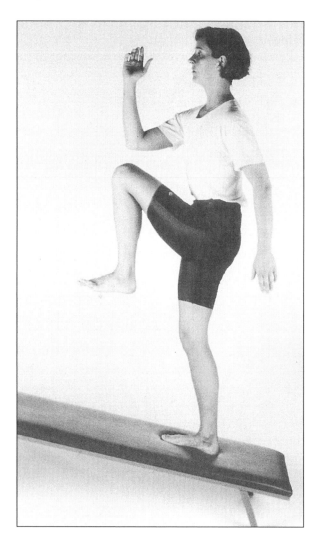

■ **Figure 22.4** Set-up of proprioceptive-coordinative training using the sloping board.

- Swinging in gait pattern in uphill position in order to activate the ventral chain (figure 22.4)

- Swinging in gait pattern in downhill position in order to activate the dorsal chain

- Standing on tiptoe during rest and motion: the minimal support surface requires a strong equilibrium response

Stability Ball

The stability ball (figure 22.5) facilitates sensomotory exercises with partial relief of strain.

Possible stability ball exercises include the following:

- Jumping while sitting on the ball, while intermittently increasing pressure on the sole of the foot; the increase in pressure promotes preparation for elevation.

- Alternating between heel and toe, which leads to a stimulation of the coordinative joint play of the feet.

- Jumping from standing onto tiptoe. Because of the reduction of the support area, the ability for concentric footwork is to a certain degree strained while the heel is raised.

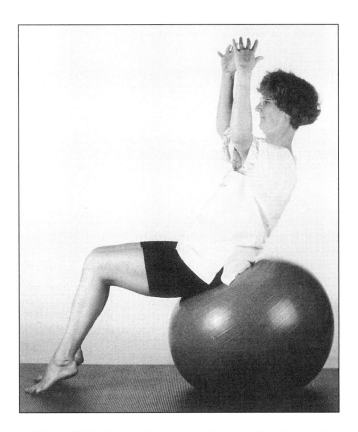

Figure 22.5 Set-up of proprioceptive-coordinative training using the stability ball.

- Jumping and stopping the movement. When stopping the heels just above the ground, excentric footwork is used.

- Moving in gait-typical rhythm.

- Lifting arms, which leads to tightening of the entire ventral chain and the opening of the kinetic chain, therefore leading to increased muscle activity (figure 22.5).

- Alternating between training of the flexors of the free leg and training of the support activity of the standing leg.

Associated Areas to be Addressed in Therapy

The following are frequent local joint-typical muscular interferences:

- Weakening of the peroneal muscles

- Weakening of the tibial anterior muscle

- Weakening of the extensor hallucis longus muscle

- Shortening of the extensor hallucis longus muscle

- Shortening of the tibial posterior muscle

- Shortening of the flexor hallucis muscle

- Shortening of the extensor digitorum longus muscle

- Shortening of the medial venter of the triceps surae muscle

The pathologically changing foot dynamic results not only in local effects, but also in effects in remote joints. At the hip, the iliopsoas muscle and the medial gluteal muscle are affected; at the hip and knee, the ischiocrural muscle and the tensor fasciae latae muscle are affected; and at the knee joint, the popliteal muscle and the vastus medialis muscle are affected. Strength training of the muscles should have the following aims:

- Intermuscular coordination

- Neuromuscular strength quality

- Local strength endurance

- Enlargement of the cross-section of the muscle

- Situation-adapted synergisms of diverse strength components

Ergometers (cycle, rowing), isokinetic machines, stepping machines, leg press, treadmill, cross-country skiing simulators, and aquajogging are used as support apparatus.

■ References

Berenberg RA, Sheffner JM, Sabol JJ. 1987. Quantitative assessment of position sense at the ankle: a functional approach. Neurology 37:89–93.

Bullock-Saxton, J.E., Janda, V., and Bullock, M. Reflex Activation of Gluteal Muscles on Walking. Spine 18 (6):704-707, 1993.

Freeman, M.A.R., Dean, M.R.E., and Hanhan, I.W.F. The Etiology and Prevention of Functional Instability of the Foot. The Journal of Bone and Joint Surgery 47B (4): 678-85, 1965.

Freeman, M.A.R. Instability of the Foot After Injuries to the Lateral Ligament of the Ankle. Journal of Bone and Joint Surgery 47-B: 669-77, 1965.

Gleitz M, Rupp T, Hess T, Hopf T. 1993. Bei instabilen Sprunggelenken: Reflextraining und Stabilisierung. Orthopädie und Schuhtechnik 5:65–68.

Janda V, Bullock-Saxton JE. 1994. Zur Frage der Stabilität der Bewegungsmuster in bezug auf die Proprioception. Dtsch Z Sportmed 45:S67–S68.

Janda, V. and Va'Vrova, M. Sensory Motor Stimulation. In Rehabilitation of the Spine. Leibenson, C. editor. Williams and Wilkins, 1996. pp 319-28.

Jerosch J, Hoffstetter I, Bork H, Bischoff M. 1995. The influence of orthoses on the proprioception of the ankle joint. Knee Surg Sports Traumatol Arthroscopy 3:39–46.

Konradsen, L., Ravn, J.B., and Sorenssen, A.I. Proprioception at the Ankle: The Effects of Anesthetic Blockade of Ligament Receptors. The Journal of Bone and Joint Surgery 75-B:433-36, 1993.

Leanderson, J., Eriksson, E., Nilsson, C., and Wykman, A. Proprioception in Classical Ballet Dancers. The American Journal of Sports Medicine 24 (3):370-74, 1996.

Lephart, S.M., Pincivero, D.M., and Rozzi, S.L. Proprioception of the Ankle and Knee. Sports Medicine 25 (3):149-55, 1998.

Lephart, S.M., Pincivero,D.M., Giraldo, J.L., and Fu, F.H.: The Role of Proprioception in the Management and Rehabilitation of Athletic Injuries. The American Journal of Sports Medicine 25 (1):130- 37, 1997.

Lofvenberg, R, Karrholm, J., Sundelin, G., and Ahlegren, O. Prolonged Reaction Time in Patients with Chronic Lateral Instability of the Ankle. The American Journal of Sports Medicine 25 (4):414-17, 1995.

Regis, D., Montanari, M., Magnan, B., Spagnol, S., and Bragantini, A. Dynamic Orthopaedic Brace in the Treatment of Ankle Sprains. Foot and Ankle International 16 (7):422-26, 1995.

Renström PA, Beynnon B, Haugh L, MacDonald L. 1997. A prospective randominzed outcome study of acute first time ankle sprains, grade I and II [abstract]. First Biennial Congress of the International Society of Arthroscopy, Knee Surgery and Orthopaedic Sports Medicine; 1997 May 11-16; Buenos Aires, Argentina.

Robbins, S., and Waked, E. Factors Associated with Ankle Injuries. Sports Medicine 25 (1):63-72, 1998.

Sheth,P., Yu, B., Laskowski, E.R., and An, K-N. Ankle Disk Training Influences Reaction Times of Selected Muscles in a Simulated Ankle Sprain. The American Journal of Sports Medicine 25 (4):538-43, 1997.

Sommer HM, Schreiber H. 1993. Die früh-funktionelle konservative Therapie der frischen fibularen Kapsel-Band-Ruptur aus sozioökonomischer Sicht. Sportverletz-Sportschaden 7:40–46.

Tropp, H., Askling, C., and Gillquist, J. Prevention of Ankle Sprains. The American Journal of Sports Medicine 13:259-262, 1985.

Chapter 23

Return to Sport After Delayed Surgical Reconstruction for Ankle Instability

Steven I. Subotnick, DPM, ND, DC

Ankle sprains are the most common lower extremity injury and one of the most common injuries overall. It is estimated that each year, 1 million people in the United States experience acute ankle injuries, most commonly plantarflexion inversion sprains (Chu & Davies 1998; Subotnick 1998).

Acute ankle sprains account for at least 15% of all sport injuries (Haas & Levine 1998). Peri et al. (1993) reported that 48% of patients with an acute first ankle sprain will develop recurrent sprains, and 26% will have frequent sprains. One wonders why more delayed reconstructions aren't necessary, or demanded. Certainly there is no universal agreement regarding the long-term consequences of ankle injury, or regarding chronic lateral instability of the ankle, with or without concurrent subtalar joint instability. However, experienced orthopedic and podiatric sport surgeons are increasingly finding that the old notion of instability leading to osteochondral lesion and early arthrosis or arthritis is more theory than fact (Robbins & Waked 1998).

As Stan James, MD, past orthopedic surgeon for the University of Oregon, once told me, "If we operated on every unstable ankle we'd never leave the operating room. Only symptomatic ankles require surgery."

Types of Instability

Three types of instability are recognized: mechanical, functional, and subtalar (Sitler & Horodysky, 1995).

■ **Mechanical instability** is characterized by ankle mobility beyond the physiologic range of motion, with increased talar tilt and anterior drawer. Symp-

toms, however, do not correlate with the degree of laxity.

■ **Functional instability** is the chronic disability characterized by a subjective feeling of "giving way." Factors include proprioception, reflex and muscular reaction time, strength, balance, and power. Other factors include chronic synovitis, adhesions, and functional imbalance.

■ **Subtalar instability and sinus tarsi syndrome** are the result of subtalar inversion sprains with subsequent synovitis, sinus tarsi inflammation, painful subtalar joint adhesions, joint dysfunction, and reduction of subtalar mobility.

The rehabilitation of the various types of instabilities, with or without surgical reconstruction, is essentially the same, except for the timing of the activities during physical rehabilitation, which is dictated by the strength and the stability of the healing tissues. Thus, the return to sport is dictated by the same parameters following injury, with or without surgery.

Of the three types of instability—mechanical, functional, and subtalar and sinus tarsi syndrome—the mechanical instability has an easily demonstrable talar tilt and anterior drawer sign, whereas the functional instability "feels" unstable to the athlete despite the fact that there is no demonstrable instability. Because it is the symptoms, and not the instability, that really count, the distinctions are more useful in predicting surgical needs at the time of surgery, if surgery is planned, than in deciding which patient should be operated on. In gross instability, ligaments are repaired, whereas with functional instability, the joint is explored for osteochondral lesions, meniscoid lesions, adhesions, or other intra-articular pathologies. Arthroscopic synovectomy decreases the dissection during open reconstruction and usually allows for adequate joint inspection and gutter debridement, when needed.

Most severe plantarflexion inversion lateral sprains or ruptures involve the subtalar joint as well as the ankle joint. The middle lateral collateral ligament, the calcaneofibular ligament, crosses both joints. The interosseous subtalar ligament is often injured, and the calcaneocuboid and cuboidmetatarsal joints may be sprained, with volar ligamentous damage and subsequent joint instability. A 3- or 4-week postoperative cast immobilization thus protects the healing ligaments or tenodesis and allows the lateral column foot joints a chance to rest and heal.

When surgery is decided on for a symptomatic unstable ankle, most authorities prefer the anatomical modifications of Broström's delayed primary ligamentous repair (1965). Certainly it is easy to perform, allowing for earlier return to function with less motion limitation. It is, however, more easily reinjured than the modified Evans or Chrisman-Snook type of procedure.

I still favor the functional repair for highly unstable ankles with multiple past injuries, especially if poor tissue for repair is present. A modified Evans procedure, passing the whole peroneal brevis tendon through an oblique drill hole in the fibular malleolus, then re-anastamosing it to the muscle proximal to the posterior superior drill hole, is my procedure of choice. Disrupted ligaments are also repaired, and bone anchoring, or a similar technique, is used to anatomically repair them.

■ Rehabilitation and Return to Sport

Rehabilitation and return to sport follow the guidelines for return from injury, focusing on proprioception, strength, flexibility, balance, power, and improved skills and reaction time, as well as protective dynamic bracing. Biodynamic custom foot orthotics help to correct foot imbalances, such as cavus or forefoot valgus, which predispose to lateral instability of the foot and ankle and reinjury of the ankle, subtalar, or calcaneocuboid joints.

Basic Principles

The rehabilitation goal is to rapidly regain strength, flexibility, balance, power, and endurance within the physiologic and tissue strength limits. The patient must do just enough exercise to stimulate functional adaptation and realignment of healing collagen within the capsule and ligaments, as well as subcutaneous and cutaneous tissue, and still maintain tensile strength and tissue integrity. The rehabilitation program should allow just enough exercise without risking a rupture or failure of anchoring fixation devices or ligamentous re-anastomosis. This is termed **supervised return to activity,** and eventually leads to unrestricted activity. Exercise thus becomes a prescription and is equally, if not more, important than the actual surgical technique, which admittedly is not technically very demanding.

It has been said, and certainly observed over and over again, that injured athletes return to full activity in far better overall condition than they were before the injury. One wonders whether many injuries could be eliminated if the postoperative rehabilitation and sport-specific "work hardening" were provided in the preseason or intraseason physical conditioning program.

Prevention of ankle ligamentous reinjury demands good proprioception, balance, flexibility, and strength. The rehabilitation of the peroneal muscle groups is of special importance in preventing subsequent ankle lateral ligament complex injuries. An important aspect of flexibility is the range of motion. Adhesions and fibrosis of the ankle joint, as well as adhesions of the subtalar joint, midtarsal joint, knee and hip joints, or even the lower back, place proportionately unusual motion and functional demands on the ankle.

The biomechanics of the ankle ("the superior ankle joint") are essentially those of a hinged joint with a small amount of inversion at the ends of motion ranges in dorsiflexion and plantarflexion. The subtalar, or "inferior ankle joint," as the late Vern Inman, MD, termed it, is a universal torque and rotational conversion joint. In concert, these two joints allow for complex multidirectional degrees of freedom of motion. When limitation of motion occurs in the subtalar joint, inversion and eversion motion and torque are forced on the ankle and midtarsal joints. This stretches the lateral ankle ligaments and predisposes them to failure. It also places greater demands on surgically repaired lateral ankle and subtalar ligaments. With limitations as discussed, return to multidirectional activity, or sport activities on uneven surfaces, is not without inherent risk.

Prevention of Reinjury

Prevention relies on taping or bracing in high-risk sports, especially basketball, and often soccer and football, and is essential after surgery. Fortunately, there are many functional braces to choose from, ranging initially from air casts and stirrups, then to lace-up braces (with or without double upright metal reinforcement), and finally to high-top shoes with more elastic anatomic wraps (Barrett & Bilisko 1995; Robbins & Waked 1996; Sitler & Horodyski 1995). Semirigid ankle braces reduce the incidence of ankle sprains in players with a history of sprains, but possibly not in those with no such history (Surve et al. 1994). Ankle braces do lower the incidence, although not the severity, of sprains in basketball players.

High-top athletic shoes increase proprioception, but their ability to reduce the incidence or severity of reinjury of the ankle is not supported by research (Barrett & Bilisko 1995).

Abnormal ability to control postural sway after injury or surgery is thought to be equivalent to functional instability and is a predictable parameter for risk of reinjury (Lephart et al. 1998). The patient's specific sport, position in team sport, age, weight, and past injury history are all factors. Risk factors for ankle injuries have been discussed by Barker et al. (1997).

Postoperative Management Protocol

In general, I place my patients in a below-knee, slightly pronated cast with an anterior univalve (to control any swelling). The cast is covered with bias cut stockinettes or an Ace wrap to prevent scratching of the other leg, or scratching of a partner's leg while in bed. The cast is applied in the operating room. It is left on for 3 weeks. The patient elevates the leg, which is nonweightbearing for 5 days, at which time a cast check is carried out. If all is going well, the patient may proceed with partial, and finally full, weight bearing to tolerance. At 3 weeks, the cast is removed, sutures removed, and the patient is provided with a short leg cam walker or air cast, depending on the extent of repair, amount of protection desired, reliability of the patient, and all of the factors discussed previously.

Physical therapy then begins with range of motion, both active-assisted and passive, first supervised by the physical therapist, then at home four or five times per day. Patients begin with the sagittal plane motions of dorsiflexion and plantarflexion, followed later by rotation, within the physiologic tolerance of the repair. Surgical overcorrection (too much valgus) by delayed primary or tendon reinforcement requires more vigorous range-of-motion exercises and manipulative techniques.

At 3 weeks, the ligaments are still easily stretched or damaged, and anchors can pull loose, so patients should be told to go easy. Motion encourages parallel collagen and pliable scar tissue.

At 4 weeks more active motion takes place, and supervised figure-of-eight walking and balance exer-cises are initiated. Kinesthetic rehabilitation takes place with the aid of the Babst rocker board, and computerized balance and hopping devices (again supervised by the therapist and trainer), with protective hand rails to prevent overstretching or falls, are used.

At 5 weeks, light running with flexible brace protection is initiated. Hopping and more vigorous Babst board exercises are undertaken. Strength as well as fitness is maintained from day to day with ergometer machines, such as an exercise bicycle or rowing machine.

At 6 weeks, figure-of-eight movements, backward shuffling and hopping, running, and exercise are stepped up. Lunging and plyometric power jumps are incorporated. At this point, many patients can return to supervised sport participation, but not competition.

Between 7 and 8 weeks, balance, proprioception, sway, and kinesthetic rehabilitation should be complete, and protected return to participation and competition is allowed. Braces or taping are used for 6 months during high-risk activities. In high-risk sports, or in injury-prone athletes, it may be wise to maintain prophylactic taping or braces throughout the athlete's career.

From the third week onward, electrical modalities—ultrasound, or interferential or medium- to high-intensity galvanic stimulation—are used to promote healing and decrease inflammation and fibrosis. Manual techniques—massage, mobilization, or joint-specific adjustment—are helpful.

As with any return to activity after surgery, this protocol is a suggestion based on experience. Most patients will logically require rehabilitation catering to their unique demands.

Often, with delayed repairs, when osteochondral lesions are present, they are drilled and **chondroplasty** is carried out. Anterior impingement exostoses are removed, ankle gutters debrided, and joint mice removed, when indicated.

Of course, nonweightbearing for 6 weeks is mandatory for any restorative procedures on the weightbearing ankle joint surfaces in order to give the weaker fibrocartilage a chance to heal in the cartilage defects. Decisions regarding high-impact loading must then seriously be made, in as much as the new fibrocartilage is only 60% as strong and able to bear load as the original healthy articular cartilage was. Repetitive high-impact loading will hasten osteoarthritis of the joint, with cartilage failure. Low-intensity activity, however, will help preserve the joint.

For athletes over 40, the decision is easy: walk, don't run or jump. For the college or professional athlete, the decision is more difficult and involves many factors.

Postoperative Pain

Postoperative pain is controlled with Tylenol with codeine 30 mg, Vicodin E.S.

Ultram, 50 mg, one to two every 4 to 6 hours, is usually effective and has the advantage of being neither a nonsteroidal anti-inflammatory drug (NSAID) nor a narcotic.

Short-term use of NSAIDs may be helpful. Long-term use of NSAIDs, other than the newer Cox II inhibitors, should be discouraged because they decrease proteoglycans, which are essential for proper chondrocyte function. Most currently available NSAIDs are nonspecific suppressors of the desired prostaglandin E-1, as well as the inflammatory prostaglandin E-2. The newer Cox II inhibitors are more specific for inflammation suppression, and do not appear to interfere with the synthesis of chondrocyte, or with the digestive prostaglandin.

Nontraditional Accessories to Treatment

Most athletes are interested in doing anything safe and "natural" to maintain health and enhance healing. They usually welcome nutritional and biological complements of standard medications used for pain and inflammation in the postoperative phase and often ask for advice and support regarding the use of these components.

■ **Nutritional support** of the healing tissues begins a few days before the operation and is maintained for 2 months or longer. Glucosamine sulphate, 300 mg per day, and chondroitin sulphate, 300 mg per day, provide nutrition for repairing cartilage, bone, and ligaments. Vitamin C, 2 or 3 g per day, calcium and magnesium in a two-to-one ratio with about 1200-1500 mg of calcium, and trace minerals, are all supportive for soft tissue repair. Zinc, 50 mg per day, aids in tissue repair. After return to high-intensity anaerobic activity, free radical production is countered with antioxidants: vitamin C, 2-3 g/day; selenium, 200 mg/day; vitamin A, 50 mg/day; vitamin E, 800 mg/day; and coenzyme Q10, 300 mg/day. Nutritional and phytochemical preparations enhance collagen synthesis and may decrease mild to moderate pain.

■ **Homeopathic remedies** are gaining more acceptance, and commercially available combinations can be easily prescribed using allopathic indications with no fear of side effects or interference with prescription drugs. Many athletes prefer more "natural" approaches and welcome the nutrition and remedies. I have found that Traumeel in oral or topical form helps reduce hematomas, while also decreasing pain. Zeel, orally or topically, reduces stiffness. Lymphomyosot helps to reduce postoperative edema, as well as more chronic edema. These preparations may be used three or four times a day, all mixed together, five or ten drops of each in a glass of water, to form a "therapeutic cocktail."

■ **Herbal preparations** containing Boswellia, 200 mg, and Curcumin, 200 mg, are anti-inflammatory and a safe and often effective natural anti-inflammatory adjunct.

References

Barker, H.B., Beynon, B.D., and Renström, P.A.F.H. Ankle injury risk factors in sports. Sports Med. 23:69-74 (1997).

Barrett, J., and Bilisko, T. The role of shoes in prevention of ankle sprains. Sports Med. 20:277-280 (1995).

Broström, L. Sprained ankles. Acta Chir Scand 130:560. (1965).

Chu, D., and Davies, G.J. Chapters on physical therapy and rehabilitation. In Subotnick, S.I. Sports Medicine of the Lower Extremity. 2nd ed. Churchill Livingstone, Philadelphia 1998.

Haas and Levine. Selected Aspects of Nutrition and Physical Performance. In Subotnick, S.I. Sports Medicine of the Lower Extremity. 2nd ed. Churchill Livingstone, Philadelphia, 1998.

Lephart, S.M., Pincivero, D.M., and Rozzi, S.L. Proprioception of the ankle and knee. Sports Med. 25:149-155 (1998).

Peri, H., Mann, G., Matan, Y., Frankl, U., Nyska, M., Milgrom, M., and Finsterbush, A. Ankle sprain: occurrence of chronic functional instability and its chronic relation to mechanical instability—a prospective study. 9th International Jerusalem Symposium on Sports Injuries, 11-12 January 1993, Jerusalem, Israel.

Robbins, S., and Waked, E. Factors associated with ankle injuries: preventive measures. Sports Med. 25:63-72 (1998).

Sitler, M.R. and Horodyski, M. Effectiveness of prophylactic ankle stabilisers for prevention of ankle injuries. Sports Med. 20:53-57 (1995).

Subotnick, S.I. Sports Medicine and Surgery of the Lower Extremity. 2nd ed. W.B. Saunders, New York, 1998.

Surve, I., Schwellnus, M.P., Noakes, T., and Lombard, C. A fivefold reduction in the incidence of recurrent ankle sprains in soccer players using the Sport-Stirrup orthosis. Am. J. Sports Med. 22:601-606 (1994).

Chapter 24

Functional Testing As the Basis for Ankle Rehabilitation Progression

George J. Davies, MEd, PT, SCS, ATC, CSCS, and James W. Matheson, MS, PT, CSCS

Rehabilitation following ankle injuries is vital to returning patients to normal activity as quickly and safely as possible. Few prospective, longitudinal, randomized, controlled clinical trials that examine the efficacy of treating ankle injuries in a large number of patients are present in the literature. However, a study published in the *Journal of Bone and Joint Surgery* (Povacz et al. 1998) that met the aforementioned criteria clearly demonstrated the importance of the rehabilitation of ankle injuries. In addition, this investigation illustrated that in subjects with isolated fibular collateral ligament injuries of the ankle, nonoperative treatment yielded results that were comparable with those of operative repair. Shorter recovery times were also apparent in the nonoperative group when compared to the operative group.

Thacker et al. (1999) recently reviewed 113 studies reporting the risk of ankle sprains in sport, methods to provide support, the effects of these interventions on performance, and comparison of prevention efforts. They determined that the most common risk factor for an ankle sprain in sport was a history of a previous sprain. Furthermore, based on this review, it was recommended that athletes should complete a supervised rehabilitation program before returning to practice or competition.

When rehabilitating a patient with an ankle injury, one must approach testing and rehabilitation systematically (Davies 1995b). To assist the clinician in systematically progressing a patient's ankle rehabilitation program, an ankle functional testing algorithm (FTA) approach should be used (Davies 1995a; Davies et al. 1997; Davies & Zillmer 1999). Based on the results of the ankle FTA, an individualized rehabilitation program can be developed that is predicated on the injury, surgery (or lack of surgery), soft tissue healing time constraints, patient's goals, and preinjury level of activity and function. Many approaches to the rehabilitation program have been taken, and there are

not enough meta-analyses featuring long-term outcome studies to demonstrate the most efficacious methods. Thus, we will describe one method that has proven successful for us in many years of clinical application. Thus, this chapter will describe the ankle FTA and discuss the different treatment and exercises that are used as the patient progresses through the testing algorithm.

■ Rationale and Definition

It is important to establish both why it is important to use the FTA, and what the FTA is.

Rationale

There exists a consensus in the literature that there is a need for a method of evaluation and systematic progression of patients through a rehabilitation program (Davies 1995b; Kannus & Renström 1991; Kegerreis 1983; Kegerreis et al. 1984). However, how one should perform this progression is elusive, because there are as many methods and techniques as there are clinicians. The need for a logical evaluation and testing instrument is the rationale behind functional testing algorithms. An FTA may be designed for any orthopedic condition. The ankle FTA, described in this chapter, is one method of assessing a patient with an ankle injury in an efficient manner and allows practitioners to base the progression of the rehabilitation on objective results. It also ensures that patients with similar injuries receive similar standards of care.

The ankle FTA testing paradigm is based on the principles of progression and control. Each test in the progressive testing sequence involves different levels of increasing stress to the patient with less clinical control. Progression to the next higher level of testing is predicated on passing each test in the FTA sequence at a minimal level of performance. The criteria used for the progression through the FTA are currently based on limited research published in the literature, many years of clinical experience, and our empirically based clinical guidelines (Davies 1995a; Davies et al. 1997; Davies & Zillmer 1999). Table 24.1 provides the current empirical guidelines used for clinical decision making regarding the functional progression of exercise during the rehabilitation program.

What the FTA Involves

Figure 24.1 presents a schematic representation of the ankle FTA. This figure summarizes and illustrates how stepwise testing and program design interact. The ankle FTA may be divided into three objective categories or classes of tests. Basic measurements, consisting of a visual analog pain scale, ankle joint anthropometrics, range-of-motion assessment, and the assessment of balance, provide the initial criteria in the ankle FTA. The second category of tests includes open and closed kinetic chain isokinetic testing. These tests examine either single- or multi-joint strength and power. The final test category in the ankle FTA includes several functional and sport-specific tests. These tests are performed when the athlete or patient has neared the completion of formal skilled rehabilitation and is preparing to return to sport or occupation.

The remainder of this chapter will present components of the three testing categories that make up the ankle FTA, and will demonstrate how they are integrated into the progression of rehabilitation of ankle injuries. These discussions will clarify the scheme shown in figure 24.1.

■ History and Subjective Examination

Initially, the clinician must determine where the patient or client requiring ankle rehabilitation will enter the ankle FTA. Typically, this initial decision is based on the results of a detailed and comprehensive history, as well as a neurological and musculoskeletal examination.

The history is important in determining whether the injury is acute or chronic. Furthermore, if surgery has been performed, soft tissue healing constraints will dictate the testing and progression of the patient. The clinician also must be aware of additional injuries that may slow progression of the rehabilitation. For example, injuries to the chondral surfaces of the ankle joint will delay full weight bearing and slow progression to higher forms of impact loading. Often, the physician will decide where the postsurgical patient may enter the FTA, based on the quality of the tissue at surgery, type and efficacy of any fixation, and duration of immobilization. Thus, good communication and a team approach between all members of the health care team are critical in order to optimize patient outcome.

Table 24.1 Criteria for Progression in the Ankle Functional Testing Algorithm (FTA)

Tests	Empirical guidelines
Subjective pain rating	< 3 (0-10 visual analog scale)
Figure-of-eight anthropometrics	< 0.5-1.0 cm difference
Active and passive range of motion (AROM/PROM)	< 10% bilateral comparison
FASTEX force platform system	< 10% bilateral comparison
Supine closed kinetic chain (CKC) test	< 30% bilateral comparison
Open kinetic chain (OKC) test	< 25% bilateral comparison
Standing closed kinetic chain (CKC) test	< 25% bilateral comparison
Functional jump test	< 20% normative (height) data
Functional hop test	< 10% bilateral comparison
Lower extremity functional (LEFT) test	< 90 secs (males) < 120 secs (females)
Sport-specific drills and testing	Replication of desired sports activity without pain or instability

Ankle Functional Testing Algorithm	**If Individual Fails Test** **(Does not meet stated criteria)**
Discharge/return to sports	Continue to place emphasis on drills that are very specific to the sport of the athlete involved.
< 10% difference with normative data, no apprehension or instability with replicated sports activity	
Sports specific test	Continue functional rehabilitation exercises with emphasis on agility drills involving cutting and pivoting.
Males < 90 seconds, Females < 120 seconds	
Lower extremity functional test	Continue functional rehabilitation exercises
< 10% bilateral comparison	
Functional hop test	Continue functional rehabilitation exercises involving jumping and hopping. Progress from a low to high intensity.
< 20% normative (height) data	
Functional jump test	Continue strength and power exercises
< 25% bilateral comparison	
CKC squat isokinetic test	Continue strength and power exercises
< 25% bilateral comparison	
Open kinetic chain (OKC) test	Continue strength and power exercises
< 30% bilateral comparison	
Supine closed kinetic chain (CKC) test	Continue proprioception and balance drills to improve neuromuscular control at the ankle
< 10% bilateral comparison	
FASTEX force platform system	Continue flexibility and stretching for the contractile and non-contractile structures surrounding the ankle joint
< 10% bilateral comparison	
AROM/PROM	Continue with methods to decrease inflammation and avoid stress to the ankle joint
< 0.5 to 1.0 cm difference bilateral comparison	
Figure 8 anthropometric measurement	Continue with methods to decrease inflammation and avoid stress to the ankle joint
< 3 (0-10 visual analog scale)	
Subjective pain rating	

■ **Figure 24.1** Ankle functional testing algorithm (FTA) as the foundation for a progressive rehabilitation program. From Davies, et al. 1999.

Basic Measurements

At our clinic, we have chosen four basic measurements to evaluate individual readiness to enter into the ankle FTA. It is important for the reader to note that one is not limited to these measurements alone. It is beyond the scope of this text to provide the reader with a comprehensive list of all the basic subjective and objective measurements taken during an initial ankle examination. Therefore, only the four criteria used for entrance and initial progression into the ankle FTA will be discussed.

Subjective Pain Rating Scale

The behavior of the patient's ankle symptoms should be evaluated at rest, during activities of daily living (ADLs), with vocational activities, and during recreation or sport. A visual analog scale is used to assess the patient's response to the special tests and measures completed during the examination. The visual analog scale we use is a colored scale that ranges from green to red and from 0 (no pain) to 10 (worst pain imaginable). Our empirical preset standard is for the patient to have a 0 pain rating at rest and a rating of less than 3 during activity prior to further exercise progression or testing (see table 24.1).

Anthropometric Measurements

Monitoring anthropometric measurements around the ankle using a figure-of-eight technique informs one about local effusion or edema. The figure-of-eight measurement technique has been described in detail in the literature (Esterson 1979). Several studies have also shown this measurement technique to be reliable and comparable to other standard measurement techniques (Petersen et al. 1999; Tatro-Adams et al. 1995). The clinician begins the measurement with the patient's ankle in neutral (0° dorsiflexion) with the end of the tape measure over the tibialis anterior tendon on the dorsum of the foot at the level of the ankle joint. The tape is pulled medially around the foot over the navicular tubercle, across the plantar surface of the foot, over the cuboid bone, across the dorsum of the ankle, inferior to the medial malleolus, above the dome of the calcaneus, inferior to the lateral malleolus, and back to the anterior tibialis tendon. To meet the criteria for advancement in the ankle FTA, the patient must demonstrate less than a 0.5 to 1.0 cm difference between the involved and uninvolved ankle figure-of-eight measurements. If there is intra-articular effusion, it creates a reflex inhibition to the joint (DeAndrade et al. 1965; Stratford 1981; Young et al. 1987). Therefore, the patient's progression through the FTA is slowed and the rehabilitation program is focused on decreasing the swelling. Decreasing the swelling may be accomplished by following the pneumonic PRICE. This pneumonic reminds the clinician to **protect** the ankle with a brace, to promote activities that **rest** the injured ankle but utilize the rest of the body, to use **ice** and other forms of cryotherapy, to prevent further swelling with **compression,** and to keep the ankle **elevated** higher than the heart as much as possible. By instructing the patient in the PRICE protocol and using other modalities such as electrical stimulation (Robinson & Snyder-Mackler 1995) and manual massage, swelling may be limited.

Range of Motion

Range-of-motion (ROM) measurements using a goniometer provide the clinician with an excellent way to objectively document patient progress. Range-of-motion measurements should be taken often and recorded on a data sheet in the patient's chart. This provides a simple and efficient method of documenting progress, as one can quickly determine the ROM gained over subsequent clinical visits. It also provides a record to demonstrate objective progress to insurance agencies for reimbursement. When performing ankle goniometry, clinicians should follow reproducible methods to improve intra- and inter-measurer reliability (Norkin & White 1985).

Active Range of Motion (AROM) or Flexibility Testing

Examination of the patient's AROM must demonstrate ankle plantarflexion, dorsiflexion, inversion, and eversion motion that is within 10% when compared to that of the uninvolved limb. If the patient has ankle active range-of-motion deficits due to the muscle-tendon unit, such as the gastrocnemius/soleus/Achilles complex, static stretching exercises or proprioceptive neuromuscular facilitation exercises are used to increase the flexibility of the contractile unit. There has always been controversy regarding the optimum "stretching times" for increasing muscle-tendon unit flexibility; however, recent research by Bandy et al. (Bandy & Irion 1994; Bandy et al. 1997, 1998) has demonstrated that one 30-second hold daily is as effective as longer holds or more frequent holds. Admittedly, Bandy et al.'s work was with hamstring flexibility, and we do think that there is denser fascial tissue in the gastrocnemius-soleus area. Therefore, without having definitive studies targeted to those particular muscle groups, we still use the recommendations described previously. Greater patient compliance with short-duration, single-repetition stretches may be another reason for the effectiveness of the preceding recommendations. Restoration of normal ankle joint flexibility is important to prevent reinjury, to prevent compensation patterns, and to improve performance.

Passive Range of Motion (PROM)

In contrast to motion deficits caused by tight contractile structures, limited motion may be secondary to tightness in noncontractile structures such as the joint capsule, ligaments, fascial tissue, and scar tissue. Passive mobility testing (using either physiological passive movement testing or accessory movement testing) is used to assess this type of limited joint motion. Similar to AROM testing, PROM testing must demonstrate less than a 10% difference bilaterally (see table 24.1) before the patient may progress to the next step in the ankle FTA. However, if passive mobility testing is positive, meaning joint motion is limited, it indicates hypomobility of the involved limb. To treat hypomobility, a low-load, long-duration treatment method must be employed to stretch out the noncontractile tissue. This approach creates a plastic (permanent) deformation of the collagen fibers present in the noncontractile tissue. To accomplish this goal, we primarily use an integrated approach of various techniques described in the research literature by Sapega et al. (1981) and McClure et al. (1994). We use these techniques as part of the integrated treatment formula described in the following paragraphs:

1. The patient performs an active warmup of the ankle on a suitable piece of aerobic exercise equipment. This increases the blood flow in the area that is going to be stretched.

2. The patient undergoes passive heating (ultrasound, hot pack, diathermy) while under a prolonged stretch for 20 minutes. The patient's ankle is held in this position with the use of straps or a weighted boot. This represents the patient's first dose of low-load stretch at the end range of motion. This follows the recommendations of McClure et al. (1994), who recommend a combined total end range time (TERT) of 60 minutes or more daily

3. After the first TERT, the clinician performs appropriate mobilization techniques and manual stretching methods to further stretch the collagen tissue.

4. To allow the patient to gain dynamic stability over the newly gained range of motion from the previous treatments in steps 2 and 3, the patient performs resisted exercises, such as isometric or short arc exercise, in the newly gained range of motion.

5. After the exercises in the new range of motion, the patient then completes the remainder of the rehabilitation program, including total leg strengthening and flexibility exercises.

6. Upon completion of all exercises, the patient is again placed at end range in a stretched position, and cryotherapy is applied for 20 minutes (Sapega et al. 1981). This application is not designed to get tissue to shorten, but rather to get the scar tissue or collagen to contract in the elongated position from the previous treatments. This also satisfies the requirements of the patient's second TERT session.

7. The patient's final TERT session is accomplished with the use of a home program of heating, stretching, and bracing.

Balance, Proprioception, and Kinesthesia Testing

The measurement of balance, kinesthesia, and proprioception is the fourth and final basic measurement test in the ankle FTA. Over three decades ago, Freeman et al. (Freeman 1965; Freeman et al. 1965; Freeman and Wyke 1967) demonstrated the importance of evaluating and treating the functionally unstable ankle with proprioceptive rehabilitation techniques. There are numerous methods of evaluating the ankle for joint proprioception and kinesthesia, and most clinical settings utilize the equipment and technology they have available (DeCario & Talbot 1986; Gross 1987; Tropp et al. 1984). It is important that the equipment used be reliable and the techniques used be reproducible and valid. It is beyond the scope of this chapter to discuss all of the different techniques for assessing balance or proprioception, so the reader is referred to the review article by Guskiewicz and Perrin (1996).

Because of the availability of the equipment in the authors' clinic, balance and proprioception are measured using the FASTEX computerized neuromuscular assessment system. The FASTEX system allows one to measure both static and dynamic balance simultaneously. The current test protocols are described in the reproducible forms, "FASTEX Static Balance Test" and "FASTEX Dynamic Balance Test." (Readers may photocopy and use the reproducible forms for patient care and education purposes.) If the patient is nonweightbearing, then angular joint replication testing can also be performed. Criteria for passing the static and dynamic balance tests are based on empiric guidelines we have generated internally. A test-retest reliability study conducted by Johnson-Stuhr (unpublished research, 1997) demonstrated that the FASTEX system was a reliable balance assessment device under the test conditions examined. If, when testing on the FASTEX, the patient demonstrates significant deficits, the emphasis of rehabilitation becomes improving neuromuscular control.

There are numerous articles in the literature that describe various methods of training for ankle proprioception and kinesthesia (Davies & Chu 1998; Garn & Newton 1988; Glencross & Thornton 1991; Hoffman & Payne 1995; Irrgang et al. 1994; Laskowski et al. 1997; Lephart et al. 1997; Sheth et al. 1997; Tropp et al. 1985). In addition to tilt board training, various functional activities performed in a progressively more difficult manner later in the ankle FTA will also enhance the patient's balance/proprioception (Kegerreis 1983; Kegerreis et al. 1984). For additional information on proprioception training, please see chapters 5 and 20-22.

There are no absolute rehabilitation protocols that are universally accepted as the most effective methods to restore proprioception, so the clinician must once again rely on the published research and empirically based clinical experiences (Davies 1992; Davies & Chu 1998; Davies & Ellenbecker 1998). Therefore, we primarily use a "superset" concept in

Static Balance Test
FASTEX

Name _____ DOB _____ Gender M / F

Clinic _____ PT _____ MD _____

Injury/surgery _____ DOS/DOI _____

Procedure:

1. Patient stands on uninvolved leg facing away from the computer, with head and eyes looking straight forward focusing on an object.
2. Nonweightbearing knee is flexed to approximately a 90° angle and the shin is held parallel to the floor.
3. Nonweightbearing knee is abducted and not touching opposite leg.
4. Hands are clasped behind the back.
5. Allow one practice test for 20 seconds.
6. Each test is 20 seconds.
7. Repeat the test 3 times with a 20 second rest period in between each test.
8. Record the Total Stability Index for each trial.
9. Repeat 1-8 on involved leg.

Date	Uninvolved L/R	Involved L/R	% Deficit
Trial 1			
Trial 2			
Trial 3			
Average			
Date	Uninvolved L/R	Involved L/R	% Deficit
Trial 1			
Trial 2			
Trial 3			
Average			
Date	Uninvolved L/R	Involved L/R	% Deficit
Trial 1			
Trial 2			
Trial 3			
Average			

From Meir Nyska and Gideon Mann, eds., 2002, *The Unstable Ankle* (Champaign, IL: Human Kinetics).

Dynamic Balance Test
FASTEX

Name _____ DOB _____ Gender M / F

Clinic _____ PT _____ MD _____

Injury/surgery _____ DOS/DOI _____

Procedure:

    1. Patient stands on both legs.

    2. Patient jumps side to side between two platforms, with the arms left free.

    3. Allow one set of submax (easy side to side) warm ups.

    4. Each set will consist of 20 jumps, with a 20 second rest period in between each set.

    5. The objective is for the patient to complete the 20 jumps as quickly as possible.

    6. The patient will complete 3 sets of 20 jumps for the test. For each set the Total Elapsed Time will be recorded.

Date	Total Elapsed Time
Trial 1	
Trial 2	
Trial 3	
Average	

Date	Total Elapsed Time
Trial 1	
Trial 2	
Trial 3	
Average	

Date	Total Elapsed Time
Trial 1	
Trial 2	
Trial 3	
Average	

Date	Total Elapsed Time
Trial 1	
Trial 2	
Trial 3	
Average	

Date	Total Elapsed Time
Trial 1	
Trial 2	
Trial 3	
Average	

Date	Total Elapsed Time
Trial 1	
Trial 2	
Trial 3	
Average	

From Meir Nyska and Gideon Mann, eds., 2002, *The Unstable Ankle* (Champaign, IL: Human Kinetics).

training the patient for balance and proprioception. In other words, the patient will perform a balance exercise for 1 minute and then will alternate with other exercises, such as static stretching of the Achilles/gastrocnemius/soleus complex.

Like all the steps in the ankle FTA, the patient undergoes balance retesting on a regular basis to determine when rehabilitation progression may occur.

Muscular Strength and Power Testing

After successful completion of all the basic measurement tests in the ankle FTA, the patient should undergo testing of muscular strength and power (Davies 1992; Davies et al. 1995; Davies & Ellenbecker 1998). Strength and power tests make up the second main category of tests in the functional testing algorithm. Although the majority of strength and power testing done in our clinic involves isokinetic testing, one should not feel limited if this equipment is unavailable. Handheld dynamometers, isotonic exercise machines, resistive tubing, and free weights may be substituted during strength and power testing. In all cases, a logical, stepwise progression is essential if the principles of the functional testing algorithm are to be upheld.

Closed Kinetic Chain (CKC) Isokinetic Testing—Semi-Sitting or Supine Position

With the increasing emphasis on CKC exercises in rehabilitation, there is obviously a need for objective testing of this component. We begin the testing using a Linea (Loredan Biomedical) Closed Kinetic Chain Computerized Isokinetic Dynamometer. Research by Davies and Heiderscheit (1997) has demonstrated that this is a reliable device to test lower extremity CKC muscular power. This allows us to assess the patient's total functional lower extremity patterns and muscle groups, including the hips, knees, and ankle plantarflexors. If the patient demonstrates deficits with this testing, follow-up testing must be performed to find the weak link of the kinetic chain in the system (Davies 1992; Davies 1995b; Davies et al. 1997; Davies & Heiderscheit 1997; Davies & Ellenbecker 1998). In the absence of CKC isokinetic equipment, the clinician may be creative and develop supine partial weightbearing strength tests using supine leg press machines or exercise devices such as the Total Gym. For this to be successful, the clinician should develop a patient database and determine specific criteria to operationally define and standardize the new test.

If weaknesses are identified during supine CKC testing, then partial weightbearing exercises, such as

leg press pattern exercises or isolated plantarflexion exercises, are performed to strengthen the muscle groups about the ankle. Currently, we use the empirically based guidelines of a bilateral comparison of less than 30% in peak force, total work, and total work as a percentage of body weight as cutoffs for patient progression in the ankle FTA (see table 24.1).

Open Kinetic Chain Testing

If a muscle does not function normally in an isolated pattern, then a muscle cannot function normally in an integrated pattern. Therefore, isolated testing must be performed to identify particular weaknesses in the kinetic chain (Davies 1992; Davies 1995b; Davies et al. 1995, 1997; Davies & Ellenbecker 1998). These weaknesses may then be specifically addressed in the rehabilitation program. Interestingly, Davies (1995b) and Feiring and Ellenbecker (1995) compared CKC to OKC testing and found similar results. Both studies demonstrated that when testing multiple muscles and joints as a unit, isolated muscle deficits are often missed. Apparently, various muscles compensate for or mask the isolated weak muscles in the extremity being tested. Thus, if only CKC testing is performed, these weak links in the kinetic chain may be missed.

The fact that isolated joint testing is a necessary part of an FTA has been shown by several authors (Davies 1992, 1995b; Davies et al. 1995; Davies & Ellenbecker 1998; Feiring & Ellenbecker 1995; Gleim et al. 1978; Nicholas et al. 1976). Furthermore, Nicholas et al. (1976) and Gleim et al. (1978) have demonstrated the need for creating a composite score for total leg strength. Specifically, Nicholas et al. (1976) found that patients who had ankle injuries also had statistically significant weaknesses of the ipsilateral hip adductors and hip abductors. Consequently, in the rehabilitation program we perform total leg strength rehabilitation training with specific isolated training of the hip adductors and hip abductors, as well as the other exercises described.

In the ankle FTA, we recommend performing isolated testing of the ankle joint plantarflexors and dorsiflexors, as well as the subtalar joint invertors and evertors. Tables 24.2 and 24.3 list the normative data (Davies 1992) for OKC isokinetic testing of the ankle joint.

If weaknesses are identified with this testing, specific rehabilitation strengthening and functional rehabilitation exercises are used to address these deficits. When designing the exercise program, we use the resistive exercise progression continuum advocated by Davies (Davies 1992; Davies et al. 1995) (see figure 24.2). The continuum is based on use of the exercises that the patient can tolerate, based on clinical examination and signs and symptoms. Then the

Table 24.2 Open Kinetic Chain Isokinetic Normative Data for Ankle Inversion and Eversion

Test motion	60°/sec isokinetic speed	120°/sec isokinetic speed
Inversion	12% BW*	10% BW
Eversion	11% BW	9% BW
Inversion/eversion ratio	91%	90%

*BW = body weight. Individuals should have peak torque results that are a certain percentage of their body weight.
From Davies 1992.

Table 24.3 Open Kinetic Chain Isokinetic Normative Data for Ankle Plantarflexion and Dorsiflexion

Test motion	60°/sec isokinetic speed		120°/sec isokinetic speed	
	Males	Females	Males	Females
Plantarflexion (PF)	65% BW*	50% BW	38% BW	40% BW
Dorsiflexion (DF)	12% BW	12% BW	9% BW	8% BW
PF/DF	25%	25%	33-40%	33-40%

*BW = body weight. Individuals should have peak torque results that are a certain percentage of their body weight.
From Davies 1992.

patient is progressed from the easier to the more difficult exercises in order to apply the principles of overload and progression. Finally, the isolated exercises are integrated along with the functional exercises for the specificity training response.

Closed Kinetic Chain Isokinetic Testing— Standing (Full Weight Bearing)

This testing follows a similar procedure as the sitting CKC testing, with the exception of the fact that the patient is fully weight bearing (Davies & Zillmer 1999). At our clinic, the Linea (Loredan Biomedical) CKC Isokinetic Dynamometer is placed in an upright position. The patient is tested in the CKC squat position using two legs. This test may be progressed by having the patient perform single-leg squats. If greater than a 20% deficit exists between the involved and uninvolved extremity, rehabilitation exercises are performed in the weightbearing position and follow the guidelines as previously described.

Functional Tests

The transition from strength and power testing to functional testing represents a major change in the emphasis of the algorithm testing sequence. The focus of the testing is now on functional testing activities. Here, the stresses that occur during testing should reach levels that the patient or athlete will experience during sport or recreation activities. The degree of control the clinician has during testing is

significantly reduced from the control that was available during the strength and power tests. Therefore, we also recommend using appropriate bracing and taping techniques as preventive measures during testing. Thacker et al. (1999) has recommended that ankle braces be worn 6 months after injury during high-risk activities in order to help prevent a recurrent ankle sprain.

Functional Jump Test

The first functional test in the ankle FTA is the functional jump test. This test is an excellent way of checking the patient's physiological and psychological readiness to progress to uncontrolled activities. Now the patient is ready to perform uncontrolled reactive eccentric exercises as part of the testing. The purpose of the functional jump test is to measure bilateral leg power by performing a standing long jump for distance (Davies & Zillmer 1999). To prevent the patient from obtaining assistance from the arms, neck, and trunk, we have the patient perform the jump test with hands clasped behind the back. To ensure safety, the patient performs four submaximal to maximal warmup jumps. These are completed at 25%, 50%, 75%, and 100% effort. At least one maximal jump during practice is necessary to create a positive transfer of learning to the actual test activity (Davies & Zillmer 1999). After the four graded warm-up jumps, the patient performs three maximal effort jumps. The average of the three jumps is then normalized by dividing by

Stages

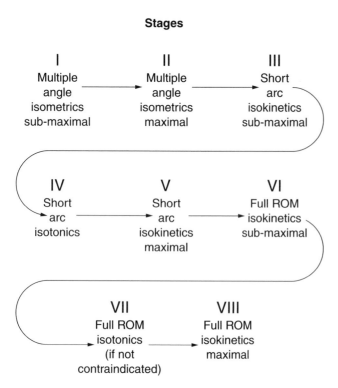

I Multiple angle isometrics sub-maximal	**II** Multiple angle isometrics maximal	**III** Short arc isokinetics sub-maximal
IV Short arc isotonics	**V** Short arc isokinetics maximal	**VI** Full ROM isokinetics sub-maximal
	VII Full ROM isotonics (if not contraindicated)	**VIII** Full ROM isokinetics maximal

■ **Figure 24.2** Stages of exercise progression.
From Davies 1992.

the patient's height. The reproducible form, "Functional Standing Long Jump and Hop Test," is an example of the data sheet we use in our clinic. The normative data we have gained in the clinic is shown at the bottom of this data form. If the patient demonstrates weaknesses, then the rehabilitation program is focused on specific bilateral proactive and reactive exercises.

Functional Hop Test

This is a unilateral hop test for distance that tests the patient's ability to hop on the involved ankle. Comparisons are made to the distance the patient can hop with the uninvolved lower extremity (table 24.1). This is a very difficult test for patients with residual ankle weakness to perform. Consequently, it once again tests for physiological and psychological readiness to use the extremity in functional ways. The warmup and procedures of this test are identical to those of the jump test. Clinicians should instruct the patient to keep from driving the nonweightbearing lower extremity forward during the hopping. The form, "Functional Standing Long Jump and Hop Test," also illustrates how hop test scores are recorded at our clinic. If deficits exist, then proactive and reactive activities (similar to those described in the previous section) are performed with both legs, but

now the functional rehabilitation is primarily focused on single-leg activities.

Lower Extremity Functional Test

The final stage of the formal testing with the ankle FTA is the Lower Extremity Functional Test (LEFT) (Davies & Zillmer 1999; Tabor et al. 1999). This agility test represents the terminal phases of the rehabilitation program, and is typically performed near the time of discharge. A recent study by Negrete and Brophy (2000) has demonstrated the validity or correlation of the LEFT with other tests used to measure performance. A recent reliability study (Tabor et al. 1999) demonstrated that this functional test had an intraclass correlation coefficient of 0.953, which is excellent for a functional clinical test. The LEFT is designed around a diamond shape that is 30 feet in length and 10 feet in width. This allows the test to be performed in an indoor setting. The test is designed as a progression of agility drills, each more demanding than the previous one. The sequence of agility drills required during the LEFT is listed in the form, "Lower Extremity Functional Test." When the patient is performing the LEFT, the clinician should examine both the quantity (time in seconds to complete the test) and the quality of the performance. The LEFT is also a very stressful test for the anaerobic cardiovascular system. It therefore also tests this component of the patient. Normative LEFT data for males and females is shown at the bottom of the form. The LEFT test incorporates many functional movement patterns that are used in everyday sporting activities, which allows for specificity in identifying where the patient is still having problems. If the patient does not pass the LEFT test quantitatively or qualitatively, then the rehabilitation program focuses on the component or components with which the patient is having difficulty.

Sport- or Ergonomic-Specific Testing

The final phase of the ankle FTA is the sport- or ergonomic-specific testing. Because the patient will have to return to certain conditions in athletic activities or work, it is important to replicate these activities in a controlled manner in the clinical setting. Then, the patient's response to the stresses can be tested and monitored. In a controlled and progressive manner, the rehabilitation program can safely stress the patient with the same stresses the patient will encounter in the sport or ergonomic setting. This applies the principle of specific adaptation to imposed demands (SAID principle). Examples include having a gymnast perform 10 handsprings, or having a construction foreman climb up and down a ladder 20 times. In

**Functional Standing Long Jump
and Hop Test Data Form**

Patient _____ Clinic # _____ DOB _____

MD _____ PT _____ DOS/DOI _____

Diagnosis _____ Dominant R / L   Ht _____ in   Wt _____ lbs

Date _____
Status/post (weeks) _____

Trial	1	2	3	Avg	%
R U / I					
L U / I					
Both					

Date _____
Status/post (weeks) _____

Trial	1	2	3	Avg	%
R U / I					
L U / I					
Both					

Date _____
Status/post (weeks) _____

Trial	1	2	3	Avg	%
R U / I					
L U / I					
Both					

Date _____
Status/post (weeks) _____

Trial	1	2	3	Avg	%
R U / I					
L U / I					
Both					

Date _____
Status/post (weeks) _____

Trial	1	2	3	Avg	%
R U / I					
L U / I					
Both					

Date _____
Status/post (weeks) _____

Trial	1	2	3	Avg	%
R U / I					
L U / I					
Both					

Date _____
Status/post (weeks) _____

Trial	1	2	3	Avg	%
R U / I					
L U / I					
Both					

Date _____
Status/post (weeks) _____

Trial	1	2	3	Avg	%
R U / I					
L U / I					
Both					

Long jump norms (% of height)

	Female	**Male**
Hop Right	80% of Ht	90% of Ht
Hop Left	80% of Ht	90% of Ht
Jump Both	90% of Ht	100% of Ht

From Meir Nyska and Gideon Mann, eds., 2002, *The Unstable Ankle* (Champaign, IL: Human Kinetics).

Lower Extremity Functional Test

Patient _____ Clinic # _____ DOB _____

MD _____ PT _____ DOS/DOI _____

Diagnosis _____ Gender M / F

Dominant L / R   Involved L / R   Ht _____ in   Wt _____ lbs

Procedure:

  1. Forward sprint (A-C-A)

  2. Retro sprint (A-C-A)

  3. Side shuffle right—face in (A-D-C-B-A)

  4. Side shuffle left—face in (A-B-C-D-A)

  5. Cariocas right—face in (A-D-C-B-A)

  6. Cariocas left—face in (A-B-C-D-A)

  7. Figure 8s right (A-D-C-B-A)

  8. Figure 8s left (A-B-C-D-A)

  9. 45° cuts right—plant outside foot (A-D-C-B-A)

10. 45° cuts left—plant outside foot (A-B-C-D-A)

11. 90° cuts right—plant outside foot (A-D-B-A)

12. 90° cuts left—plant outside foot (A-B-D-A)

13. Crossover 90° cuts right—plant inside foot (A-D-B-A)

14. Crossover 90° cuts left—plant inside foot (A-B-D-A)

15. Forward sprint (A-C-A)

16. Retro sprint (A-C-A)

C

30 ft

B ●———┼ 10 ft ● D

A

Data

Date _____   Date _____   Date _____

Time _____ sec   Time _____ sec   Time _____ sec

Date _____   Date _____   Date _____

Time _____ sec   Time _____ sec   Time _____ sec

Norms

Males	Females
90 sec—good	120 sec—good
100 sec—avg	135 sec—avg

From Meir Nyska and Gideon Mann, eds., 2002, *The Unstable Ankle* (Champaign, IL: Human Kinetics).

contact sports, progression of sport-specific activities may include having the patient perform the activity first without an opponent, followed by performing the activity with an opponent.

Summary

This chapter describes an ankle functional testing algorithm (FTA) as the basis for testing and designing ankle rehabilitation programs. Various steps and criteria in the FTA are described, and particular examples of exercises to address the limitations are provided. To those unaccustomed to the FTA approach, this type of serial stepwise testing may seem impractical. Based on our experience, it actually assists the patient to progress more quickly through a rehabilitation program (Davies & Zillmer 1999). This is because the patients are frequently tested and monitored, allowing them to know exactly where they are in their rehabilitation. It also gives the patient and clinician objective measures from which to set goals and make decisions. This allows the clinician to modify home and clinical programs on a regular basis to address specific rehabilitation needs and goals.

Ankle functional progression also improves communication between physicians, therapists, trainers, parents, and coaches, because everyone is more aware of where the patient is in the recovery phase. This type of "evidence-based" practice is critical in today's clinical environment of managed care and limited patient visits.

References

Bandy, WD, Irion, JM. The effect of time on static stretch on the flexibility of the hamstring muscles. Phys Ther 74:845-850, 1994.

Bandy, WD, Irion, JM, Briggler, M. The effect of time and frequency of static stretch on flexibility of the hamstring muscles. Phys Ther 77:1090-1096, 1997.

Bandy, WD, Irion, JM, Briggler, M. The effect of static stretch and dynamic range of motion on the flexibility of the hamstring muscles. J Orthop Sports Phys Ther 27:295-300, 1998.

Davies, GJ. A Compendium of Isokinetics in Clinical Usage and Rehabilitation Techniques, 4th ed. S & S Publishers, Onalaska, WI, 1992.

Davies, GJ. Functional Testing Algorithm for patients with knee injuries. (Abst) Proceedings of the 12th International Congress of the World Confederation for Physical Therapy, Washington, DC, p. 91, June 1995a.

Davies, GJ. Descriptive study comparing open and closed kinetic chain isokinetic testing of the lower extremity in 200 patients with selected knee pathologies. (Abst) Proceedings of the 12th International Congress of the World Confederation for Physical Therapy, Washington, DC, p. 906, June 1995b.

Davies, GJ, Chu, D. Physical therapy. In Subotnick, S, ed. Sports Medicine of the Lower Extremity, 2nd ed. Churchill Livingstone, Philadelphia, 1998.

Davies, GJ, Ellenbecker, TS. Application of isokinetic testing and rehabilitation. In Andrews, JR, Harrelson, GL, Wilk, KE, eds. Physical Rehabilitation of the Injured Athlete. W.B. Saunders, Philadelphia, PA, 1998.

Davies, GJ, Heiderscheit, BC. Reliability of the Lido Linea closed kinetic chain isokinetic dynamometer. J Orthop Sports Phys Ther 25:133-136, 1997.

Davies, GJ, Heiderscheit, B, Clark, M. Open kinetic chain assessment and rehabilitation. Athletic Training: Sports Health Care Perspectives 1:347-370, 1995.

Davies, GJ, Wilk, K, Ellenbecker, TS. Assessment of strength. In Malone, TR, McPoil, T, Nitz, AJ, eds. Orthopaedic and Sports Physical Therapy, 3rd ed. Mosby, St. Louis, MO, pp 225-257, 1997.

Davies, GJ, Zillmer, DA. Functional progression of exercise during rehabilitation. In Ellenbecker, TS, ed. Knee Ligament Rehabilitation. Churchill Livingstone, New York, 1999.

DeAndrade, JR, Grant, C, Dixon, A. Joint distension and reflex muscle inhibition in the knee. J Bone Joint Surg 24:313-332, 1965.

DeCario, MS, Talbot, RW. Evaluation of ankle joint proprioception following injection of the anterior talofibular ligament. J Orthop Sports Phys Ther 8:70-75, 1986.

Esterson, PS. Measurement of ankle joint swelling using a figure-of-eight. J Orthop Sports Phys Ther 1:51-52, 1979.

Feiring, DC, Ellenbecker, TS. Open versus closed kinetic chain isokinetic testing with ACL reconstructed patients. Med Sci Sports Exerc 27:S106, 1995.

Freeman, MA. Instability of the foot after injuries to the lateral ligament of the ankle. J Bone Joint Surg 47(B):669-677, 1965.

Freeman, MA, Dean, MR, Hanham, IW. The etiology and prevention of functional instability of the foot. J Bone Joint Surg 47(B):678-685, 1965.

Freeman, MA, Wyke, B. Articular reflexes at the ankle joint: an electromyographic study of normal and abnormal influences on ankle joint mechanoreceptors upon reflex activity in the leg muscles. Br J Surg 54:990-1001, 1967.

Garn, SN, Newton, RA. Kinesthetic awareness in subjects with multiple ankle sprains. Phys Ther 68:1667-1671, 1988.

Gleim, GW, Nicholas, JA, Webb, JN. Isokinetic evaluation following leg injuries. Phys Sports Med 6:74-82, 1978.

Glencross, D, Thornton, E. Position sense following joint injury. J Sports Med Phys Fitness 21:23-27, 1991.

Gross, MT. Effects of recurrent lateral ankle sprains on active and passive judgments of joint position. Phys Ther 67:1505-1509, 1987.

Guskiewicz, KM, Perrin, DH. Research and clinical applications of assessing balance. J Sport Rehab 5:45-63, 1996.

Hoffman, M, Payne, VG. The effects of proprioception ankle disc training on healthy subjects. J Orthop Sports Phys Ther 21:220-226, 1995.

Irrgang, J, Whitney, S, Cox, E. Balance and proprioceptive training for rehabilitation of the lower extremity. J Sports Rehab 3:68-83, 1994.

Johnson-Stuhr, P. Reliability of the FASTEX during static and dynamic balance. Unpublished master's degree project, 1997.

Kannus, P, Renström, P. Current concepts review. Treatment of acute tears of the lateral ligaments of the ankle. Operation, cast, or early controlled mobilization. J Bone Joint Surg 73(A):305-312, 1991.

Kegerreis, S. The construction and implementation of functional progression as a component of athletic rehabilitation. J Orthop Sports Phys Ther 5:14-19, 1983.

Kegerreis, S, Malone, T, McCarroll, J. Functional progression: an aid to athletic rehabilitation. Phys Sports Med 12:67-71, 1984.

Laskowski, ER, Newcomer-Aney, K, Smith, J. Refining rehabilitation with proprioception training. Phys Sports Med 5:89-102, 1997.

Lephart, SM, Pincivero, DM, Giraldo, JL, Fu, FH. The role of proprioception in the management and rehabilitation of athletic injuries. Am J Sports Med 25:130-137, 1997.

McClure, PW, Blackburn, LG, Dusold, C. The use of splints in the treatment of joint stiffness: biological rationale and an algorithm for making clinical decisions. Phys Ther 74:1101-1107, 1994.

Negrete, R, Brophy, J. Predicting performance of single leg hop, single leg vertical jump and a speed and agility test using isokinetic devices. J Sport Rehab 9:46-65, 2000.

Nicholas, JA, Strizak, AM, Veras, G. A study of thigh muscle weakness in different pathological states of the lower extremity. Am J Sports Med 4:241-248, 1976.

Norkin, CC, White DJ. Measurement of Joint Motion: A Guide to Goniometry, F.A. Davis Co., Philadelphia, PA, 1985.

Petersen, EJ, Irish, SM, Lyons, CL, Miklaski, SF, Bryan JM, Henderson, NE, Masullo, LN. Reliability of water volumetry and the figure-of-eight method on subjects with ankle joint swelling. J Orthop Phys Ther. 29:609-615, 1999.

Povacz, P, Unger, SF, Miller, WK, et al. A randomized, prospective study of operative and non-operative treatment of injuries of the fibular collateral ligaments of the ankle. J Bone Joint Surg 80:345-351. 1998.

Robinson, AJ, Snyder-Mackler, L. Clinical Electrophysiology: Electrotherapy and Electrophysiological Testing, 2nd ed. Williams and Wilkins, Baltimore, MD, 1995.

Sapega, AA, Quedenfeld, TC, Moyer, RA, Butler, RA. Biophysical factors in range-of-motion exercises. Phys Sports Med 9:57-65, 1981.

Sheth, P, Yu, B, Laskowski, E, et al. Ankle disc training influences reaction times of selected muscles in a simulated ankle sprain. Am J Sports Med 25:538-543, 1997.

Stratford, P. Electromyography of the quadriceps femoris muscles in subjects with normal knees and acutely effused knees. Phys Ther 62:279-283, 1981.

Tabor, MA, Paterson, AM, Davies, GJ, et al. Test re-test reliability of the Lower Extremity Functional Test. MS Project. Research paper submitted for presentation, APTA National Meeting, Washington, DC, 1999.

Tatro-Adams, D, McGann, SF, Carbone, W. Reliability of the figure-of-eight method of ankle measurement. J Orthop Phys Ther 22:161-163, 1995.

Thacker, SB, Stroup, DF, Branche, CM, Gilchrist, J, Goodman, RA, Weitman, EA. The prevention of ankle sprains in sports: a systematic review of the literature. Am J Sports Med 27:753-760, 1999.

Tropp, H, Askling, C, Gillquist, J. Prevention of ankle sprains. Am J Sports Med 13:259-262, 1985.

Tropp, H, Ekstrand, J, Gillquist, J. Stabilometry in functional instability of the ankle and its value in predicting injury. Med Sci Sports Exerc 16:64-66, 1984.

Young, A, Stokes, M, Iles, JF. Effects of joint pathology on muscle. Clin Orthop 219:21-27, 1987.

Part VI

Surgical Treatment

The main indication for operative treatment is giving way of the ankle, causing major interference in daily activity, accompanied by pain. After failure of conservative treatment, surgical treatment is indicated. The combination of mechanical and functional instability is the most commonly reported indication for surgery.

The vast number of surgical procedures may be classified into nonanatomic and anatomic procedures. The nonanatomic procedures are augmentation techniques using endogenous tendons or ligaments tenodesed from the fibula to the talus and calcaneus or exogenous. The Watson-Jones procedure and the Chrisman-Snook operation are described in detail.

Anatomic repair includes direct suturing, imbrication, and repair to bone or using local tissue as augmentation. The Broström procedure, which is based on direct suturing of the capsule, and the Williams procedure, which is based on imbrication of the extensor digitorum brevis, are described in detail.

Chapter 25

Overview of the Operative Treatment of Ankle Instability

Meir Nyska, MD, and Gideon Mann, MD

Not all recurrent ankle sprains will need operative treatment such as that described in chapters 26 through 31.Conservative methods, such as soft supports (Guskiewicz & Perrin 1996), high shoes (Ottaviani et al. 1995; Richard et al. 1997), taping (Karlsson & Andreasson 1992), ankle braces (Leanderson & Wredmark 1995; Sitler & Horodyski 1995; Thonnard et al. 1996), physical therapy, development of peroneal muscle strength and proprioception, and activity modification will often suffice as the sole treatment (Freeman 1965; Kannus & Renström 1991; Tropp et al. 1985; Wester et al. 1996). When ankle sprains continue to occur despite conservative treatment, degenerative changes of the ankle joint could eventually occur (Lofvenberg et al. 1994), and the athlete may be severely disabled (Yeung et al. 1994). In these cases, operative treatment should be considered.

■ Indications for Operative Treatment

There has been a long-standing debate concerning the indications for operative treatment of acute ankle sprain. Older literature favored the operative treatment for acute ankle sprain. After reviewing the literature, Kannus & Renström (1991) demonstrated no advantage of operative treatment in acute ankle sprains. When chronic mechanical and functional instability occurs, surgical treatment should be considered. Unless the patient suffered overt dislocation of the talus, it is the authors' opinion that immediate surgical stabilization has no place, even in the worst ankle sprains.

Nilsonne (1932) was the first to report good results of reconstruction of the lateral ligaments of the ankle using the peroneus brevis tendon. In Nilsonne's technique the tendon is transposed into a subperiostal groove behind the lateral malleolus. Since Nilsonne published his technique more than 50 procedures and modifications have been described (Peters et al. 1991), The vast number of procedures indicate that there was no one good solution that gave consistently good results with no complications.

As a result, practitioners must be familiar with the various types of procedures, and should have an understanding of the indications for choosing a specific procedure. The main indication for operative treatment is repeated "giving way" of the ankle that causes major interference in daily activity, accompanied by pain and the failure of conservative treatment. This combination of mechanical and functional instability is the most commonly reported indication for surgery. Mechanical instability, proven by a stress test, may not in itself be a sufficient criterion for operative treatment if there is no accompanying functional instability. There is a debate in the literature and among surgeons regarding whether functional instability without proven mechanical instability is an indication for operative treatment. Ahlgren and Larsson (1989) found that radiological examination was negative even in ankles with functionally and clinically severe instability, despite the fact that radiography was performed under epidural anesthesia, which reduces pain and thus overcomes muscle resistance. In their study, stress radiography was abandoned and the indications for surgery were based strictly on symptoms and clinical evidence of instability. The development of anatomic repair, which maintains the normal physiology of the ankle and subtalar motion, expanded the indications for surgery to include functional instability without mechanical instability.

■ Anatomic and Nonanatomic Surgical Procedures

In order to evaluate the large number of surgical alternatives, Peters et al. (1991) suggested a classification of the surgical procedures into **nonanatomic** and **anatomic** procedures. Anatomic repair is based on the fact that the torn ligaments usually recover by forming a scar of dense, fibrous tissue. This feature was noted by Broström (1965), who was the first to suggest direct suturing of the torn ligaments even many years after the initial injury. Nonanatomic procedures are augmentation techniques that form a tenodesis of the fibula to the talus and calcaneus. These could be endogenous, using ligament, tendons, or other tissue from the operated patient, or exogenous, using biological or artificial material recruited from other sources. These procedures are further described in the following sections.

Nonanatomic Procedures

Endogenous tendons or ligaments, or exogenous tendons, ligaments, or foreign materials can be used for nonanatomic repair. Accordingly, the nonanatomic procedures are divided as mentioned above into endogenous and exogenous operations.

Endogenous Operations

The endogenous operations are basically tenodesis procedures, and are based on the use of the lateral tendons: the peroneus brevis as a whole or divided (Anderson et al. 1962; Druart & Simons 1982; Castaing et al. 1961; Chrisman & Snook 1969; Evans 1953; Gallie 1913; Good et al. 1975; Kiaer 1946; Kristiansen 1982; Leach et al. 1980; Lee 1957; Lucht 1989; Lauttamus 1982; Nilsonne 1932; Silver & Deutsch 1982; Watson-Jones 1940, 1960; Windfeld 1953), the peroneus longus (Hambley 1945; Pouzet 1954; Watson-Jones 1952), the Achilles tendon (Stören 1959), the plantaris (Anderson 1985; Sefton et al. 1979), fascia lata (Elmslie 1934; Rosendahl-Jensen 1952), fascia lata combined with peroneus brevis (Lee 1957), the corium under the skin (Francilion 1961; Gschwend 1958), the anterior tibiofibular ligament (Haig 1950), or a periosteal flap (Glas et al. 1988). The various tenodesis operations are reported to give results in the range of 80-95% "good" to "excellent" results.

Probably the most widely practiced procedure to date is the Watson-Jones operation, which uses the peroneus brevis (Anderson & Lecocq 1954; Anderson et al. 1962; Gillespie & Boucher 1971; Hedoba & Johannsen 1979; Watson-Jones 1940, 1960) and is reported as having from 80% (Gillespie & Boucher 1971) to 93% (Stewart 1980) "good" to "excellent" results, although unsatisfactory results and deterioration over time have also been reported (Boszotta & Sauer 1989). The Chrisman-Snook method (Chrisman & Snook 1969; Rechtine et al. 1982), using half the peroneus brevis, has been reported as giving 82% "good" to "excellent" results (Rechtine et al. 1982). The Evans operation (Bjorkenheim 1988; Canale 1988; Evans 1953; Kristiansen 1981, 1982; Karlsson et al. 1988; Lauttamus 1982), using the peroneus brevis as a single tendon, has shown 80% to 96% "good" to "excellent" results (Bjorkenheim 1988; Canale 1988; Evans 1953; Good et al. 1975; Kristiansen 1981). As with the Watson-Jones procedure, results with the Evans procedure are not always consistent: In the Evans procedure the drawer sign may be reduced (Orava et al. 1983) and overall, a 78% improvement can be expected (Kristiansen 1981, 1982). It is interesting to observe that eventually only 33% of patients who underwent the Evans procedure resumed athletic activity (Kristiansen 1982), and only 50% had a satisfactory result 14 years after operation (Karlsson & Andreasson 1988).

Numerous problems accompany the tenodesis operations (Broström 1966a, 1966b). Most of the procedures are somewhat complicated, healing is prolonged, the anatomy is not accurately restored, the peroneal tendons are damaged, and the active muscular stabilization system is disabled. These procedures cannot be used in children because of possible muscle imbalance and damage to the distal fibular growth plate. The surgical incisions are 12-20 cm long, causing further damage to the skin and cutaneous nerves.

One in three cases in Chrisman-Snook operations (Rechtine et al. 1982) has been reported to exhibit one or another surgical complication: sural nerve damage, skin necrosis, or scar hypersensitivity. All the tenodesis operations limit the subtalar mobility, as shown in the Elmslie procedure, Watson-Jones, Chrisman-Snook, and Evans operations (Anderson & Lecocq 1954; Chrisman & Snook 1969; Coutts & Woodward 1965; Evans 1953; Good et al. 1975; Kristiansen 1981; Silver & Deutsch 1982). Return to full activity will be prolonged and discouraging, ranging from 3 (Anderson & Lecocq 1954) to 6 months (Leach et al. 1980; Rechtine et al. 1982). Probably the most disturbing observation is the late occurrence of arthritic changes in over 60% of the surgical population (shown in the Watson-Jones procedure) as a result of disturbance of the normal complex physiology of the foot and ankle joints (Boszotta & Sauer 1989).

Exogenous Operations

The exogenous augmentation materials include carbon fiber (Burri & Neugebauer 1985; Freedman 1988; Jenkins & McKibbin 1980), dacron, or bovine collagen. Using exogenous augmentation has the advantage of preserving subtalar mobility. Dacron substitution gave 88% "good" to "excellent" results (Park 1982), and carbon fiber gave "good" to "excellent" results in 3 of 5 cases (Jenkins & McKibbin 1980), 49 of 51 cases (Burri & Neugebauer 1985), and 35 of 37 cases (Freedman et al. 1988). Thirteen patients in this last series needed carbon fiber extraction because of local difficulties. Carbon extraction resulted in loss of stability (Freedman et al. 1988).

Anatomic Repair

Anatomic repair includes direct suturing, imbrication, and repair to bone (Petersen 1981) or using local tissue, if needed, as augmentation (Broström 1966a). The Broström procedure (1966b) is based on direct suturing of the capsule and ligaments and, if needed, augmenting the anterior talofibular ligament (ATFL) with a section of the calcaneofibular ligament (CFL). Gould (1980) added a modification that includes augmentation using the extensor retinaculum. Petersen (1981) described a deviation of the anterolateral capsuloligamentous complex, rerouting the distal part to the fibula and reefing it over the proximal part. Ahlgren and Larsson (1989) suggested proximal advancement of an osteoperiostal flap that includes all the lateral ligaments. He reported good results in 86% of the patients at 2-year follow-up, and the results were unchanged at 5-year follow-up. Mukherjee and Gangopadhyay (1983) used advancement of the extensor digitorum brevis as a sole procedure, with excellent results, probably by achieving resumption of the proprioceptive sensation. Langstaff and Handley (1991) and Williams (1988; Mann et al. 1994) suggested imbrication techniques and advancement of the extensor digitorum brevis. Others reported anatomic techniques, including capsulorraphy combined with peroneus brevis advancement (Barlett & Wilson 1988), and shortening and sewing the ligament back into the fibula and reefing the remaining ligament (Althoff et al. 1981; Fieres 1983).

■ Summary and Conclusions

Offering surgical treatment to an acutely sprained ankle is probably not justified. Surgical treatment could be suggested in chronic functional instability in patients with (and probably also without) concurrent mechanical instability. Surgical procedures can be divided into anatomic procedures, which aim to restore the anatomic construction of the ankle, and to nonanatomic procedures, which utilize active stabilizers of the ankle or other body connective tissue, and achieve mechanical stability at the price of losing normal ankle subtalar or foot anatomy and physiological function. The nonanatomic procedures are often divided into endogenous procedures, which use body tissues, and generally include the tenodesis operations, and exogenous procedures, which use artificial materials or bovine connective tissue (allografts).

Though good results have been reported in most procedures, foreign materials carry inherent risks of hypersensitivity, local reaction, or infection. The tenodesis procedures are accompanied by numerous complications arising from the disturbance of normal anatomy, removal of the active stabilizers, overstabilization (especially of the subtalar joint), and various skin and sensation disturbances. The anatomic procedures, which are all endogenic by nature, aim to restore the normal anatomy and utilize minimal incisions. These tend to restore both mechanical and functional stability. Thus, when surgical reconstruction of ankle instability is indicated, one of the anatomic procedures should be advised.

■ References

Ahlgren O, Larsson S. Reconstruction for lateral ligament injuries of the ankle. J Bone Joint Surg 1989;72:300-303.

Althoff B, Peterson L, Renström P. Enkle plastik av inveterade. Ladbandsskador ifitleden (Simple plastic surgical repair of inveterate ligament damage in the ankle joint). Lakartioningen 1981;78:2857-2861.

Anderson KJ, Lecocq JF. Operative treatment of injury to the fibular collateral ligament of the ankle. J Bone Joint Surg 1954;36-A:825-832.

Anderson KJ, Lecocq JF, Clayton ML. Athletic injury to the fibular collateral ligament of the ankle. Clin Orthop Rel Res 1962;23:146-160.

Anderson ME. Reconstruction of the lateral of injury to the fibular collateral ligament of the ankle. J Bone Joint Surg 1985;76-A:930-934.

Barlett RJ, Wilson PJ. Dynamic reconstruction for chronic lateral instability of the ankle. Proceedings of English-Speaking Orthopedic Societies. 1988.

Bjorkenheim JM. Evans' procedure in the treatment of chronic instability of the ankle. Injury 1988;19:70-72.

Boszotta H, Sauer G. Chronic fibular ligament insufficiency at the upper ankle joint. Late results after modified Watson-Jones plastic surgery. Unfallchirurg 1989;92(1):11-16. (In German; English abstract.)

Broström L. Sprained ankles III. Clinical observations in recent ligament ruptures. Acta Chir Scand 1965;130:560.

Broström L. Sprained ankles V. Treatment and prognosis in recent ligament ruptures. Acta Chir Scand 1966a;132:537.

Broström L. Sprained ankles VI. Surgical treatment of chronic ligament ruptures. Acta Chir Scand 1966b;132:551-565.

Broström L, Sundelin P. Sprained ankles IV. Histological changes in recent and chronic ligament ruptures. Acta Chir Scand 1966;132:248.

Burri C, Neugebauer R. Carbon fiber replacement of the ligaments of the shoulder girdle and the treatment of lateral instability of the ankle joint. Clin Orthop 1985;19:112-117.

Canale, ST. Ankle injuries. In Canale ST, ed. Campbell's Operative Orthopaedics, 6th ed. C.V. Mosby Co., St. Louis, MO, 1988, p. 1079-1112.

Castaing J, LeChevallier PL, Meunier M. Entorse a repetition ou recidivante de la tibiotarsienne. Une technique simple de ligamentoplastique extern. Rev Chir Orthop 1961;47:598-608.

Chrisman, OD, Snook GA. Reconstruction of lateral ligament tears of the ankle. J Bone Joint Surg 1969;51A:094-912.

Coutts B, Woodward PE. Surgery and sprained ankles. Clin Orthop Rel Res 1965;42:81-90.

Druart ML, Simons M. Ankle sprains. Clinical review of 25 surgically treated cases. Acta Orthop Belg 1982;48(6)871-879.

Elmslie, R.C. Recurrent dislocation of the ankle joint. Ann Surg 1934;100:364-367.

Evans DL. Recurrent instability of the ankle. A method of surgical treatment. Proc R Soc Med 1953;46:343-344.

Fieres AWFM. The unstable ankle—giving way and a method of operative therapy. Acta Orthop Scand 1983;54:675.

Francilion MR. Distorsio pedis. Schweiz Med Ascher 1961;91:117-122.

Freedman LS, Jenkins AIR, Jenkins DHR. Carbon fiber reinforcement for chronic lateral ankle instability. Injury 1988;19:25-27.

Freeman MAR. The etiology and prevention of functional instability of the foot. J Bone Joint Surg 1965;47-B:678-685.

Gallie WE. Tendon fixation—an operation for the prevention of deformity in infantile paralysis. Am J Orthop Surg 1913;11:151-155.

Gillespie HS, Boucher P. Watson-Jones repair of lateral instability of the ankle. J Bone Joint Surg 1971;53-A:920-924.

Glas E, Paar O, Bernett P. Periosteal flap for reconstruction of the ankle ligaments. Follow-up results. Unfallchirurg 1988;88:219-212.

Good CJ, Jones MA, Livingstone BN. Reconstruction of the lateral ligament of the ankle. Injury 1975;7:63-65.

Gould N, Seligson D, Glassman J. Early and late repair of lateral ligament of the ankle. Foot Ankle 1980;1:84-889.

Gschwend N. Die fibularen bandlesionen mit der haufig verkannten folge der fussverstauchungen. Praxis 1958;47:809-813.

Guskiewicz KM, Perrin DH. Effect of orthotics on postural sway following inversion ankle sprain. J Orthop Sports Phys Ther 1996;23(5):326-331.

Haig H. Repair of the ligaments in recurrent subluxation of the ankle joint. J Bone Joint Surg 1950;32-B:751-755.

Hambley E. Recurrent dislocation of ankle due to rupture of external lateral ligament. Br Med J 1945;1:413.

Hedoba JL, Johannsen A. Recurrent instability of the ankle joint. Surgical repair by the Watson-Jones method. Acta Orthop Scand 1979;50:337-340.

Jenkins DHR, McKibbin B. The role of flexible carbon fiber implants as tendon and ligament substitutes in clinical practice. J Bone Joint Surg 1980;62-B:497-499.

Kannus P, Renström P. Treatment for acute tears of the lateral ligaments of the ankle. J Bone Joint Surg 1991;73-A:305-312.

Karlsson J, Andreasson GO. The effect of external ankle support in chronic lateral ankle joint instability: an electromyographic study. Am J Sports Med 1992;20(3):257-261.

Karlsson J, Bergstern T, Peterson L. Lateral instability of the ankle treated by Evans' procedure. J Bone Joint Surg 1988;70-B:476-480.

Kiaer S. Bristning af fodleddets udvendige sideligamenter behandlet med. Tenodese Ugeskr Laeg 1946;110:373-375.

Kristiansen B. Evans' repair of lateral instability of the ankle joint. Acta Orthop Scand 1981;52:679-682.

Kristiansen B. Surgical treatment of ankle instability in athletes. Br J Sports Med 1982;16(1):40-45.

Langstaff RJ, Handley CH. Functional ankle instability in members of the armed forces: the results of the extensor digitorum brevis transfer operation. Injury 1991;22(2):105-107.

Lauttamus L, Korkala O, Tanskanen P. Lateral ligament injuries of the ankle. Surgical treatment of late cases. Ann Chir Gynaecol 1982;71(3):164-167.

Leach, RE, Namiki O, Paul ER, Stockel J. Secondary reconstruction of the lateral ligaments of the ankle. Clin Orthop Rel Res 1980;160:201-211.

Leanderson J, Wredmark T. Treatment of acute ankle sprain. Comparison of semi-rigid ankle brace and compression bandage in 73 patients. Acta Orthop Scand 1995;66:529-531.

Lee, HG. Surgical repair in recurrent dislocation of the ankle joint. J Bone Joint Surg 1957;39A:828-834.

Lofvenberg R, Karrholm J, Lind B. The outcome of non-operated patients with chronic lateral instability of the ankle: a 20-year follow-up study. Foot Ankle Int 1994;15(4):165-169.

Lucht U, Vang PS, Termansen NB. Lateral ligament reconstruction of the ankle with a modified Watson-Jones operation. Acta Orthop Scand 1981;52(3):363-366.

Mann G, Elishuv MD, Lowe J, Finsterbush A, Frankl U, Nyska M, Matan Y. Recurrent ankle sprain: Literature review. Isr J Sports Med January 1994;104-108.

Mukherjee K, Gangopadhyay P. Extensor digitorium brevis transfer in chronic unstable ankles. J R Col Surg Ed 1983;28:250-255.

Nilsonne H. Making a new ligament in ankle sprain. J Bone Joint Surg 1932;14:380-381.

Orava S, Jaroma H, Suvela M. Radiological instability of the ankle after Evans' repair. Acta Orthop Scand 1983;54:734-738.

Ottaviani RA, Ashton-Miller JA, Kothari SU, Wojtys EM. Basketball shoe height and the maximal muscular resistance to applied ankle inversion and eversion moments. Am J Sports Med 1995;23(4):418-423.

Peters JW, Trevino SG, Renström PA. Chronic lateral ankle instability, Foot Ankle 1991;12:182.

Petersen L. Enkel plastik av invetererade ledbandsskador i fotleden (Simple plastic surgery of inveterate ligament damage in the ankle joint). Lärkartidningen 1981;78:2857-2861.

Pouzet F. Plastic ligamentaire externe de l'articulation tibiatarsienne. Lyon Chir 1954;49:618-619.

Rechtine GR, McCarrol JR, Webster DA. Reconstruction for chronic lateral instability of the ankle: A review of twenty-eight surgical patients. Orthop 1982;5:46-50.

Richard et al. Natl Athletic Trainers Assoc J (NATA) 1997;32(suppl):S 13 Abs. 207.

Rosendahl-Jensen S. Behandlingen av laterale ligamentrupturer I fod leddet. Nord Med 1952;47:903-904.

Sefton GK, George J, Fitton JM, McMullen H. Reconstruction of the anterior talofibular ligament for the treatment of the unstable ankle. J Bone Joint Surg 1979;61B:352-354.

Silver CM, Deutsch SD. Evans repair of lateral instability of the ankle. Orthopedics 1982;5(1):51-56.

Sitler MR, Horodyski M. Effectiveness of prophylactic ankle stabilisers for prevention of ankle injuries. Sports Med 1995;20(1):53-57.

Stewart MJ. Personal communication, quoted by Canale ST. In Edmonson AS, Crenshaw AH. Campbell's Operative Orthopaedics, 6th ed. C.V. Mosby Co., St. Louis, MO, 1980, p. 880.

Stören H. A new method for operative treatment of insufficiency of the lateral ligaments of the ankle joint. Acta Chir Scand 1959;117:501-509.

Thonnard JL, Bragard D, Willems PA, Plaghki L. Stability of the braced ankle. A biomechanical investigation. Am J Sports Med 1996;24:356-361.

Tropp H, Askling C, Gillquist. Prevention of ankle sprains. J Am J Sports Med 1985;13(4):259-262.

Watson-Jones R. 1940. Fractures and other bone and joint injuries. Edinburgh: Livingstone.

Watson-Jones R. 1952. Recurrent forward dislocation of the ankle joint. J Bone Joint Surg Br 34:519.

Watson-Jones R. 1960. Fractures and joint injuries, vol. 2, 4th ed. Edinburgh: Livingstone, p. 821-823.

Wester JU, Jespersen SM, Nielsen KD, Neumann L. Wobble board training after partial sprains of the lateral ligaments of the ankle: a prospective randomized study. J Orthop Sports Phys Ther 1996;23(5):332-336.

Williams JGP. Application of the anterolateral capsule of the ankle with extensor digitorum brevis transfer for chronic lateral ligament instability. Injury 1988;19:65-69.

Windfeld P. Treatment of undue mobility of the ankle joint following severe sprain of the ankle with avulsion of the anterior and middle bands of the external ligament. Acta Chir Scand 1953;105:299-304.

Yeung MS, Chan KM, So CH, Yuan WY. An epidemiological survey on ankle sprain. Br J Sports Med 1994;28(2):112-116.

Chapter 26

Watson-Jones Operation for Ankle Instability

Moshe (Perry) Pritsch, MD, and Moshe Salai, MD

The Watson-Jones operation for ankle instability was first described in 1955 (Watson-Jones 1955). The operation is a combination of tenodesis and ligament reconstruction, using the peroneus brevis tendon. Since the operation was instituted, it has gained popularity and has been performed in many medical centers. Although in recent years several other operative methods for ankle instability have been described, and the Watson-Jones operation has become less popular, it is still the gold standard for many orthopedic surgeons.

■ Surgical Technique

The patient is placed in a lateral decubitus position. A vertical incision is made behind the lower shaft of the fibula, is carried distally past the tip of the lateral malleolus, and is then curved medially towards the neck of the talus. The peroneal sheet is divided and retracted, and the peroneus brevis is identified.

The peroneus brevis tendon is dissected from its muscle belly, starting from the lateral malleolus and moving proximally as far as possible. The annular fibers holding the tendon in position behind the lateral malleolus should not be disturbed. The muscle fibers are sutured to the tendon of the peroneus longus, so that the power of active eversion will not be impaired. The tendon is cleaned from residual muscle fibers, and a nonabsorbable holding suture is put through its tip.

The distal part of the incision is dissected, elevating a flap that includes the periosteum of the lateral malleolus and exposing the lateral aspect of the ankle joint and the talar neck.

The fat pad in the sinus tarsi is excised to enable exposure of the lateral aspect of the talar neck. A 5-mm tunnel is drilled horizontally from the posterior to the anterior margin of the malleolus, emerging at the point where the anterior band of the lateral ligament

is normally attached. A second tunnel is drilled vertically in the outer margin of the neck of the talus, starting from the roof of the sinus tarsi and emerging adjacent to the articular surface.

A third tunnel is drilled approximately 1 cm proximal to the malleolar tip. It is advisable to create the tunnels first by using a 3.5-mm power drill, and then to enlarge the tunnels gradually and carefully with the aid of a hand drill in order to prevent breakage of the tunnel walls.

Using the holding suture, the tendon is guided through the tunnels, first through the proximal tunnel in the lateral malleolus, then through the talar neck tunnel, and finally through the distal malleolar tunnel (figure 26.1). After applying tension to the tendon to achieve proper tension throughout its length, it is sutured together behind the malleolus, while the ankle joint is held in the neutral position.

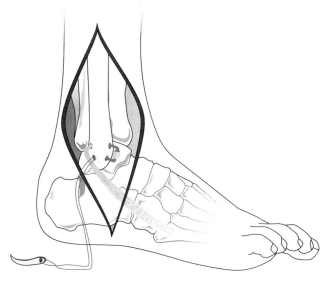

■ **Figure 26.1** The tendon passing through the bony tunnels.

The peroneal sheet is closed with absorbable stitches, the wound is closed, and the foot and ankle are immobilized in a plaster cast for 3 months. Weight bearing is permitted after the change of plaster at 6 weeks. After removal of the plaster, a rehabilitation program is initiated.

■ Personal Experience

The Watson-Jones operation for ankle instability has been performed at the Chaim Sheba Medical Center since 1965.

In order to assess our results, we reviewed 34 patients, 7 women and 27 men, who were available for follow-up. The average age at the time of the operation was 21 years (range 19 to 28 years).

The duration of symptoms before surgery was 3 to 60 months. Twenty-eight of the patients were involved in nonprofessional sport activity before surgery; the average follow-up period was 9.5 years (range 4 to 15 years).

The patients were asked to complete a detailed questionnaire, including ratings of pre- and postoperative functional ability and grade of satisfaction. Examination of each patient included assessment of gait, local tenderness or swelling, stability of both tibia talar and subtalar joints, eversion power, and modified Romberg test (the ability to stand on one foot with eyes closed for 5 seconds). In addition, every patient underwent a series of radiographs, including inversion and anterior drawer stress radiographs.

The results in our series indicated that most patients were satisfied with their operations and regained their preinjury functional level, with most regaining full range of motion and normal eversion power postoperatively. Only three patients felt that their results were poor.

In six cases, there was a mild decrease in subtalar motion, and four cases were found to have increased subtalar motion. Two of these had generalized laxity.

The postoperative stress radiographs demonstrated very good postoperative static stability. However, the modified Romberg test, which represents functional stability (Freeman & Hanham 1965), was less encouraging. Nevertheless, in the patients who were followed up for more than 9 years, the results of the Romberg test were excellent.

It appears that the Watson-Jones operation provides very good static stability, which is the basis on which functional stability is achieved over time.

In the search for the development of arthritic changes, we found that three patients with arthritic changes in the ankle joint prior to surgery had the same changes 4, 6, and 8 years after surgery. Eight patients who had no changes prior to surgery had mild asymptomatic arthritic changes at a mean period of 9 years after surgery; the nonoperated ankles in these patients were normal. This finding cannot support the belief that one of the purposes of reconstructive surgery for unstable joints in general, and the ankle joint in particular, is to prevent early osteoarthritis (Harrington 1979). It is possible that in some cases the operation may actually be the cause of early osteoarthritis. Conversely, the arthritis may be the final result of initial articular changes that occurred prior to surgery (Hoy & Henderson 1994).

A point of interest was the identification of optimal sites for the tunnels in the fibula. In our study, we found that the best static stability is achieved when the distal tunnel is sited between 6 mm and 13 mm from the fibular tip, and the distance between the tunnels is between 8 mm and 14 mm.

■ Complications

Three patients had postoperative superficial wound infection, and two suffered from a transient sural nerve injury.

The results in this series, in comparison with those of other known series, are good (Cass & Morreg 1984; Gillespie & Boucher 1971; van der Rigt & Evans 1984) and do not support the claim that the operation inevitably restricts subtalar motion (Kjaersgaard-Andersen et al. 1989).

Our results support the claim that instability is corrected and stability maintained with no deterioration over time (Hoy & Henderson 1994; Lucht et al. 1981; Younes et al. 1988).

■ References

Cass JR, Morreg BF. 1984. Ankle instability: current concepts, diagnosis and treatment. Mayo Clin Proc 59:165-170.

Freeman MAR, Hanham WF. 1965. The etiology and prevention of functional instability of the foot. J Bone Joint Surg Br 47:678-685.

Gillespie HS, Boucher P. 1971. Watson-Jones repair of lateral instability of the ankle. J Bone Joint Surg Am 53:920-924.

Harrington KD. 1979. Degenerative arthritis of the ankle secondary to long standing lateral ligament instability. J Bone Joint Surg Am 61:354-361.

Hoy GA, Henderson IJP. 1994. Results of Watson-Jones ankle reconstruction. J Bone Joint Surg Br 76:610-613.

Kjaersgaard-Andersen P, Sjoberg JO, Wethelund JO, Helmig P, Madsen F. 1989. Watson-Jones tenodesis for ankle instability: a mechanical analysis in amputation specimen. Acta Orthop Scand 60:477-480.

Lucht U, Vang PS, Termansen NB. 1981. Lateral ligament reconstruction of the ankle with a modified Watson-Jones operation. Acta Orthop Scan 52:363-366.

van der Rigt AJ, Evans GA. 1984. The long term results of Watson-Jones tenodesis. J Bone Joint Surg Br 66:371-376.

Watson-Jones R. 1955. Fractures and joint injuries. 4th ed. Volume II. Edinburgh: Livingstone.

Younes C, Fowles JV, Fallaha M, Antoun R. 1988. Long term results of surgical reconstruction for chronic lateral instability of the ankle: comparison of Watson-Jones and Evans technique. J Trauma 28:1330-1334.

Chapter 27

Lateral Chronic Instability of the Ankle: Chrisman-Snook Technique

Alberto Macklin Vadell, MD

The incidence of chronic symptoms after acute lateral ankle injuries is approximately 20%. Complaints vary but include functional instability, frank mechanical instability, recurrent swelling, pain, and stiffness. Causes of chronic ankle symptoms include ligament rupture, proprioceptive damage, peroneal tendon subluxation, and tibiotalar or talofibular bony impingement; any of these may be associated with ligament instability. Approximately 20% of symptomatic patients may eventually require surgery. Most instabilities are caused by trauma, but cavus feet, calcaneus varus, or os subfibular may contribute to the functional or mechanical instability. High success rates have been reported with various surgical procedures for repair or reconstruction of the lateral ligaments. Our preferred approach for a reconstructive procedure is the Chrisman-Snook technique, which uses the peroneus brevis tendon to stabilize the lateral aspect of the ankle.

■ Surgical Anatomy and Biomechanics

For more details on surgical anatomy and biomechanics, see chapters 2 through 4.

The ankle is a modified hinge joint. Its motion includes upward and downward movement of the foot about a single axis that is oriented obliquely to the long axis of the leg.

The lateral malleolus is located at the distal end of the fibula. It is positioned approximately 1 cm distal and posterior to the medial malleolus. It has two facets: one for the talus and a posterior sulcus of the peroneal tendons.

Three majors groups of ligaments provide stability to the ankle joint: the lateral ligaments, the tibiofibular syndesmosis, and the medial ligaments. The lateral ligaments consist of the anterior talofibular, calcaneofibular, and posterior talofibular ligaments (see chapter 2).

The axis of the ankle joint in relation to the knee joint is approximately 25° of external tibial torsion. The ankle joint is inclined laterally and posteriorly.

Both the anterior talofibular ligament (ATFL) and the calcaneofibular ligament (CFL) are positioned in a parasagittal plane. The TFL is anterior fibular with a clear anterior position, and the CFL is directed backward and downward, attaching to the lateral side of the calcaneus. Thus, the CFL is biarticular, crossing the tibiotalar and subtalar joints. The posterior talofibular ligament (PTFL) is an extremely strong structure and is rarely injured with simple inversion ankle injuries. Between the ATFL and the CFL, there is an angle of 70-140° (average 105°). The ATFL is the major lateral ligament in plantarflexion, for it lines up with the fibula as the talus moves to a plantarflexed position. In dorsiflexion, the CFL takes up a similar vertical position. In a planterflexion of approximately 25°, both ligaments are lax, a situation which may contribute to occurrence of ankle sprain in this position. The ATFL is the most frequently injured ligament of the ankle, followed by the CFL. An isolated CFL tear may occur when a varus force is applied to the neutral or dorsiflexed ankle.

■ Diagnosis

See chapters 6 through 11 for further details on diagnosis.

A patient with chronic lateral ankle instability usually has a history of acute inversion ankle injury that in many cases was treated inadequately. The patient will complain of recurrent ankle sprains and a feeling of giving way. Some patients have a recorded history of recurrent inversion injuries that occur when walking on uneven surfaces.

The examination may disclose increased excursion of the talus and peroneal muscle weakness. A positive anterior drawer sign and talar tilt stress radiographs may be apparent (figure 27.1).

In 1979, Cox published a paper based on the ankles of 404 navy cadets who had never suffered from ankle instability. He found 396 individuals with talar tilt stress radiograph between 0-5°. Cox suggested that this tilt of 5° would thus be considered normal.

Anderson and Le Coq, in 1954, suggested a classification of instabilities based on angular tibiotalar values. This study was conducted on 50 cadaverous ankles. According to the results, instabilities could be classified in three different grades:

- Grade 1: Lateral tilt is absent or not larger than 5° and anterior drawer is always present.

- Grade 2: Lateral tilt measuring between 7° and 10°.

- Grade 3: Talar tilt is measured between 15° and 30°, or even more.

If all the external system is destroyed, the talus luxates from the joint. The three grades would correspond to damage of one, two, or three components of the lateral ligament.

According to this classification, the therapeutic plan would be the following: sprains of grade 1 and 2 respond to conservative methods or to surgical procedures that correct the insufficiency of the anterior components. Sprains of grade 3 are always accompanied by severe symptomatology. These lesions can only be corrected with techniques that replace the anterior and medial ligaments and reproduce, at the same time, their normal orientation.

■ Treatment

In cases of chronic functional instability, especially if accompanied by mechanical instability, surgical treatment would be considered after failure of conservative measures. Conservative measures include peroneal strengthening, proprioceptive training, and taping or bracing as discussed in chapters 20 through 24 in this book.

Surgical Procedures

High success rates have been reported with various surgical procedures for reconstruction of the lateral ligaments. The preference of one method over another is essentially in accordance with the technical complexity and biomechanical advantages of each specific procedure as assessed by the surgeon.

We use the Chrisman-Snook procedure for patients with combined tibiotalar and subtalar instability or patients with generalized laxity of all ligaments.

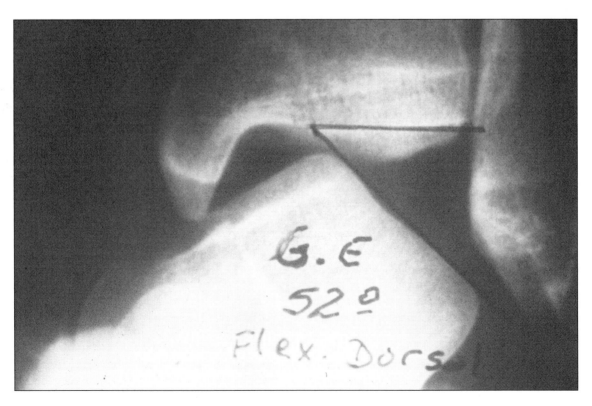

■ **Figure 27.1** A radiograph showing positive anterior drawer sign and talar tilt stress.

Historical Overview of Surgical Treatment

Over the past 80 years, various surgical procedures have been described and good results have been reported with most procedures. The preferences for one method or the other would depend on the technical complexity, inherent risks, and biomechanical advantages of each procedure, as viewed by the surgeon. We will briefly review the techniques, as published in the medical literature since 1913. (See also the general overview in chapter 25.)

In 1913, Gallie described, for the first time, the tenodesis with the short peroneal tendon in a case of paralytic clubfoot. Nilsonne modified the procedure, adapting it to a specific case of ankle instability and using, essentially, the technique that Evans would describe later in 1953. Elmslie (1934) proposed the reconstruction of the ATFL and CFL with the fascia lata, passing it through drill holes in the lateral malleolus, talar neck, and calcaneus.

Watson-Jones criticized the use of fascia lata but adopted the idea of tunneling the talar neck, using the peroneus brevis tendon. In Argentina in 1977, Girardi published a modification of Elmslie's technique performed by Vidal, pointing out that it reconstructs the ankle instability without limiting the hindfoot.

Kelikan, in 1980, introduced a method of reconstruction using the plantaris tendon. The tendon was passed through a drill hole in the calcaneus and to the talus among the course of the CFL.

Chrisman-Snook Procedure

Elmslie, in 1934, proposed the reconstruction of the TFL and CFL with the fascia lata, passing it through drill holes in the lateral malleolus, talar neck, and calcaneus. Returning to Elmslie's ideas in 1969, Chrisman and Snook published a modification of the technique using the anterior half of the peroneus brevis tendon (figure 27.2). This procedure has the advantage of reproducing the orientation and angular values between both components of the lateral ligament. The most important factor leading to a successful surgical procedure is the success in forming the angle between the anterior and medial branch of the transplant. This angle must be 105°. Thus, the subtalar motion will be minimally affected.

Surgical Technique

A curved incision is made over the peroneus brevis tendon beginning 8 cm proximal to the tip of the fibula and ending at the base of the 5th metatarsal. Care must be taken to avoid injuring the sural nerve. The peroneal sheath is opened and the peroneus brevis tendon is split lengthwise from its insertion at the bone of the fifth metatarsal to the musculotendinous junction. Half of the tendon is detached from the muscle and pulled distally.

The joint is inspected. A drill hole is then made about 2 cm proximal to the fibular tip, from anterior

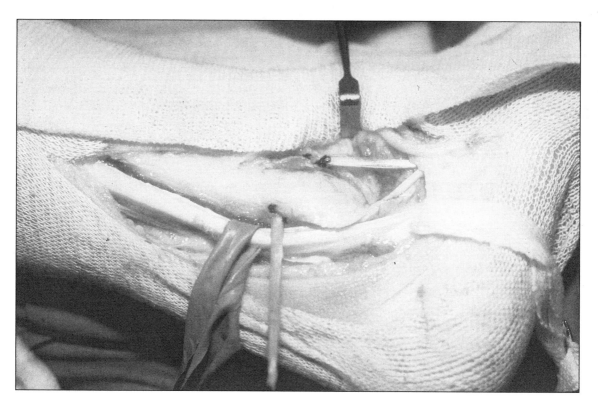

■ **Figure 27.2** Surgical technique.

to posterior and downward with a 4.5 drill. The tendon is passed from anterior to posterior and is fixed to the periosteum of the lateral malleolus. It is important to ensure that the motion of the ankle is maintained (figure 27.3).

The lateral aspect of the calcaneus is exposed at the insertion of the calcaneofibular ligament. Two oblique drill holes are made with a 4.5 drill, two cm apart in the horizontal plane, and then connected. The graft is passed superficial to the peroneal tendons and then from posterior to anterior through the calcaneus before being sutured under tension to the periosteum. The reconstruction is accomplished using 3.0 absorbable sutures. The wound is then irrigated and the peroneal tendon sheath is closed. The skin is closed with subcuticular sutures.

Postoperative Treatment

A short leg cast or walker boot is used for about 6 weeks, with weight bearing as tolerated. Then the cast is removed and the patient is started on an aggressive rehabilitation program. The level of activity allowed progresses over time, with sport usually permitted in the fourth month after surgery.

Author's Experience

From March 1975 to June 1991, the author operated on and followed 27 patients who formed the basis for this report. The group consisted of 13 males and 14 females whose age ranged from 15 to 43 years old (average 23.6). The right ankle was affected in 16 patients and the left in 11. The talar tilt stress test ranged from 12-30° with an average of 21.3°. All the patients recalled that the original accident had taken place between from 6 months and 5 years before. They received symptomatic treatment only, or a cast for no longer than 3 weeks. Only one case had a cast on for 6 weeks. This patient presented a tilt of 10°, which 1 year later increased to 25° as the result of an additional injury. All the patients were evaluated after surgery according to the score that Pace published in 1990. This score takes five items into account: pain, mobility, laxity, swelling, and activity level. Evaluating each of these items between 0 and 10 points, a score from 0 to 4 is considered as a good result, a score of 5 to 8 is considered a fair result and a score over 9 is considered a poor result. We had 22 patients with a good result (81.4 %) and 5 with a fair result (18.6%).

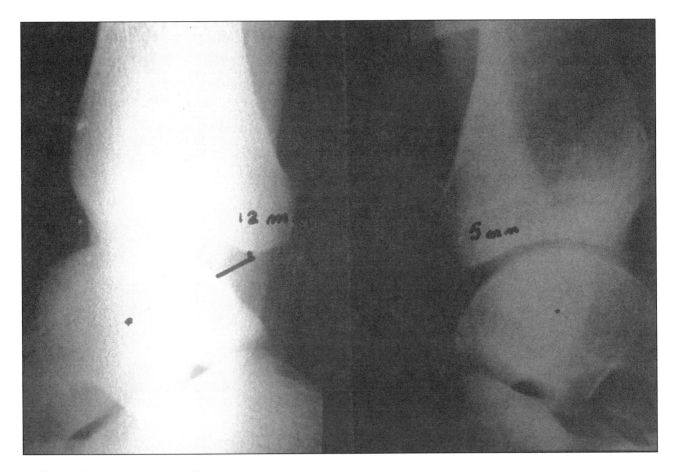

■ **Figure 27.3** Placement of drill holes.

Complications

We observed the following complications:

1. Persistent swelling: 7 cases
2. Difficulty of returning to full physical activity: 3 cases
3. Stiffness of the subtalar joint: 1 case
4. Feeling of instability: 1 case
5. Residual laxity: 1 case with a tilt of 9°
6. Dehiscence of surgical wound: 1 case

■ Conclusions

When deciding on surgical intervention, we use the clinical history and apply the Anderson and LeCoq classification.

- For grade 1, we recommend conservative treatment.
- For grade 2, the decision depends on the patient's age and athletic activity, and the degree of instability and security that the patient experiences.
- For grade 3, we recommend surgical treatment.

Of the surgical techniques described in the literature, we feel that the Chrisman-Snook technique comes the closest to reproducing the normal ankle anatomy in relation to the position and direction of the components building the lateral ligament complex. We believe that this is a reliable and simple technique, the results of which have entirely met our expectations. In most of the patients we have treated, we obtained stable ankles with good tibiotalar and subtalar mobility, and no degenerative signs have been observed during 9 to 25 years of follow-up.

■ References

Anderson R, Le Coq J: Operative treatment of injury to the fibular collateral ligament of the ankle. JBJS 36-A (4): 827-832, 1954.

Chrisman H, Snook G: Reconstruction of the lateral tears of the ankle. JBJS 51-A (5): 904-911, 1969.

Cox J, Hewes T: "Normal" talar tilt angle. Clin Orthop 140: 37-41, 1979.

Elmslie RC: Recurrent subluxations of the ankle joint. Ann Surg 100:364,1934.

Evans DL: Recurrent instability of the ankle—a method of surgical treatment. Proc R Soc Med 46:343, 1953.

Gillesie H, Boucher P: Watson-Jones repair of the lateral instability of the ankle. JBJS 53-A (5): 920-924, 1971.

Girardi H: Técnica de Elmslie modificada para corregir la inestabilidad del tobillo. Bol y Trab SAOT 6: 400, 1977.

Kelikan H, Kelikian AS: Disorders of the ankle. Philadelphia: WB Saunders, 1980.

Watson-Jones R: Recurrent forward dislocation of the ankle joint. J Bone Joint Surg 34B:519, 1952.

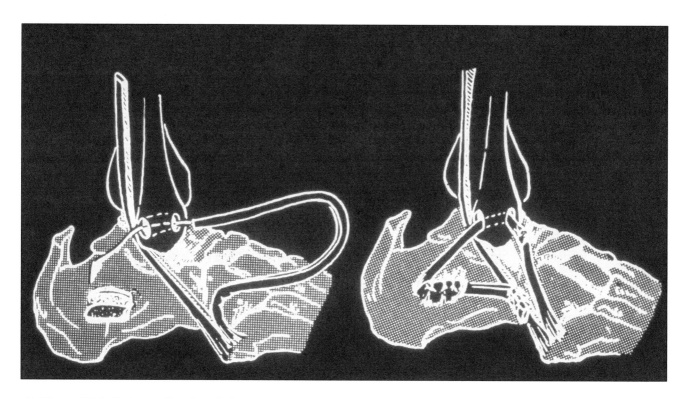

■ **Figure 27.4** Chrisman-Snook technique.

Chapter 28

Ankle Ligament Reconstruction: The Broström Procedure

Roger A. Mann, MD, and Jeffrey A. Mann, MD

■ Decision Making

The decision to surgically repair an unstable ankle joint should be based on the patient's history, physical examination, radiographic findings, and physical activities. Patients should have undergone prior conservative management, including peroneal strengthening, possible shoe modifications such as lateral heel or sole lift or both, and occasionally bracing with a stirrup brace or lace-up brace. Unless there is a moderate degree of instability, reconstruction is usually not indicated. If an element of subtalar joint instability is present in addition to ankle instability, it should also be repaired.

If the patient has a cavus type foot, then one must decide whether the major problem is the postural deformity or whether it is ligamentous instability. If a patient only has a varus deformity of the calcaneus, a Dwyer or lateral closing wedge osteotomy of the calcaneus should be considered. If a forefoot valgus with a plantarflexed first metatarsal is present, then a dorsiflexion osteotomy of the first metatarsal is indicated. If an anatomic deformity is present, a reconstructive procedure without correction of the bony deformity will usually not produce a satisfactory long-term result.

For ligamentous instability of the anterior talofibular ligament, with or without calcaneofibular ligament involvement, I believe the Broström procedure to be the procedure of choice (Broström 1966). This procedure consists of a ligamentous and capsular repair of the anterior talofibular ligament. The Gould modification utilizes the extensor retinaculum to correct calcaneofibular ligament laxity or subtalar joint instability (Gould et al. 1980). The Broström procedure is an anatomic repair of the ligaments and results in excellent stability without violating the peroneal tendons. It will usually ensure satisfactory

postoperative motion (Clanton 1999) (figure 28.1, a-d).

■ Modified Broström Procedure for Ankle Ligament Reconstruction

1. The patient is placed supine with a large bolster under the ipsilateral hip in order to simplify visualization of the lateral aspect of the ankle joint.

2. The incision begins 1-2 cm anterior to the fibula, at the level of the ankle joint. It is carried distally and posteriorly along the skin crease over the lateral aspect of the ankle, crossing over the tip of the fibula. Extreme caution must be taken at both ends of the incision to avoid injuring the superficial branches of the peroneal nerve dorsally and the sural nerve posteriorly.

3. The incision is deepened through the joint capsule and remnants of ligament, exposing the entire lateral aspect of the ankle joint and creating an anterior and posterior flap. The anterior flap contains the part of the ligament attached to the talus, and the posterior flap contains ligament remnants attached to the fibula.

4. The articular surface of the ankle is carefully inspected for evidence of pathology, especially along the dorsolateral aspect of the talus. If a chondral defect is present, any irregular edges or loose cartilaginous flaps should be debrided. Also, any loose bodies should be searched for and removed.

5. The ligamentous tissue remaining on the distal fibula is then peeled off and retracted posteriorly. The bone beneath this flap is curetted to produce a raw surface of bleeding bone.

6. The anterior flap of the ligamentous tissue that was created is now sutured over the raw bone surface

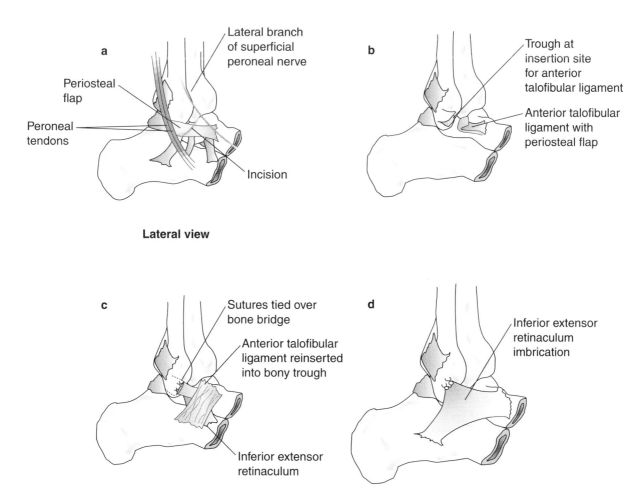

a

Lateral branch of superficial peroneal nerve

Periosteal flap

Peroneal tendons

Incision

Lateral view

b

Trough at insertion site for anterior talofibular ligament

Anterior talofibular ligament with periosteal flap

c

Sutures tied over bone bridge

Anterior talofibular ligament reinserted into bony trough

Inferior extensor retinaculum

d

Inferior extensor retinaculum imbrication

■ **Figure 28.1** Modified Broström direct repair with imbrication. *(a)* Lateral exposure and creation of a lateral periosteal flap continuous with the anterior talofibular ligament. *(b)* Creation of a trough in the anterior part of the fibula for insertion of the anterior talofibular ligament. *(c)* Insertion of the anterior talofibular ligament into the fibular trough and sutures tied over the bony ridge. *(d)* Imbrication of the inferior extensor retinaculum to reinforce the repair and provide subtalar joint stability. It should be noted that an alternative method to making the trough in the anterior talofibular ligament is simply to cut and plicate the lateral joint capsular tissue with a pants-over-vest type repair as described in the text.

Reprinted from Clanton and Schon 1999.

along the distal fibula. The sutures are begun in the periosteum of the fibula, placed through the anterior cuff of the ankle ligament, and then brought back through the periosteum. Usually, five or six sutures are placed. If there is involvement of the calcaneofibular ligament, the sutures are extended distally into this area. Care must be taken not to inadvertently place a suture through the peroneus brevis tendon.

7. Once this suture has been placed, the sutures are tightened, pulling the anterior flap to the fibula and tucking it under the posterior flap. As this is done, the ligamentous instability about the lateral aspect of the ankle is noted to disappear. The sutures are tied while the leg is resting on a block of soft material so that the heel can be easily displaced posteriorly, ensuring that the ligament reconstruction is under no tension. The posterior portion of the flap is now sutured over the

anterior flap with a series of interrupted sutures, thereby reinforcing the initial repair. This having been carried out, there should no longer be any evidence of anterior instability of the ankle joint. If there is, the sutures have not been properly placed.

8. Occasionally, at the time of surgery, it is noted that the ligamentous tissue is of very poor quality and does not seem strong enough to maintain a repair. We have found that even such tissue can essentially always effect a satisfactory repair. The reconstructed ligaments seem to hypertrophy in reaction to the surgery and to reconstitute tissue for a sufficiently firm reconstruction.

9. If there is any element of subtalar instability or calcaneofibular insufficiency, it must be addressed at this time. The Gould modification of the original Broström repair brings the extensor retinaculum across

the repair and sutures it into the fibula (Clanton 1993). The extensor retinaculum at times is difficult to identify, but is always present and is a fairly stout structure. It can be found by dissecting subcutaneously in the distal part of the incision and observing that there is a heavy band of tissue that obliquely crosses the ankle almost in the same line as the incision. This is the extensor retinaculum.

10. Once the extensor retinaculum is identified, it is carefully developed, with caution not to detach it distally. This sheet of tissue is then brought up across the ankle joint as the subtalar joint is held in an everted position. As the retinaculum is attached, the physician may note that it provides excellent stability to the subtalar joint. This layer is then sutured into the periosteum of the fibula over the previous repair. Immediately after the repair, a 50% to 75% restriction of subtalar joint motion should be noted.

11. The patient's wounds are closed in a routine manner, and the patient is placed into a short leg nonweightbearing compression dressing incorporating plaster splints.

12. The patient is kept in a short leg nonweightbearing cast for 4 weeks and then in a short leg removable cast for another 4 weeks, at which time strengthening exercises are begun.

13. It requires approximately 2 months of intense physical therapy to reestablish normal ankle function. Initially, there is some restriction of subtalar joint motion at times, but this usually loosens over a short period of time. The Broström repair does not produce the overall tightness or hard fixed end points observed with repairs using a tendon, such as the Elmslie, Watson-Jones, or Chrisman-Snook procedures. The excessive tightness of such procedures sometimes appears to cause the patient pain.

■ Complications

The main complication associated with this procedure is entrapment of either a peroneal or sural nerve. In most cases, this can be avoided by careful dissection at the ends of the incision. We have not personally had a patient whose ligament repair has failed, although I have been told of a few instances of failure in heavy linemen playing American football.

■ References

Broström L. 1966. Sprained ankles VI. Surgical treatment of "chronic" ligament ruptures. Acta Chir Scand 132:551-565.

Clanton TO. and Schon LE. 1993. Athletic injuries to the soft tissues of the foot and ankle. In Mann RA, Coughlin MJ, editors. Surgery of the foot and ankle, vol. II, 6th ed. St. Louis, MO: Mosby.

Clanton TO. 1999. Athletic injuries to the soft tissues of the foot and ankle. In Coughlin MJ, Mann RK, editors. Surgery of the foot and ankle, vol. II, 7th ed. St. Louis, MO: Mosby. p. 1126-1129.

Gould N, Seligson D, Gassman J. 1980. Early and late repair of lateral ligament of the ankle. Foot Ankle Int 1:84-89.

Chapter 29

The Williams Procedure

Gideon Mann, MD; Eli London, DPM; G. Chaimsky; and Meir Nyska, MD

The Williams procedure is intended to treat mechanical and functional instability resulting from an old injury. Broström first reported that previously injured ligamentous tissue remained intact, or encased in scar tissue, and could be used for ligament repair (Broström 1966). Other authors agreed that ligamentous material remains present after injury. The ends of the ligaments are not necessarily easy to find and have often healed together. The ligament might be attenuated or only scarred. Therefore, there are few possibilities of performing direct repair. The Williams procedure is based on imbrication of the scar tissue or the attenuated ligaments; hence, it stabilizes the ankle mechanically. Functionally, it is based on advancement and reattachment of the extensor digitorum brevis (EDB) muscle to the capsule of the ankle joint. The EDB muscle belly lies close to the ankle joint capsule, and the extensor retinaculum lies just on its fascia. The EDB can be mobilized and stretched easily. By this method, the mechanoreceptors of the muscle belly itself react to tension on the ankle joint capsule. The Williams technique of lateral ligament repair was first reported in 1988 by Williams, and we adopted and modified his technique (Lindman et al. 1994; Mann et al. 1993; Williams 1988)

■ Operative Technique

Under ankle block anesthesia and supramalleolar tourniquet, a lateral approach to the sinus tarsi is performed. The skin incision is oblique, about 7 cm, starting from the peroneal tuberosity of the calcaneus, extending between the fibula and the base of the extensor digitorum brevis 1 cm anterior and parallel to the fibula, and ending at the extensor digitorum longus (EDL) tendons (figure 29.1). The fat of the sinus tarsi is undermined down to the extensor retinaculum. The fat is dissected from the area of the base of the EDB toward the anterior border of the fibula. A deep incision 3-5 mm anterior and parallel to the

fibula is made through the extensor retinaculum and the capsule of the ankle joint, including the anterior talofibular ligament, which is usually fibrotic. The incision extends from the long extensor tendons to the peroneal tendons, including the outer tendon sheath. Care is taken not to harm the branch of the superficial peroneal nerve at the area of the EDL.

When the ankle joint is approached, synovectomy and exploration of the lateral process of the talus is done, if necessary. Another parallel cut 1.5 cm distally at the base of the EDB is performed, extending down to the calcaneus and dissecting 2-3 mm of the EDB, creating a flap (figure 29.2). One suture of Vycril 0 is inserted, starting from the tissue just anterior to the fibula, passes under the bridge of soft tissue that has been created by the two parallel incisions, and is taken out at the fascia of the EDB (figure 29.3). Then it is inserted again to the fascia of the EDB, passed under the bridge, and pulled out close to the anterior border of the fibula, where the

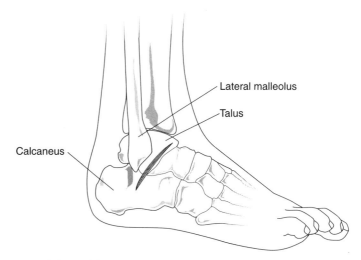

■ **Figure 29.1** The skin incision for reefing of the lateral ligament of the ankle.

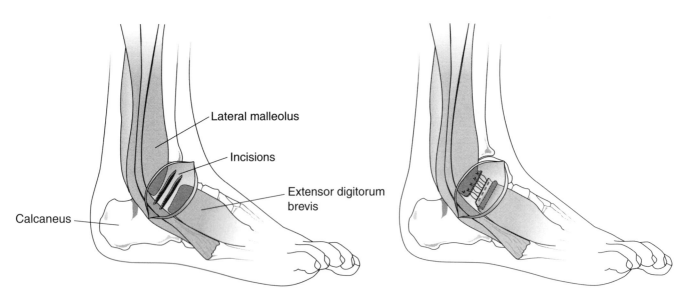

■ **Figure 29.2** Two parallel incisions in the lateral ligament close to the anterior side of the fibula and at the insertion of the extensor digitorum brevis.

■ **Figure 29.4** Reefing the lateral ligaments by tying the suture and stretching of the extensor digitorum brevis.

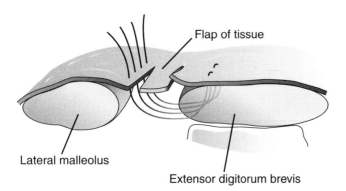

■ **Figure 29.3** Placement of the sutures from the anterior area of the fibula to the base of the extensor digitorum brevis under the bridge over the sinus tarsi.

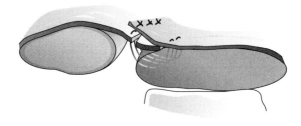

■ **Figure 29.5** Outer layer of sutures from the extensor digitorum brevis to the anterior area of the fibula.

suture was originally inserted. At least five sutures are inserted starting from close to the EDL, and the last suture is inserted close and under the peroneal tendon parallel to the calcaneofibular ligament. Then the sutures are tightly tied while the foot is held in slight eversion and plantigrade (figure 29.4). After tightening the sutures, the ankle stability and range of motion is checked. In order to augment the repair, the edges of the bridge are sutured to the fascia of the EDB and to the anterior side of the fibula, creating a second layer of soft tissue that contains the bridge and extensor retinaculum (figure 29.5). The subcutaneous tissue and the skin are closed in the usual manner.

■ Postoperative Management

The leg is immobilized in a cast for 6 weeks. The sutures are removed at 2-3 weeks and full weight bearing is encouraged from 2-3 weeks, as tolerated. At 6 weeks, the cast is removed and an intensive course of physiotherapy is taken.

■ Clinical Follow-Up

Our first experience with the modified Williams procedure included 15 patients with an average follow-up of 24 months. The average age of the patients was

22 years (range 18-33 years), and duration of the complaints after the first inversion injury was from 8 months to 15 years. The patients complained of giving way, recurrent sprains, and a feeling of insecurity and pain on the lateral side of the ankle. Stress radiography on TELOS demonstrated mechanical instability in 5 ankles. Although 10 were stable radiographically, they qualified as functionally unstable ankles. In all the patients, the initial treatment was conservative, lasting at least 6 months. Operation was suggested after failure of conservative treatment. According to a scoring system for evaluation of instability of the ankle (see chapter 7), surgical patients had less than 60 points (out of 100) before the operation, and had 77 points after the operation. (The objective score after the operation was 89 and the subjective was 72). The stress radiographic examination demonstrated significant improvement from 6.9° to 4.3° in lateral tilt of the talus, and from 5.7 mm to 5 mm in the posterior opening of the tibiotalar joint. The latter was not statistically significant. After the operation, two patients still suffered from occasional sprains, but were improved compared to their situation before the operation. This caused the lower score of 72 in the subjective evaluation. We concluded that the Williams procedure was a physiological repair that was effective in treating mechanical and functional instability.

■ References

Broström L. 1966. Sprained ankles VI. Surgical treatment of chronic ligament ruptures. Acta Chir Scand 132:551-565.

Lindman Y, Nyska M, Lowe J, Elishuv O, Finsterbush A, Mann G. 1994. The Williams capsular plication for recurrent ankle sprain. Presented at the Tenth International Jerusalem Symposium on Sports Injuries, 1994, Jerusalem, Israel.

Mann G, Elishuv O, Nyska M, Chaimsky G, Finsterbush A, Perry C. 1993. Recurrent ankle sprain: Experience with modification of William reefing technique. J Orthop Tech 8(3):361-376.

Williams JGP. 1988. Application of the anterolateral capsule of the ankle with extensor digitorum brevis transfer for chronic lateral ligament instability. Injury 19:65-69.

Chapter 30

Arthroscopic Reconstruction of the Unstable Ankle

Charles C. Southerland Jr., DPM, FACFAS, FACFAOM, DABDA

In the United States, lateral ankle injuries lead the ICD-9 coding index for all emergency room admissions (Garrick 1977; McMaster 1943). Although the vast majority of lateral ankle sprains do not result in serious lateral ankle instabilities, a significant number are seen clinically by foot and ankle specialists. Many grading method nomenclatures have been proposed for this malady (Reichen & Marti 1974; Rubin & Witten 1960). Most have already been discussed in this text. It is not the intent of this discussion to go into considerable detail on the nature and disposition of ankle injury, except as it applies to arthroscopic lateral ankle stabilization (ALAS) procedures.

■ Role of Arthroscopy

Arthroscopy in general has been well established both in literature and education. First described by Takagi in 1939 (Lundeen 1987), confirmatory outcomes were reported by Watanabe and Chen (van Dijk & Scholte 1997) based on 10 cadaveric investigations and in vivo outcomes on 75 patients reported in 1970. As a result of the Watanabe and Chen paper, arthroscopes of 2-4 mm in diameter were identified as optimal for ankle joint visualization. Four-millimeter scopes are generally considered to offer the best proportion between field of view and cannula size, particularly for anterior articular visualization (Ferkel & Fischer 1989). Although they significantly limit the field of view, 2.7-mm scopes have become quite popular for deeper penetrations into the joint. Smaller 2.2- to 1.7-mm scopes are capable of being inserted over the dome of the talus, but sacrifice field of view and sweeping manipulation for a rather limited view of the posterior ankle joint. Most arthroscopists prefer either a posterocentral (through the Achilles tendon) or posterolateral (between the Achilles tendon and the sural nerve) approach for posterior ankle joint visual-

izations with either a 4.0- or 2.78-mm scope (Lundeen 1985). In 1983, Lundeen et al. offered the first dedicated seminar in ankle joint arthroscopy, at Indiana Arthroscopy Associates (Lundeen et al. 1983). From that time forward, numerous manufacturers have produced a wide variety of excellent instruments.

The fundamental advantages of ankle joint arthroscopy include early, accurate diagnosis of osteochondral talar dome and tibial plafond lesions, synovial impingement syndromes, and intra-articular exostoses. A more sophisticated application includes repair of grade II or mild grade III ankle instabilities. For purposes of this discussion, we shall classify optimal arthroscopic indications for ankle sprains as represented objectively by radiographic talar tilt angles of 10-15° greater than those of an unaffected ankle (Glick et al. 1990). Ankle joint sprains with a 10-20° difference in inversion stress views as contrasted with views of an unaffected ankle are classified as grade III and their eligibility for arthroscopy remains controversial (Glick et al. 1990). Although some question the validity of inversion stress testing, it remains the only proposed method of quantifying or grading the degree of injury in severe ankle sprains. All grade IV (>20°) ankle instabilities should be considered beyond the scope of reliable outcomes in arthroscopic interventions.

The ideal patient profile is that of a symptomatic, healthy, young, physically active patient. Athletes with moderate lateral ankle instability are primary candidates, as the procedure permits a relatively fast recovery with minimum incursion, as well as the potential for rapid return to peak performance.

Any such intervention should only be attempted after a reasonable amount of time in conservative therapy. This typically represents 3-6 months of therapy directed toward increasing range of motion (ROM), with strengthening of peroneal and extensor musculature (Bassewitz & Shapiro 1997). There should also be a history of repetitive sprains with continuing symptoms. Instability should be confirmed with an anterior ankle drawer sign on clinical examination (see figure 12.6 on page 106). To review briefly, this simple test is performed by placing the patient in a supine position and flexing the knee of the affected extremity as much as possible. The foot should then be placed plantigrade on the examining table and secured with one hand, while the other hand grasps the ankle joint medially and attempts to move the joint forward/backward. The result will be positive if there is a dramatic protrusion of the lateral malleolus against the soft tissue sleeve of the ankle. Without an intact anterior talofibular ligament, the lateral malleolus will demonstrate a much greater dimpling of forward movement. This should be quite evident, particularly in comparison with the unaffected opposite side. Additional tests that may be useful for determining injury to the anterior talofibular ligament include the syndesmotic squeeze test, the external rotation stress test, and the tibiotalar shuck test (Cotton test) (Lassiter et al. 1989; Marder 1995). Although the latter three are primarily used to evaluate an initial injury, the drawer sign is usually more consistent with chronic injury. Arthroscopic lateral ankle stabilization (ALAS) should not be done in place of primary open capsular repair, in the event that a patient opts for primary repair of an acute ankle injury (Kannus & Renström 1991).

■ Practical Applications of Ankle Anatomy

The ankle joint is a delicate soft tissue envelope in which many anatomic structures coalesce, all of which must be well understood by the capable arthroscopist. Starting from the medial malleolar tangent of the anterior ankle, from medial to lateral, one encounters the following in sequence:

1. Saphenous nerve
2. Saphenous vein
3. Tibialis anterior muscle tendon
4. Extensor hallucis longus muscle tendon
5. Anterior tibial artery and vein
6. Deep peroneal nerve
7. Common tendons of the extensor digitorum longus
8. Medial dorsal cutaneous nerve
9. Intermediate dorsal cutaneous nerve

From the lateral malleolar tangent, progressing around the ankle, the following soft tissue structures are encountered sequentially, from posterolateral to posteromedial:

1. Sural to lateral dorsal cutaneous nerve
2. Lesser saphenous vein
3. Peroneus brevis muscle tendon in common tendon sheath with longus
4. Peroneus longus muscle tendon in common tendon sheath with brevis
5. Terminus of peroneal artery (lateral calcaneal artery)
6. Achilles tendon with plantaris muscle tendon insertions
7. Flexor hallucis longus muscle and/or tendon
8. Posterior tibial nerve (or branches of medial and lateral plantar nerves)
9. Posterior tibial artery
10. Posterior tibial veins (venae commitantes)
11. Flexor digitorum longus muscle tendon
12. Tibialis posterior muscle tendon

We will now also review some gross articular anatomy of the lateral ankle joint. The ankle joint capsule is a thick, reinforced structure that, on its lateral extremity, demonstrates three ligaments, two of which are intrinsic, one extrinsic. The anterior and posterior talofibular ligaments (ATFL and PTFL) are intrinsic structures. That is to say, they are represented as thickenings within the ankle joint capsule that cannot be separated from the structure of the tunica externa, or fibrous capsule. The calcaneofibular (CFL) ligament is an extrinsic ligamentous structure that can be visibly separated from the ankle joint capsule. It is invested by the common peroneal tendon sheath in the midst of its span, and ultimately forms a calcaneal attachment that is dorsal and posterior to the peroneal tubercle.

Peculiarities of Arthroscopic Anatomy

Arthroscopy poses anatomic definitions that are peculiar to this surgical form. In the arthroscopic ankle joint, as viewed anteriorly, the following features are identified arthroscopically as normal anatomy (figure 30.1; features are shown left to right in the same order as the following list):

1. Medial gutter (medial malleolar-talar facet articulation)
2. Medial shoulder or medial bend of the talar dome
3. Dorsal tangential plane of the talar dome, medial aspect (talotibial articulation)
4. Median sagittal groove of the talar dome
5. Syndesmotic tibiofibular synovial fringe

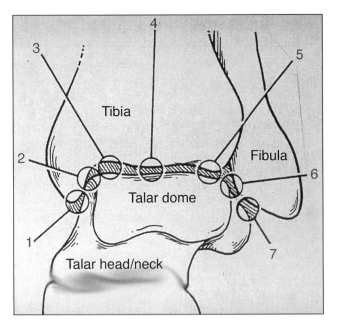

■ **Figure 30.1** Arthro-anatomic features of the arthroscopic ankle joint.

6. Lateral shoulder or lateral interval of the talar dome

7. Lateral gutter (area of visible transluscence of anterior talo-fibular ligament)

■ Mechanism of Injury

The most common mechanism of injury for lateral ankle sprains is forced plantarflexion with inversion. As the foot supinates, the orientation of tibia and fibula support moves away from an anterolateral quadrant of the ankle joint complex. This results in tension over the anterolateral capsule, wherein the anterior talofibular ligament is invested. As tension force increases beyond a soft tissue strain limit, the capsule tears. Once this tear begins, there is a "snap rebound" injury, which causes a circular rip to form. Tension forces on the joint capsule are quickly dispersed as the capsule angles forward and medially; however, tension forces acting laterally are accelerated by rebound as the foot is driven into greater amounts of inversion with lessening resistance of the lateral soft tissue complex. As these forces reach an apogee along the rip line, they start to dissipate. This dissipation is resisted by the extrinsic placement of the calcaneofibular ligament. If inversion ankle strain forces are substantial, the calcaneofibular ligament may also be torn, which causes a concomitant tear in the peroneal tendon sheath. In severe injuries, there may also be peroneal subluxation. During physi-

ologic healing, the intrinsic component of the anterior talofibular ligament may repair without integrity, forming a span of poorly organized, loose, collagenous fibers without proprioceptive elements. The resulting laxity sans perception lends to repeated episodes with similar movements of plantarflexion and inversion. As time goes on, the simple process of stepping down off a curb, or walking down stairs, can turn the ankle joint complex with progressively less resistance.

■ Operating Room Set-Up and Surgical Technique

Following is an overview of optimal operating room set-up and surgical technique.

Operating Room Set-Up

In performing an ALAS procedure, instrumentation must be carefully checked by the surgeon prior to making the first incision. Arthroscopic equipment is highly technical and often involves several different brand name manufacturers with interchangeable or noninterchangeable pieces. If the surgeon fails to do such a check—especially if working with a less experienced operating room team—he or she will often discover equipment incompatibilities only after the patient anatomy has already been violated by surgical intervention for portal placement (Brazytis & Hergenroeder 1992). The following checklist is recommended for completion by the surgeon prior to inflation of the tourniquet and/or first incision:

1. ☐ Video console power source is functional and compatible (i.e., U.S. 110-Hertz vs European 220-Hertz circuits).

2. ☐ Video console adapters are compatible with all connectors and cables.

3. ☐ Cathode ray tube (CRT) or television monitor is functional and online.

4. ☐ Fiber optic light cable is functional and compatible with arthroscopic connector. Operating room personnel are warned not to kink or sharply bend fiber optic cables. The surgeon should warn everyone in the operating room not to look directly into the light source, as it is potentially powerful enough to damage a retina.

5. ☐ If intended, any photographic imaging devices are on line with the power and video consoles. Circulating personnel in the room understand clearly how the imaging device works, and are capable of taking a picture at

the surgeon's direction from outside the sterile field.

6. ☐ The video connector mount for the arthroscope must be correctly oriented. Most manufactures have gone to the convention of placing a bend in the electrical cable connection as it comes out of the connector. This bend should be directed distally relative to the patient, or toward the toes. If the video connector is not oriented correctly, the image will be sterotactically incorrect. On the monitor screen, what is up may appear to be down, and what is left may appear to be right. A good way to check stereotaxis of the equipment is to place a small mark with a sterile skin marker on the medial palmar aspect of the proximal phalangeal portion of a gloved middle finger. Then, by placing gloved index and middle fingers together, an arthroscopic image of the dot will permit correct stereotactic confirmation.

7. ☐ The angle of the arthroscope is oriented to video and fluid line connections. For example, most 4.0-mm arthroscopes are optimally angled at 30°. This permits rotation of the scope to extend a field of view diameter by up to 100%. Most 2.7-mm scopes only support a 15° angle, which extends the field of view diameter up to 50% via rotation. Occasionally, a 70° angled 4.0-mm scope has been found to be useful for visualization down into the lateral gutter. These 70° scopes produce central blind spots when rotated and do not actually extend a field of view. They are only useful for acute angle viewing. Normally, the angle will be directed downward as the arthroscope is first inserted into the joint. This permits visualization of the dome and anterior mortise as a landmark anatomy encounter.

8. ☐ Whatever ingress fluid system is to be used should be checked. This may be either a gravity system or a pressure pump system. Make certain that cannula connectors are compatible and there is a quick valve for turning the flow on or off. Also, ensure that backup fluid reservoirs are in the room and available should the primary reservoir run dry.

9. ☐ Make certain that all arthroscopes, cannulas, obturators, and trochars are compatible. In the event that more than one size scope is to be used during the procedure (i.e., 4.0 plus 2.7 mm), assure that video and light source

cables as well as fluid lines are interchangeable.

10. ☐ Most arthroscopic procedures will require use of a power shaver handpiece with vacuum. Although several different shavers are available, at least two will be required for arthroscopic ankle stabilization. One should be a synovial shaver, such as a 3.5-mm full-radius shaver. The other must be an abrader, such as a 4.0-mm ball abrader. Both should be interchangeable with the same shaver power console and cable. Handpieces for this instrumentation normally have an irregular lane on at least one side of an otherwise circular surface. When inserting disposable shaver stems on the handpiece, it is best to orient the distal open face of either full-radius cutter or abrader stems opposite this irregular surface, so that the surgeon can orient movement within the joint from a known plane of reference outside of the joint. A scaled vacuum control knob or switch should be easily accessible and the vacuum system should be checked for proper function.

In addition to primary arthroscopic instrumentation, secondary arthroscopic instrumentation should be available. This includes nonpowered hand instruments, such as probes, microtomes, rasps, scissors, ring instruments, basket cutters, bucket cutters, graspers, and jaw cutters. Finally, some form of anchoring system must be available. This can take the form of either small staples, such as the Acuflex 5.5-mm arthroscopic staple set, or bone anchors, such as the Mitek G-2 system.

A number of distraction systems are commercially available for ankle joint arthroscopy. These include both invasive as well as noninvasive systems. Ankle joint distraction systems *should not* be used for lateral ankle stabilization procedures. They place stress and strain on ligamentous and capsular structures. Mechanical distracters will resist a tight appositional repair of lateral ligaments. All essential structures for this procedure can be easily viewed via manual manipulation of the ankle without any mechanical joint distraction adjunct.

Surgical Technique

Anesthesia for this procedure may be either general or monitored anesthesia control (MAC) with combined IV sedation and local anesthesia. In the event MAC is used, tourniquet use is limited to the lower leg. A tourniquet is quite useful in field visualization during the procedure. The leg should be prepped and positioned in accordance with normal ankle arthroscopic processes. It is quite useful to use a fluid collection drape system in order to limit spillage onto the operating room floor. The joint should be insufflated with approximately 20 cc of lactated Ringer's or normal saline. Local anesthetic is also acceptable for this purpose, so long as the accumulation does not exceed guidelines regarding the toxic dose for peripheral compartment. After insufflation, a medial portal is formed at the joint line, directly medial and parallel to the tibialis anterior where it crosses the ankle. This is a relatively safe portal, as the nearest vital structures are the saphenous vein and nerve, which are normally separated by a distance of about 15 mm posterior and medial to the tibialis anterior.

Unlike the knee, which can easily be entered using an 11 blade, the ankle joint should only be perforated with careful, layered dissection. Using a 15 blade, a 1-cm incision is made in the outer skin, centered over the insufflation injection site. This incision should only be deep enough to penetrate to the bottom of the dermis. A curved mosquito hemostat is then used to bluntly dissect and retract down to capsule. At that point, a trocar and cannula are used to lightly puncture the tunica externa. The trocar is then removed from the sleeved cannula and replaced with a blunt obturator. Sharp trocars should never be used to enter the joint, as they pose considerable potential for scoring articular cartilage. Once the obturator has pierced the tunica intima and is clearly protruded into the joint, it should be removed from within the cannula. If the joint has been successfully entered, there will be a fluid return from the cannula after removal of the obturator. Anticipating this, the surgeon should be prepared to place a fingertip or thumbtip over the cannula lumen to prevent complete extravasation of the joint. The arthroscope can then be placed into the cannula and used to obtain a quick look at the joint. Without an egress, there will be backflow stasis from fluid ingress through the cannula. Therefore, the view

may not be ideal, particularly if there is considerable synovial hypertrophy (figure 30.2).

Using the arthroscope within the first portal for transillumination, additional portals may be placed anterocentrally, through the conjoined tendon of the extensor digitorum brevis, and/or anterolaterally. Particular care should be taken on the lateral portal to avoid contact with either medial or intermediate dorsal cutaneous nerves. These represent purely sensory branches of the musculocutaneous or superficial peroneal nerve. In the event they are cut, nicked, or impinged by scar tissue, they pose the potential to cause postoperative sensory problems. As soon as a second portal is placed, egress will considerably improve the visual field, and a thorough examination of the joint complex can be conducted. Frequently, lateral ankle instabilities will be associated with other forms of intra-articular pathologies, such as hypertrophic synovitis and/or osteochondral injury, which are easily addressed by arthroscopic intervention at this point.

It will be necessary to use the full-radius power shaver to clear out excessive hypertrophic synovium (figure 30.3). Villinodular synovitis will be increasingly apparent as the lateral gutter is approached (figure 30.4). This is an intimal articular capsular response to the chronic nature of lateral ankle instability. As the field becomes clearer, it will be possible to visualize the ATFL as a reflected structure through the tunica interna.

Once the lateral gutter has been adequately evacuated to visualize the lateral talar facet (figure 30.5), another portal should be placed on the lateral aspect of the ankle joint, almost directly over the ATFL. Again, the arthroscope can be used for transillumination to greatly facilitate this process. Using the lateral portal, the power shaver stem can then be inserted into an area directly over the lateral talar facet, as visualized from the arthroscope inserted through the

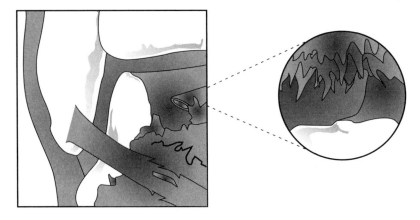

■ **Figure 30.2** Initial visualization of lateral gutter with hypertrophic synovium.
Adapted from Lundeen 1992.

anterocentral portal and placed from directly dorsal, with the scope now viewing down into the lateral gutter (figure 30.6). The full radius shaver on the power synovial shaver handpiece should at this point be replaced by a sleeved ball burr abrader. The abrader will then be used to disarticulate an oval area of about 6 × 8 mm in oval diameter, located about 10 mm distal to the fibular malleolar articular surface with the foot held in neutral position at 90° to the leg. This abrasion should be carried out down to bleeding bone (figure 30.7). Thereafter, it is often helpful to use the 3.5 full-radius synovial resector to smooth down the edges of the ligamentodesis crater that has been formed by the abrader (figures 30.8 and 30.9).

After forming this crater, a ligamentodesis should be performed using either staple or bone anchor. In the case of a staple, the staple should be placed in such a way as to catch the ATFL between the tangs of the staple (figure 30.10). The ligament and associated capsule should then be twisted, as when tuning a guitar string, while holding the rearfoot everted and maintaining the foot at 90° to the leg (figure 30.11). This will result in a "tweaking" or tightening of capsule and remnant intrinsic ligament over the anterior talofibular area. As the staple is driven, care must be taken to make it tight and drive it deep enough, but not to permit the body of the staple, where the tangs come together, to cut through bunched fibrous capsule and ligament.

In the event the surgeon chooses to use a bone anchor instead of a staple, one of two systems may be employed. The traditional method called for two bone anchors into the talus, one anterosuperior and the other posteroinferior to the crater (figure 30.12). After insertion of the bone anchors, with allowance of a 10-second lag time for setting of each anchor, 2-0 Ethibond monofilament suture is tied over capsule and ATFL, binding capsular soft tissue down into the ligamentodesis crater site. A second method is to place one bone anchor into the talus and a second into the fibula, tying the two ends together directly over the ATFL in order to, again, bind the substance of the anterolateral ankle joint capsular complex down onto the ligamentodesis crater site.

Closing the Portals

After securing capsules and ligament over the ligamentodesis crater, the ankle joint should be flushed with a mix of 5 cc bupivicaine with epinephrine and 1 cc dexamethasone phosphate. A short-acting phosphated corticosteroid resists synovial inflammation, and should prevent recurrence of synovial hypertrophy.

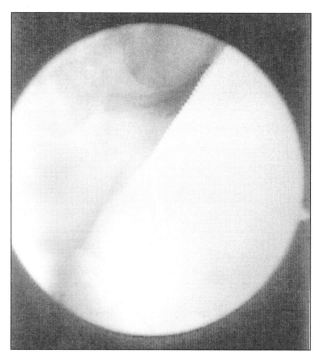

■ **Figure 30.3** Initial visualization of lateral gutter with hypertrophic synovium.

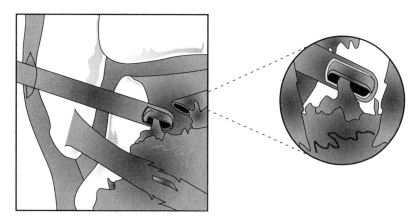

■ **Figure 30.4** Arthroscopic synovectomy for lateral gutter visualization.
Adapted from Lundeen 1992.

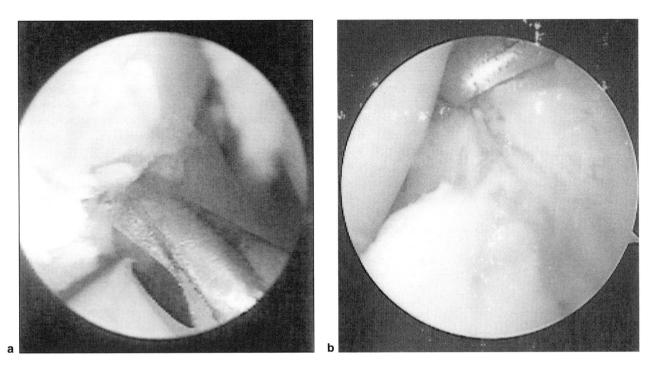

■ **Figure 30.5** *(a)* Examples of inflamed synovial villa. *(b)* Progress of shaving out villinodular protrusions into the lateral gutter.

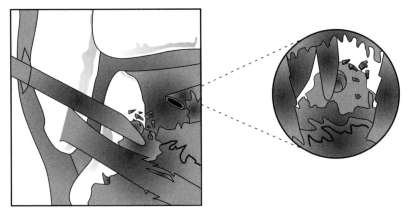

■ **Figure 30.6** Power shaver stem inserted into an area directly over the lateral talar facet.
Adapted from Lundeen 1992,

It is important not to use acetated or longer-acting corticosteroids, which carry a remote risk of avascular necrosis. In addition, some arthroscopists add to the mix 1 cc (10 mg) of Duromorph or Astromorph, morphine derivatives that bind to endomorphic joint complex receptors and extend reduction of postoperative pain. Each of the portal sites are then closed in sequence with one or two simple interrupted prolene sutures. No deep approximation is indicated. The anterolateral ankle joint portal should not be sutured, but should be approximated dorsally with a steri-strip. This leaves a site of egress for any bleeding that follows dropping of the tourniquet. The patient should be placed in a posterior splint with the foot maintained at 90° to the leg, incorporated into a Jones compressive dressing.

Postoperative Treatment

Passive range of motion should be started in a constant passive motion (CPM) device around 48-72 hours postoperatively. On the first day of CPM, no more than 2 hours is recommended, with a maximum range of dorsiflexion to perpendicular and maximum range of plantarflexion to 10°. The foot should always be maintained in a slightly everted position while in this device. CPM should be increased over a 3-4 week period until the patient is spending 6 hours with 10° of dorsiflexion (knee extended) and 45-60° of plantarflexion. The patient should be kept absolutely nonweightbearing on crutches for 4 weeks, progressing through touchdown weight bearing to partial weight bearing to full weight bearing between 4 and

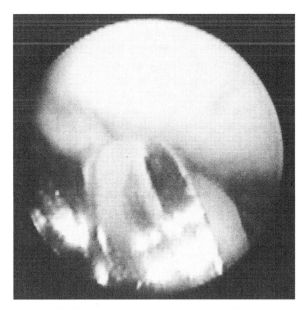

Figure 30.7 Abrasion carried out down to bleeding bone.

6 weeks postoperatively. Sutures are pulled at 10-14 days postoperatively, and the patient should be encouraged to elevate the extremity when not ambulating with crutches. At 6 weeks postoperatively, an anterior drawer test should be attempted. There should be visible evidence of lateral ankle integrity. From there, the patient should be graduated back into normal activity while being encouraged to wear an ankle brace during aggressive activities (e.g., basketball, tennis, etc.) for at least 3 months thereafter. For a more detailed discussion of postoperative rehabilitation, see chapters 22, 23, 24, and 31.

■ Experience and Follow-Up

Follow-up in our series is based on both reviews of previous studies as well as ongoing monitoring of patient outcomes within our own facilities.

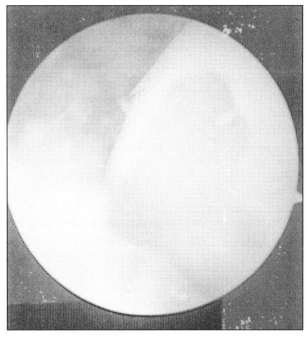

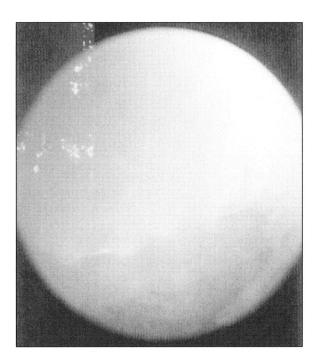

Figures 30.8 and 30.9 Smoothing down the edges of the ligamentodesis crater that has been formed by the abrader.

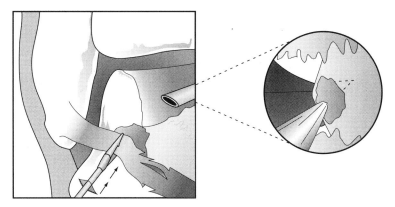

Figure 30.10 Catching the ATFL between the tangs of the staple.

Adapted from Lundeen 1992.

Follow-Up

In terms of extended follow-up, Hawkins (1987, 1988) reported on 25 consecutive procedures in 24 patients performed between 1983 and 1987. Of this group, one patient had recurrence of lateral ankle instability after recovery of ALAS, resulting from the same activity that produced the initial injury. After this, the patient had several additional recurrences. The balance of 24 patients were reported to be quite satisfied with their outcome, although several of those who received staple procedures required secondary procedures for removal because the staple position interfered with ankle joint motion.

In our own 8-year ongoing study (1993-2001), we have followed 32 patients, of whom all but 7 had staples. To date, all of these patients are subjectively

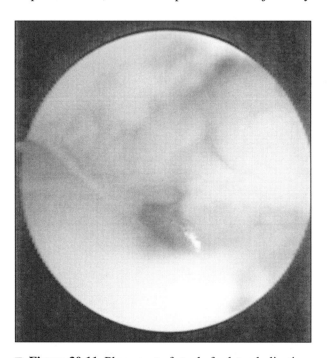

■ **Figure 30.11** Placement of staple for lateral plication.

satisfied with their outcomes. One patient developed a recurrence of anterior drawer sign in objective postoperative testing, although this was less apparent than preoperatively. Radiographs of this patient suggest that the staple was driven too deep and probably cut through the capsular/ligament complex during placement. However, the patient was satisfied with the outcome. Patient selection has played a large part in limiting the total number of procedures. We have not performed any ALAS procedures in stabilizations that demonstrated >15° or <10° difference in preoperative talar tilt radiograph stress inversion films. All patients had a history of repetitive ankle injuries and were symptomatic, with at least 3 months of continuing symptoms, despite use of ankle bracing and muscle strengthening.

Outcome Comparisons

In comparing outcomes between ALAS and traditional lateral ankle stabilization (LAS) procedures, we have contrasted outcomes between 14 ALAS and 36 open LAS procedures performed during the same period. Among the open LAS procedure set were included about eight patients who would fit the criterion (>10°, <15°) for ALAS. The balance were >15°, but were reported for technical comparatives. Total open LAS procedures included Chrisman-Snook (Chrisman & Snook 1969), Evans (Evans 1953), Broström (Broström 1966), and Williams (Williams 1988) procedures. Generally speaking, advantages and disadvantages of each procedure are shown in table 30.1. ALAS involves much less soft tissue dissection and therefore offers a decided advantage when comparing soft tissue surgical injury produced by the various procedures. Visualization of the essential components in ALAS procedures is adequate, but cannot be compared with the amount of visualization possible in open procedures. Because it leads to less soft tissue injury, ALAS procedure recuperation time

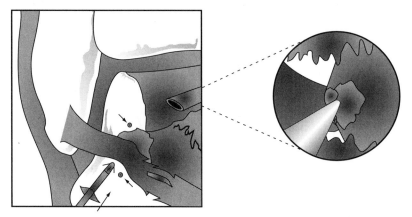

■ **Figure 30.12** Insertion of bone anchors into the talus.
Adapted from Lundeen 1992.

Table 30.1 Weighing of Advantage Between Arthroscopic Lateral Ankle Stabilization Versus Open Lateral Ankle Stabilization Techniques

	ALAS	Open LAS
Soft tissue dissection	++++	+
Visualization	++	++++
Recuperation	++++	+++
Recurrence	+++	++++
Complications	++++	++
Surgical technique	+++	+++

is generally considered to be less than that for open LAS. Potential for recurrence is theoretically greater in the ALAS procedure, although this has not been demonstrated in our exclusionary patient population set. Complications after surgery are notably less in the ALAS set. Technique is equally challenging in both methodologies, and in the author's opinion, neither methodology effectively outweighs the other.

Dealing With Complications

Complications of the ALAS technique are common to those that accompany any arthroscopic procedure. Infection in any large joint of the body is potentially catastrophic. Prophylactic antibiotics may be routinely administered in any procedure that involves placement of an implant, such as a staple or bone anchor. (Oishi et al. 1993). For example, the protocol for Cefazolin suggests 1 gram preoperatively, one gram intraoperatively, and one gram postoperatively. If a postoperative infection seems to be developing, early aggressive intervention with intravenous antibiotics in a hospital setting can often avoid more serious consequences. Should the infection linger, or if intervention is delayed, then standard protocols should be followed. These include opening (or expanding as necessary) the incision sites, as well as removal of any indwelling hardware.

Nerve damage carries perhaps the highest index of complication after ankle joint arthroscopies. The Guhl study (Guhl 1993), which covered progressive development of ankle arthroscopic techniques from 1974 through 1992, found that of 350 ankle joint arthroscopies, 11.1% reported complications ranging from minor to severe. Nerve damage accounted for the majority of reported complications from ankle joint arthroscopy (approximately 49%). Damage to the sensory cutaneous nerves (medial and intermediate dorsal cutaneous nerves) posed the highest potential for patient dissatisfaction with subjective outcomes. Careful, layered, lateral portal placement with

transillumination remains the best method of avoiding this problem.

Vascular injury to the anterior tibial artery or perforating branch of the peroneal artery is documented. Either of these incidents may cause a hemarthrosis, which can cause problems. Problems can include an increased risk of infection, hypertrophy of synovial membranes, and transient changes in the viscosity of normal synovial fluid. Perhaps the best way to avoid these problems is to maintain good visualization of all cutting instruments (i.e., power shaver and hand instruments) when cutting any tissue. The most common cause of injury to the anterior tibial artery is nicking by power shaver activation while the artery is not on the visible field. The most common cause of injury to the perforating branch is placement of the lateral portal under tourniquet without transillumination.

In addition to infection and neurovascular injury, other general arthroscopic complications reported in the series included traumas from distraction devices, granuloma, deep venous thrombosis, sinus formation, and stress fractures, although none except for trauma from distraction devices were associated specifically with complications from arthroscopic lateral ankle stabilization procedures.

■ Summary

In 1997, Ogilvie, Gilbart and Chorney reported on exactly 100 patients treated arthroscopically for symptoms of chronic ankle pain associated with sprains of the ankle. They found that limited arthroscopic intervention (without traditional open lateral ankle stabilization) demonstrated poor outcomes when contrasted with those who had osteochondral injures with stable ankles. They did not include arthroscopic lateral ankle stabilization as a factor in their study. Komenda and Ferkel reported in 1999 on the outcomes of 54 patients with chronic lateral ankle instability who were examined arthroscopically prior to traditional open surgical repair. They found a 25% incidence of associated osteochondral talar dome injuries along with a much higher incidence of hypertorphic synovitis, osteophytic formation, adhesions, and loose bodies. Komenda et al. contrasted their own findings with the 1993 study reported by Taga et al., who found an incidence of chondral injuries approaching 95% in ankles examined arthroscopically prior to open lateral ankle stabilization within a range of 31 patients. Sijbrandij et al. found an 18% incidence of chondral injuries on MRI's of patients with chronic lateral ankle instability occurring in their study reported December of 2000, surveying a range of 146 MRI ankle films.

Due to an increasingly reported prevalence of an association between lateral ankle instability with chronic ankle pain and associated intraarticular lesions amenable to arthroscopic intervention, it is likely that associated arthroscopy of the ankle will become a more common adjunct in the treatment of lateral ankle instability. While it certainly is not necessary to perform an arthroscopic stabilization procedure in conjunction with arthroscopic exploration of an ankle subject to chronic instability, the advantages of surgical intervention limited to arthroscopy are obvious. If the apparent trend will lead to examination of all lateral ankle instabilities arthroscopically, it is likely that there will be an associated trend toward arthroscopic stabilization in favor of combined arthroscopic/open surgical intervention combinations.

ALAS procedures offer an excellent option to the surgical armamentarium of foot and ankle surgeons, particularly those dealing with common sports injuries and chronic lateral ankle pain. There are now more than 20 years of follow-up available on the ALAS with adequate documentary confirmation of reliable outcomes. ALAS procedures generally demonstrate great advantages over traditional open lateral ankle stabilization procedures within selected patient populations when performed using proper instrumentation in the hands of a competent surgical team.

■ References

Bassewitz HL, Shapiro MS. 1997. Persistent pain after ankle sprain: targeting the causes. Phys Sportsmed 25(12):58-68.

Brazytis KI, Hergenroeder PT. 1992. Arthroscopic ankle surgery. Overcoming anatomic difficulties with improved techniques. AORN J 55(2):492-502.

Broström L. 1966. Sprained VI surgical treatment of "chronic" ligament ruptures. Acta Chir Scand 132:551.

Chrisman OD, Snook GA. 1969. Reconstruction of lateral ligament tears of the ankle. J Bone Joint Surg Am 51(5):904-912.

Evans DL. 1953. Recurrent instability of the ankle: a method of surgical treatment. Proc R Soc Lond 446:333.

Ferkel RD, Fischer SP. 1989. Progress in ankle arthroscopy. Clin Orthop (240):210-220.

Garrick JM. 1977. The frequency of injury, mechanism of injury, and epidemiology of ankle sprains. Am J Sports Med 5(6):241-242.

Glick J, Morgan C, Meyerson M. 1990. Arthroscopic ankle arthrodesis. Arthroscopic Association of North Carolina, Orlando, Florida, April 1990.

Guhl JF (Ed.). 1993. Foot and ankle arthroscopy, 2nd ed. Thorofare, NJ: SLACK.

Hawkins RB. 1987. Arthroscopic stapling repair for chronic lateral instability. Clin Podiatr Med Surg 4(4):875-883.

Hawkins RB. 1988. Stapling repair for chronic lateral ankle instability. In: Ankle arthroscopy: pathology and surgical techniques, Guhl JF, editor. Thorofare, NJ: SLACK.

Kannus P, Renström P. 1991. Treatment of acute tears of the lateral ligaments of the ankle: operation, cast or early controlled mobilization. J Bone Joint Surg Am 73(2):305-312.

Komenda GA, Ferkel RD. 1999. Arthroscopic findings associated with the unstable ankle. Foot Ankle Int 201(11):708-713.

Lassiter TE, Malone TR, Garrett WE. 1989. Injury to the lateral ligaments of the ankle. Orthop Clin North Am 20(4):629-640.

Lundeen GW. 1987. Historical perspectives of ankle arthroscopy. J Foot Surg 26(1):3-7.

Lundeen RO. 1985. Arthroscopic lateral ankle stabilization. J Am Podiatr Assoc 75(7):372-376.

Lundeen, RO. 1992. Manual of ankle and foot arthroscopy. NY: Churchill Livingstone.

Lundeen et al. 1983. Indiana Arthroscopy Associates. 1983. Personal communication.

Marder RA. 1995. Current methods for the evaluation of ankle ligament injuries. Instr Course Lect 44:349-357.

McMaster PE. 1943. Treatment of ankle sprain: observations of more than five hundred cases. JAMA 122(10):

Ogilvie-Harris DJ, Gilbart MK, Chorney K. 1997. Chronic pain following ankle sprains in athletes: the role of arthroscopic surgery. Arthroscopy 13(5):564-574.

Oishi CS, Carrion WV, Hoaglund FT. 1993. Use of parenteral antibiotics in clean orthopaedic surgery. A review of the literature [review]. Clin Orthop 296: 249-255.

Reichen A, Marti R. 1974. Rupture of the fibular collateral ligaments: diagnosis, surgical treatment, results [in German]. Arch Orthop Unfallchir 80(3):211-222.

Rubin G, Witten M. 1960. The talar-tilt angle and the fibular collateral ligaments: A method for determination of talar tilt. J Bone Joint Surg Am 42(2).

Sijbrandij ES, van Gils AP, Louwerens JW, de Lange EE. 2000. Posttraumatic subchondral bone contusions and fractures of the talotibial joint: occurrence of "kissing lesions." AJR Am J Roentgenol 175(6):1707-1710.

Taga I, Shino K, Inoue, M, Nakata K. Maeda A. 1998. Articular cartilage lesions in ankles with lateral ligament injury: an arthroscopic study. Am J Sports Med 21(1):120-126.

van Dijk CN, Scholte D. 1997. Arthroscopy of the ankle joint. Arthroscopy 13(1):90-96.

Williams JG. 1988. Plication of the anterolateral capsule of the ankle with extensor digitorum brevis transfer for chronic lateral ligament instability. Injury 19(2):65-69.

Chapter 31

Arthroscopy for the Injured Ankle

Wolf-Ruediger Dingels, MD, PhD

Ankle joint arthroscopy was ignored for a long time after it was first described in 1939 because the narrow joint space was impossible to inspect with the equipment then used (Takagi 1939). Now, improved and better-scaled optics allow the joint space to be viewed adequately.

■ Acute Arthroscopy

The joint can be viewed quite well with acute arthroscopy, especially after a rupture of ligamentous structures. A joint distraction can be carried out up to 8 mm with a 90-130 N force without neurovascular or ligamentous damage (Albert et al. 1992). The addi-

tional development of intra- and transmalleolar portals allows improved inspection of the joint.

Techniques

Normally, the anterior portals are sufficient to perform most of interventions in ankle surgery. External distraction has improved the arthroscopic possibilities in this joint and should be applied as a matter of routine. A sufficient distraction can also take place with stable ligaments and the aid of an assistant or a brace that does not obstruct the surgical field (figure 31.1). If it is carefully manipulated, a normal elevator can be used without complications for distraction from within the joint (Hempfling and Putz 1998).

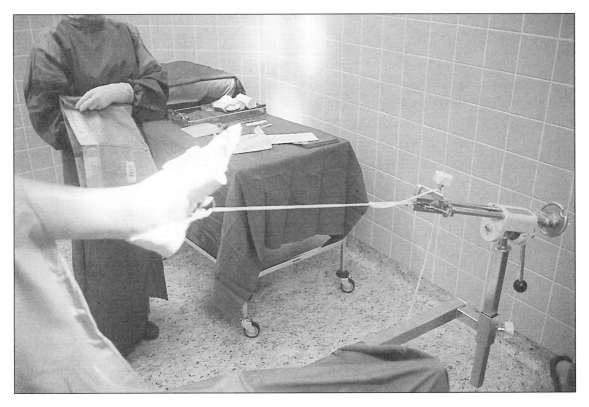

■ **Figure 31.1** Noninvasive distraction of the ankle joint with a prefabricated brace.

Arthroscopy for the Acutely Injured

Because of swelling and hematoma, the usual outline of the ankle is often obscured and the landmarks cannot be recognized, increasing the risk of injuring the dorsalis pedis artery or the superficial peroneal nerve (Sayli et al. 1998; Grechening et al. 1997). Thus it is advisable not to inflate the tourniquet during the diagnostic phase to help avoid injury to the dorsalis pedis artery and to the saphenous vein.

The patient is positioned on a knee holder in approximately 90° knee flexion. The heel can be propped up onto the operating table or the foot can be pulled beside the table for a better distraction. It is important to puncture the joint with a needle before introducing the blunt trocar. For preparation of the puncture hole, make sure that the scalpel is held vertically and only the subcutaneous tissue is incised. It is recommended to enlarge the subcutaneous tissue

bluntly with a Péan's forceps and thus penetrate the synovial membrane. This will, in most cases, prevent postoperative hemarthrosis (figure 31.2, a and b).

All arthroscopies are carried out with the conventional 5-mm arthroscope. Usually, a 30° optic is sufficient. Under sight, after rinsing out the hematoma and imaging the joint parts (figure 31.3), additional medial incisions for surgical instruments can be made. At this phase, the tourniquet can be inflated, or the procedure may continue under constant fluid pressure applied by an arthroscopy pump.

Arthroscopic Evaluation and Treatment

After removing the hemarthroses, the joint can be systematically examined. If the anterior talofibular ligament is torn (figure 31.4), the ligament stump

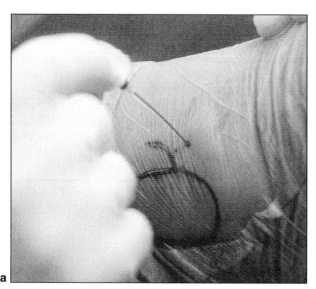

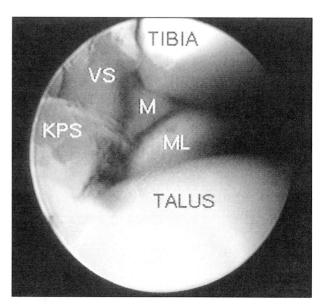

■ **Figure 31.3** Lateral part of ankle joint.

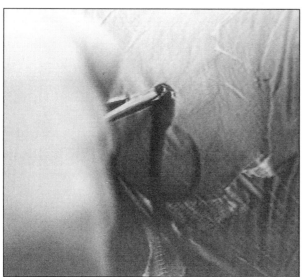

■ **Figure 31.2** (*a*) Tapping the joint with needle. (*b*) Spreading the portal to avoid nerve damage.

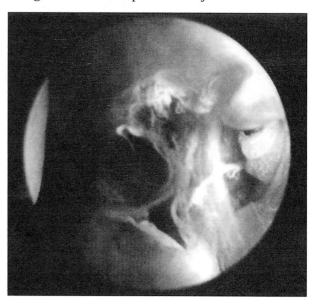

■ **Figure 31.4** Tear of the anterior talofibular ligament.

should be cleaned and sutured through the arthroscope. Torn and impinged synovial tissue and capsule fragments (figure 31.5, a and b) are resected with the aid of a punch or shaver. Cartilage lesions on the tibial edge or on the talus are inspected to determine whether they can be refixed using biodegradable pins. If they are not repairable they should be excised (figure 31.6, a and b). In superficial osteochondral lesions, the cartilage fragments are removed and the edges are smoothed (figure 31.7). In a disruption of the syndesmosis and diastasis, arthroscopically assisted repositioning will be performed and a percutaneous fixation screw inserted (figure 31.8, a-c).

Partial ruptures of the calcaneofibular ligament in its anterior part (figure 31.9) may also be approximated and refixed with a percutaneous suture.

Postoperative Course

Operative ankle arthroscopy in younger patients and athletes is performed as an outpatient procedure. In the immediate postoperative period, the patient begins active assisted range-of-motion exercises and resistive exercises. Weight bearing is protected, however, until full range of motion has returned. In this phase of treatment, the ankle is

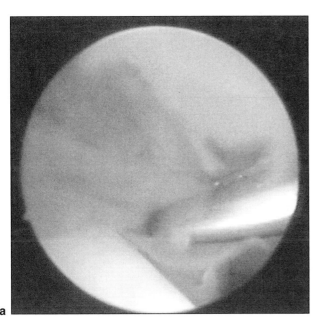
a

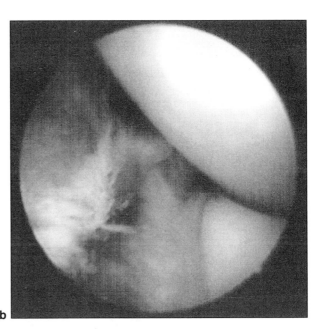
b

■ **Figure 31.5** (*a*) Impingement due to a sprained ankle. (*b*) Impingement of a torn lateral ligament.

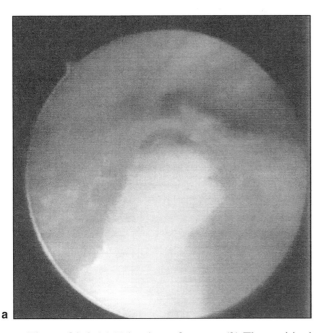
a

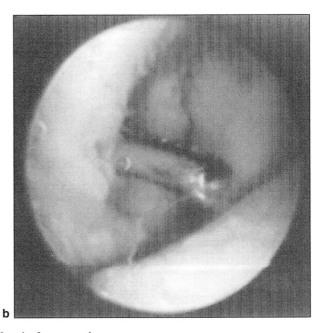
b

■ **Figure 31.6** (*a*) Talar dome fracture. (*b*) The positioning of a pin for reattachment.

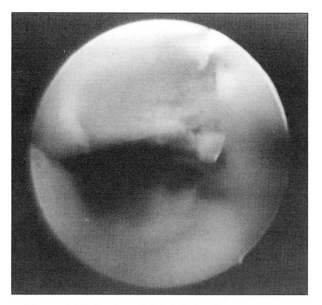

■ **Figure 31.7** Lesion of tibial plafond.

bandaged or supported by a walking brace. That can be changed later to a training brace, which is quite comfortable and will fit inside footwear. The patient may then begin unprotected weight bearing, depending on the status of the articular surface. Patients are allowed to progress in their rehabilitation program after they achieve full range of motion and return of strength without pain or swelling.

Complications

Complication rates associated with ankle arthroscopy range from 10% to 15% (Martin 1989). These complications include sensory disturbances from either temporary or permanent damage to the sensory cutaneous nerve on the lateral aspect of the ankle. Pressure of the hemarthrosis or the edema of the tissues can also cause complications. Several measures should be

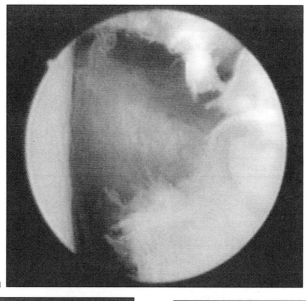

a

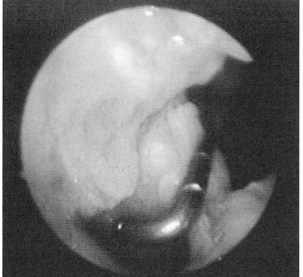

b

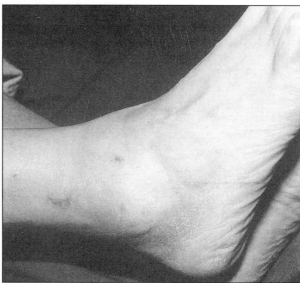

c

■ **Figure 31.8** (*a*) Rupture of distal tibiofibular. (*b*) Reposition of tibiofibular disaster. (*c*) Skin after transarthroscopic surgery.

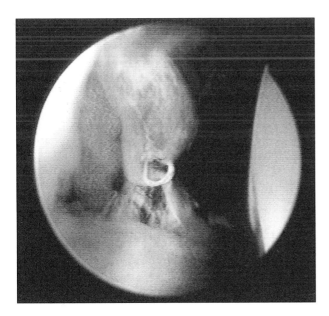

■ **Figure 31.9** Refixation of anterior talofibular ligament.

taken at the completion of the procedure to avoid these problems. The tourniquet should be deflated to ensure that hemostasis is achieved, and a padded pressure bandage should be applied after the arthroscopy.

■ Arthroscopy for Complications of Chronic Ankle Sprain

Severe sprains with hematoma or osteosynthesis after a fracture of the malleoli with deep scars of the soft tissues result in restriction of motion and stiffness. Isolated scars of soft tissues can be caught in the articular surface and result in an impingement syndrome. Articular destruction is often caused by posttraumatic conditions or primary arthrosis.

Arthroscopy for Chronic Lateral Instability

In 30% of patients, injury of the ankle joint leads to chronic lateral pain with a tendency toward repeated swelling and difficulties in sports or everyday activities. A history of insecurity, instability, and giving way along with clinical examination showing instability are vital for the diagnosis (Mann et al. 1994).

Radiographic examination for exclusion of abnormalities and osteochondritis dissecans, as well as subluxation, is prompted by the symptoms of an unstable joint. Forty percent of patients with symptoms of unstable ankles do, in fact, have one or more of these conditions. Therefore, all patients with such symptoms should be x-rayed to exclude the conditions previously mentioned (Mann et al.

1994). Pain and giving way alone are not unambiguous proof of instability. The studies of Freeman (1965) show that some of those people with symptoms of an unstable ankle in fact have only proprioceptive deficits that can be addressed with therapy rather than by surgical means of treatment.

General Considerations

Here are the targets, methods, indications, and contraindications for surgical correction of chronic ankle instability:

■ **Targets and methods:** Indications for surgical correction of chronic ankle instability are numerous. Surgery should only take place if conservative measures have failed. Most peroneus operations are based on tenodesis with part or all of the peroneus brevis tendon or the peroneus longus tendon. Other procedures utilize the Achilles tendon, plantar tendon, or fascia lata. In Europe, the periosteal flap is equivalent to the other procedures. All procedures involve damaging noninjured tissues and sacrificing noninjured tendons to repair the damaged ones. If an extensively preserved capsula or substantial fragments of the lateral ligament complex are present, an attempt should be made to repair them directly in the hope of restoring proprioceptive capacities. When the lateral ligament and capsule apparatus are badly or completely scarred, the periost of the distal lateral malleolus formed to a split Y-flap still seems to be an appropriate procedure. Editors remark: As discussed elsewhere in this book, it seems that most of these procedures are being replaced by the "anatomic" procedures, such as the Williams, Broström, or Mann procedures.

■ **Indications:** An absolute indication for operation does not exist. The indication is always relative with the aim of improving function.

■ **Contraindications:** I consider advanced arthrotic changes (especially at an advanced age) to be strongly contraindicative. In these cases, those involved must think carefully about the usefulness of an arthrodesis.

■ **Special preparations:** Special preparations are not necessary. A chisel for deperiostation is necessary.

Operative Risks and Patient Information

Patients must be made aware of the risks of any proposed operation.

■ **Intraoperative risks:** Intraoperative risks do not exist. The periosteal flap is to be prepared carefully with a sufficient attachment to the bone. A fixation with the aid of periosteal sutures is preferred because screw fixation or staples may destroy the fine rudiments of proprioception and fine motor control.

■ **Patient information:** The conversation should be focused on possible injuries of nerves, vessels, and tendons.

Arthroscopy for Revision of Scars, Capsula Ligament Reconstruction, Periosteal Flaps

The operation can be carried out in spinal anesthesia or femuropopliteal block. A tourniquet is advantageous. Prior to any stabilizing operation, a joint arthroscopy should take place to exclude further joint pathologies.

With a 3- to 4-cm longitudinal incision over the lateral malleolus (to avoid disturbance of the lymphatic paths), the lateral ligament complex can be viewed, and it can then be decided if a reconstruction of the capsule ligament apparatus can be applied or if a periosteal flap is necessary. Before finishing the operation, it is necessary to open the tourniquet for thorough hemostasis. Subsequently, if there is any delayed wound-healing, functional treatment should be postponed. For mobilization, an aircast walking brace can be applied.

Arthroscopy for Loss of Motion and Arthrodesis

Loss of motion and arthrodesis are results of distortion trauma with hemorrhage into the joint or of ankle joint osteosynthesis and postoperative scar development resulting in a fibrous alkalosis that may impede joint function. Localized scar and soft tissue impingements after distortion as well as lateral capsula ligament injuries may lead to a lateral soft tissue impingement syndrome.

General Considerations

Here are important points to think about as you consider how to correct loss of mobility:

■ **Targets and methods:** Function-improving operations include debridement of soft tissue in the upper ankle joint through arthroscopy. Resection of impinging tissue may lead to acceptable results if arthritic changes are not present. A minimally invasive operation technique with a well-aimed functional treatment is crucial.

■ **Indications:** An absolute indication for operation does not exist. The indication is always of a relative nature with the aim of improving function.

■ **Contraindications:** I consider a very advanced and terminal arthrotic stage of the ankle joint with much pain—especially at older age—to be a contraindication to attempting to restore normal function. In these cases, indication for the arthrodesis of the ankle joint must be discussed.

■ **Special preparation:** Special preparations are not necessary. Suitable resection instruments, as well as an internal distracter, are sufficient.

Operative Risks and Patient Information

Patients must be made aware of the risks of any proposed operation.

■ **Intraoperative risks:** Because of poor visibility in extensive scar development, there is some danger that the surgeon could stray from the articular surface with his or her resecting instruments, possibly damaging the nerves, tendons, and vessels that pass close to the joint.

■ **Patient information:** The discussion should concentrate on injuries of nerves, tendons, and vessels and must additionally point out that an improvement of function is not guaranteed.

Techniques

The operation can be carried out with spinal anesthesia. The anterior portals, with an anterolateral and anteromedial access, are sufficient. The dissection of the inner articular surface occurs according to the technique mentioned previously.

Because of adhesions, it may be that the inner articular surface cannot be clearly seen. In this case, changing to open synovectomy is preferred over blind resection attempts. At the end of the operation, the joint is washed out, a drain is left in the joint, and the tourniquet is released. A bulky elastic bandage and an immobilization plaster cast for 2 to 3 days are advisable.

During the period of immobilization, antithrombotic treatment should be considered.

Arthroscopy for Damage to Cartilage

Joint destruction may develop after trauma as primary arthrosis, or as a result of osseous changes at the anterior margin of the tibia.

General Considerations

Relatively minor alterations in bone quality may result in dysfunction and injury of cartilage. The etiology of cartilage lesions—aside from post-traumatic lesions—may include an endocrinologic cause, osteomalacia, or metabolic bone disease, especially in elderly people. Therefore, optimal treatment is not based only on surgical interventions but also on routine diagnostic laboratory tests.

■ **Targets and methods:** If irreparable damage of the articular surface is present and extensive functional disturbances exist, as well as severe pain, joint debridement, and, in other rare cases, arthrodesis should be considered. It depends on the grade of severity of the cartilage damage and the consequent joint destruction. Besides the noninvasive diagnostic measures, the next step is arthroscopy in the upper ankle joint to clear the joint situation with the aim (in addition to diagnosis) of carrying out the debridement. Typical resecting measures are the following:

1. Partial synovectomy
2. Arthrolith (loose bodies) removal
3. Cartilage debridement
4. Arthrodesis of the ankle joint

■ **Indications:** Indications for joint debridement include painful weight bearing with partial stiffening. A further indication is blockage (e.g., by arthroliths or by osseous impingement), which might be either ventral or dorsal. A dorsal location results in a limitation of the heel-toe walking function of the ankle; therefore, the indication for operative intervention is more often present in dorsal (or tibial) osteophytes than in ventral (or talar) osteophytes. If a radiologically visualizable joint cavity is no longer present, an arthroscopic debridement has no chance of success and the patient should be advised to have an arthrodesis. It is a matter of relative indications. The operation date is chosen according to pain status.

■ **Contraindications:** Contraindications for joint debridement arthrodesis include patients unfit for anesthesia or those who have overly optimistic expectations of the joint function. The long immobilization period in arthrodesis may also exclude patients who are not prepared for immobilization. Debridement and loose body (arthrolith) removal are not accompanied with immobilization. Infection would be a contraindication for all procedures, especially for arthrodesis.

■ **Special preparations:** For resective arthroscopic procedures in the upper ankle joint, internal or external distraction is necessary. Therefore, internal distractors as well as a suitable fixation system should be at hand. The internal distractor is a common elevator equipped with a grip, as mentioned previously. When long-lasting operations or resective measures in the medial area of the talus are planned, it is advisable to use the external distractor brought in laterally, which makes the external distraction possible using shunt screws in the talus and the tibia. The distraction is carried out under image converter control. If the articular cavity is dilated more than 7 mm, ligament ruptures are likely to occur. For resection of the articular surface, smoothing of cartilage, and synovectomy, suitable rongeurs or shaver systems are available. Arthrolith removal is possible with the aid of rongeurs or forceps. For the resection of the osseous impingement, small chisels are needed.

If an arthrodesis is planned, besides the external distraction, cannulated screws must be prepared, as well as Kirschner's wires to match them.

Operative Risks and Patient Information

The task of informing the patient about both the risks and the degree of necessity of a surgical intervention for a patient is very delicate. The more necessary a surgery is (e.g., acute abdomen with peritonitis), the less difficult the issue of imparting information is. However, if an operation is not vital (and arthroscopic operations are usually not vital—except in the case of a generally infected joint), the more thoroughly practitioners must inform their patients, even about the slightest risk. Otherwise they may have difficulties with patients or attorneys before or after the operation.

■ **Intraoperative risks:** For the joint debridement, arthrolith removal, and resection of osteophytes, risks of any surgical procedure must be mentioned. These risks include nerve, vessel, and tendon injuries, in particular when an external fixator is applied as a distractor. If this is the case, the additional risk of inducing ligament injury of the ankle joint or fractures on the insertion points of the shunt screws must be mentioned. The same is true for the arthroscopically controlled arthrodesis of the ankle joint, independent from the general risk of infection, especially if the ankle has been operated on previously. The use of distraction by an external fixator should be carefully considered in case of osteoporotic bones.

■ **Patient information:** In addition to the intraoperative risks, patients must be made aware of potential failures. Because radiographs do not always show the true condition of the cartilage when the indication for debridement is made postoperatively, the patient must be informed about the indication for arthrodesis. If the indication for arthrodesis was made in the first place, a detailed explanation is needed that conveys that function in the ankle joint is no longer possible. Total joint replacement or another method of arthroplasty could be considered if no infection is present. Other techniques of ankle joint arthrodesis should be considered, such as open-surgery techniques.

Techniques

The following must be kept in mind when approaching these procedures:

■ Preparations for surgical arthroscopy for joint debridement are the same as for treatment of soft tissue injury.

■ It is necessary to apply an internal or external distractor for longer operations.

■ Poor visibility could make it necessary to change the intervention to open arthrotomy in order to avoid complications.

■ Postoperative functional treatment and weight bearing is started right away, and the intensity of both is determined by the severity of pain and insecurity.

Osteochondritis Dissecans

Osteochondritis dissecans is a focal osteochondral separation with or without necrosis of the bone fragment. If bone reabsorption occurs, the articular cartilage loses its support. Osteochondral fractures or lesions have, in most cases, a traumatic etiology.

General Considerations

Because the clinical presentation is often identical to an ankle sprain, without a strong awareness of this condition the diagnosis of transchondral fractures is easily missed. According to Flick and Gould (1985) from their review of more than 500 cases of reported transchondral fractures of the ankle, a history of injury was found in approximately 98% of lateral lesions. A traumatic etiology was found in only 70% of the reported cases in medial dome lesions. Arthroscopy has proved to be of great value in the management of osteo-chrondritis dissecans.

■ **Targets and methods:** Arthroscopy serves for classification and for stage-dependent treatment of osteochondritis dissecans. The aim should always be to preserve a good fit between the articular surfaces. The most frequent location of the osteochondritis dissecans is on the dorsal medial talus, so that for inspecting the dorsal medial talus, internal distraction becomes necessary. Standard procedures for dissecans maintenance are subchondral drilling as well as curettage for stage IV and debridement of the necrotic bone.

■ **Indications:** The indications for an arthroscopic procedure to address osteochondritis dissecans on the talar dome are decided according to the classification of the damage (Anetzberger et al. 1998; Hempfling and Putz 1998). For stages I and II, subchondral drilling with spongious padding without further dam-

age to the cartilage lining may be useful. This procedure is almost always indicated for young patients with the aim of preserving the joint.

■ **Contraindications:** Subchondral drilling is contraindicated for stages III and IV of osteochondritis dissecans. Here other measures are necessary.

■ **Special preparations:** In addition to common arthroscopic instruments, a two-plane image intensifier (converter) is needed, and a drill or a Kirschner's wire is prepared. The preparations for surgical arthroscopy for subchondral drilling in osteochondritis dissecans tali are the same as already mentioned. The lower portion of the limb must be accessible for the image converter, the anterolateral portal for the diagnostic arthroscope, and the anteromedial portal for the internal distraction and the operating instruments. A puncture incision on the level of the lateral talar process might be necessary for the drilling. A preoperative radiographic control must be available for accurate location of the lesion. An image converter control with arthroscopically controlled assistance might become necessary intraoperatively.

Operative Risks and Patient Information

■ **Intraoperative risks:** In the process of searching for the osteochondritic lesion, the nerves, vessels, or healthy cartilage may be damaged. In a few cases of stage I, a mislocation might take place because the cartilage covers the lesion.

■ **Patient information:** Prior to operating on a patient with osteochondritis dissecans, the physician must inform the patient that the stage can only be determined intraoperatively (by the diagnostic arthroscopy) and therefore only then can the surgical procedure be determined. Assurance of healing of the lesion after drilling cannot be given, nor can it be given even when bone grafting is used. The patient must be informed about alternative procedures, including the open operation.

Technique

The Kirschner's wire is drilled into the dorsomedial osteochondritic lesion, and the curetted drill is drilled up to 5 mm into the lesion. With a pestle, the drilling channel can be padded with spongious bone graft from the surrounding distal or proximal tibia. A final radiographic control should always be carried out.

In case of complications, such as nerve, vessel, and tendon lesions, there is some danger of misplacing the Kirschner's wire. In that case, the intervention must be changed to an open procedure, perhaps including a medial malleolar osteotomy.

After the operation, the patient will use crutches to prevent weight bearing on the affected ankle. This temporary decompression will allow callus to develop. Once this has happened, postoperative treatment should begin.

■ References

Albert I, Reimann P, Njus G, Kay DB, Theken R. Ligament sprain and ankle joint opening during ankle distraction. Arthroskopie 8: 469, 1992.

Anetzberger H, et al. Sprunggelenk. Chirurgische Operationslehre, 1998.

Flick AB, Gould N. Osteochondritis dissecans of the talus (transchondral fractures of the talus): Review of the literature and new surgical approach for medial dome lesions. Foot Ankle 5: 165-185, 1985.

Freeman M. Instability of the foot injuries to the lateral ligament of the ankle. J Bone Joint Surg 47-B: 678-685, 1965.

Grechening W, Fellinger M, et al. Beeinflussen anatomische Gefäßvariationen die Wahl der Arthroskopieportale zur Sprunggelenksarthroskopie? Arthroskopie 10: 160-163, 1997.

Hempfling H, Putz, R. Klassifikation der Osteochondrosis dissecans. Chirurgische Operationslehre, 1998.

Mann G, Eliashuv O, Perry C, Finsterbush A, Frankl U, Nyska M, Mattan Y. Recurrent ankle sprain: Literature review. Israel J Sports Med 1: 104-113, 1994.

Martin DF, et al. Operative ankle arthroscopy long-term followup. Am J Sports Med 17: 16, 1989.

Sayli U, Tekdemyr Y, et al. The course of the superficial peroneal nerve: an anatomical cadaver study. Foot Ankle Surg 4: 63-69, 1998.

Takagi K. The arthroscope. I. Ipn Orthop Assoc 14: 359, 1939.

Part VII

Additional Issues

As in any field of medicine, the real heroes are not the emergency room doctors, the intensive care unit physicians, or the operating room surgeons. The real heroes are those who prevent illness. This could be done through immunizing half a continent for tetanus and diphtheria, through education to reduce road accidents, or through predicting, defining, and preventing acute injuries. These methods are not dramatic, but require long hours of hard work by the doctor, physiotherapist, coach, and athlete. Considering the fact that ankle sprains are reported by half the world population and by at least 20% of athletes, there is no doubt that effective prevention would be the best measure for reducing disability from this injury. This part examines in depth how ankle injuries might be prevented. It also includes a chapter on treating pediatric ankle injuries, highlighting what is unique in pediatric ankle injury etiology, diagnosis, and treatment.

Chapter 32

Ankle Instability in Children and Adolescents

A. Ross Outerbridge, MD, FRSC; Eliezer Trepman, MD; and Lyle J. Micheli, MD

Ankle pain, instability, and fracture are all common problems in the pediatric and adolescent age group. Ankle injuries can occur in both free play and organized sport settings. Ankle sprains are the most common injury in sport. In the adult population, ankle sprains make up 16% of all sport injuries (Maehlum & Daljord 1984). Unfortunately, the epidemiology of ankle injuries in the pediatric and adolescent age group is not clear. One source found that foot and ankle injuries made up 12% of all sport injuries presenting to a pediatric sport injuries clinic (Trott 1983). In some sports, such as basketball and soccer, ankle sprains and ankle instability can be seen in up to 70% of participants in this age group (Schmidt-Olsen et al. 1991).

As more information is gathered regarding ankle injuries in the young patient, it becomes clear that, as compared with adults, there is a different pattern of injury, a different set of factors that determine injury, and a variety of conditions that are seen only in this age group. This chapter outlines factors that account for the differences seen in the types and patterns of ankle injuries among pediatric, adolescent, and adult age groups. Important factors in the evaluation of these injuries will be defined, including investigation, treatment, and outcome for the important ankle conditions that are seen in this young population.

Pediatric Differences

The main factor that determines the differences in type and pattern of injuries in the pediatric and adolescent age group is growth. There are differences in tissue characteristics of structures involved in ankle injuries in the pediatric age group, in comparison to adults. In addition, the effects of growth also determine the pattern of injury.

The growing tissues include the physis, apophysis, and articular cartilage. All of these growing tissues lead to a different susceptibility to injury when compared to the adult. The susceptibility of these tissues to injury differs between the preadolescent and the adolescent. In the preadolescent, the physis and its attachment to mature bone are strong. An injury to a joint at this stage may more commonly result in a ligament injury than an injury to the physis. A similar mechanism of injury in the adolescent during periods of rapid growth, when the physis has become relatively weaker than the surrounding ligaments, may more likely result in a physeal injury than a ligament or bone injury (Krueger-Franke et al. 1992). Once the growth plates have fused, in late pubescence, ligament injuries once again predominate. Ossification centers may also become symptomatic in preadolescent and adolescent athletes (Stanitski & Micheli 1993).

This pattern is particularly evident with ankle injuries. The peak incidence of physeal injuries, such as the juvenile Tillaux fracture (page 267) or triplane fracture (page 267), is in the 12-15-year-old age group (Kling 1990; Krueger-Franke et al. 1992), when the physis has started to close. The pattern of closure of the distal tibial physis closely determines the pattern of injury, as the physis begins to fuse first centrally, then medially, and finally anterolaterally (McManama 1998; Outerbridge & Micheli 1995). Therefore, the mechanism of injury that causes ankle sprain in an adult may result in a distal tibial plafond fracture in the adolescent age group.

The articular cartilage is also particularly susceptible to injury in children and adolescents. Twisting or angular forces at the ankle may result in chondral or osteochondral fractures (Loomer et al. 1993).

A second factor relating to growth, and which determines the pattern of injury in children and adolescents, is flexibility. In the growing child, the growth of bone is faster than that of the soft tissues such as the muscle and tendon units that span the joints. This may result in periods of decreased flexibility during the adolescent growth spurt, and may increase susceptibility to apophyseal or tendinous injuries (Micheli 1983). This determines the age distribution of both acute and overuse injuries.

A third factor that affects the pattern of injury in the young athlete is foot deformity. The pes cavus and pes planus foot may have different susceptibilities to overuse and acute injuries. There are also specific congenital and developmental conditions observed in this age group, such as tarsal coalition and the accessory navicular, that may present with either acute injuries or chronic pain.

■ Mechanisms of Injury

Injury about the ankle from acute trauma that results in ankle instability or fracture usually involves a combination of axial loading, rotational torques, and angular stresses. These injuries can occur in both recreational and organized sport. Rotational stress applied to the ankle from a planted and fixed foot, inversion and rotation of the landing foot and ankle, excessive dorsiflexion or plantarflexion, and direct blows are all specific mechanisms that can produce ankle pain, instability, or fracture (Hergenroeder 1990). These acute injuries are the most common types seen in the general pediatric and adolescent population.

In overuse injuries of the ankle, repetitive impact (as in running) or repetitive flexion and extension (as in dance) are the major mechanisms of injury. With the increased availability of intensive and repetitive sport training programs and competitions for the young athlete, we are observing an increasing incidence of overuse injuries of the foot and ankle.

■ Evaluation

As with adults, pediatric and adolescent ankle evaluation includes a thorough history, a comprehensive physical examination, and imaging techniques as appropriate.

History

Evaluation of the child or adolescent with ankle pain or an acute ankle injury begins with a thorough history. The symptoms may be either acute or chronic. In the case of an acute injury, it is extremely important to attempt to clearly elicit the mechanism of injury, because this may suggest specific injury patterns or structures injured. In the case of chronic pain that has been present for a few weeks or longer, it is important to determine the location of the pain, as well as the specific factors that produce or relieve the pain. The presence of swelling, instability, or obvious deformity noted by the patient may also be important. The possibility of systemic illness, inflammatory arthritis, infection, or malignancy that have become manifest in the course of sport participation should also be considered (Churchill & Mazur 1995).

In the young athlete, the duration, intensity, and rate of progression of training are often the most important risk factors for overuse injury. A training schedule that has been advanced too quickly, or improper technique, can contribute to overuse injuries such as traction apophysitis (Canale & Williams 1992; Micheli & Ireland 1987), stress fractures, or tendinitis about the foot and ankle.

Types of treatment previously used by the patient, such as ice, elevation, and compression, braces or splints, physiotherapy, or previous surgical treatment are all potentially helpful factors to elicit in the history.

Physical Examination

A comprehensive physical examination is essential. A complete lower limb assessment may reveal that the complaints about the foot and ankle are the result of referred pain from another joint. Observation of alignment of the foot and ankle, deformity, and specific areas of swelling may indicate the area of involvement and diagnosis. Deformities such as pes planus, pes cavus, or residual clubfoot may be important. Range-of-motion assessment includes dorsiflexion and plantarflexion of the ankle joint, as well as inversion and eversion of the subtalar joint. It may be difficult to accurately quantify range of motion in degrees, but comparing the motion to that of the contralateral side may suggest whether motion is limited. Restriction in subtalar joint range of motion is one of the hallmarks of tarsal coalition.

Specific areas of tenderness and swelling about the ankle are noted, and provocative tests that may localize the site of pain are performed. Stability testing may also be helpful. The interpretation of the response to a stress test may depend on the position of the foot and ankle, as well as the direction of the applied stress. Inversion of the plantarflexed ankle results in tension of the anterior talofibular ligament. Inversion of the dorsiflexed ankle places tension along the calcaneofibular ligament and superior peroneal retinaculum. External rotation of the dorsiflexed ankle stresses the anterior tibiofibular ligament (syndesmosis). Anterior drawer stress of the neutral ankle also results in tension of the anterior talofibular ligament, as well as the peroneal tendons. The response to such stress maneuvers may include specific or non-specific findings, including pain localized to the structure stressed, apprehension, laxity, a click, a snap, or visible translation of the talus or peroneal tendons. A response of pain or a click may be consistent with a ligament injury or inflammation, subluxation of the ankle or subtalar joint, intra-articular derangement, or a periarticular tendon problem, all of which may be difficult to characterize with stress testing alone. Posterior ankle pain with maximal passive plantarflexion of the foot and ankle may indicate an os trigonum injury; anterior ankle pain with maximal passive dorsiflexion may suggest the presence of anterior tibiotalar impingement.

The neurovascular examination may reveal potential factors important in diagnosis and treatment. Strength testing of inversion, eversion, dorsiflexion, and plantarflexion, as well as thorough sensory testing about the distal tibia, foot and ankle, and deep tendon reflexes, will help to rule out any specific neurological involvement. Specific strength testing of the motors of the foot and ankle may also suggest tendon derangements such as flexor hallucis longus tendinitis or peroneal subluxation. Vascular assessment by palpation of pulses and observation of capillary refill of the toes should also be included.

Imaging Techniques

The imaging modalities utilized to evaluate joint instability include standard radiographs of the ankle, stress views, and special studies. Plain film radiographs are essential to help complete the basic diagnostic workup. These should include anteroposterior, lateral, and mortise views of the ankle. A mortise ankle view is completed with the foot and tibia internally rotated approximately 15-20°. Furthermore, depending on the history and physical examination, a plain radiographic series of the foot should be considered in order to evaluate for problems such as base of fifth metatarsal fracture, anterior process of calcaneus fracture, or calcaneonavicular coalition.

Stress views of the ankle can include an ankle inversion stress (mortise) view and an anterior drawer stress (lateral) view; reliability may be limited by pain and apprehension, and stress views under anesthesia may be considered. Stress views (mortise or lateral) of both ankles (injured and uninjured sides) allow for comparison. The inversion stress view, where inversion stress is placed on the ankle while a mortise view is taken, may demonstrate an increased talar tilt. The specific criterion governing the importance of this finding is controversial. Some authors have suggested that an increase in talar tilt of 6° or more in comparison to the uninjured side is suggestive of an unstable ankle joint, whereas others have suggested

values as high as 15°. The lateral stress view, in which an anterior drawer stress is placed on the neutral ankle while a lateral radiograph is done, may demonstrate anterior talofibular ligament insufficiency if there is at least 4 mm of increased anterior translation of the talus from the tibia in comparison to the uninjured side.

Depending on the conclusions from the imaging studies noted previously, further studies can be considered. These may include plain film tomography or CT scan to evaluate fracture displacement, osteochondral defect, or tarsal coalition. Contrast arthrography can sometimes be a useful adjunct to demonstrate a complete capsular tear in the case of a grade III ankle sprain. Injection of local anesthetic, with contrast confirmation, may enable localization of pain to a specific anatomic region, such as the ankle joint, subtalar joint, or peroneal tendon sheath. Magnetic resonance imaging (MRI) may be a useful modality in demonstrating longitudinal tears or subluxation of the peroneus brevis or longus tendons. MRI is not the modality of choice for acute fracture evaluation, but it can be useful to evaluate osteochondral defects (Anderson et al. 1989), lateral ligament injuries, stress fractures, or medial deltoid ligament injuries in the young patient (McConkey et al. 1991).

■ Specific Conditions

Instability problems may be manifested by obvious symptoms such as unambiguous giving way or locking, or more subtle complaints such as apprehension, clicks, or popping. Patients with various conditions involving intra-articular or extra-articular structures may present with complaints of unsteadiness or pain. The goals of evaluation include the identification of a specific anatomic etiology of the symptoms, in order to enable directed, rational treatment of the problem.

Ankle Sprain

Ankle sprains are the most common sport injuries seen in all age groups (Boruta et al. 1990). These injuries can also occur in free play situations or during daily activities. Approximately 10% to 30% of all musculoskeletal injuries involve the ankle, with ankle sprains representing the largest component of those (Maehlum & Daljord 1984; Schmidt-Olsen et al. 1991).

Mechanisms of Injury

The most common mechanism of injury, which occurs in approximately 85% of cases, is inversion (Hergenroeder 1990). This mechanism typically injures the lateral ligamentous structures of the ankle.

Eversion and rotational injuries can also occur, resulting in combination injuries, or—infrequently—isolated injuries to the deltoid ligament.

The epidemiology of ankle injuries in the pediatric and adolescent group is not as well defined as that in the adult, and in the growing child, the same mechanism of injury may produce a fracture of the physis instead of a ligamentous injury.

During most activities that involve running or jumping, the ankle is both plantarflexed and inverted or supinated when the foot is not in contact with the ground, such as near the end of the swing phase of gait. The static restraints to inversion of the ankle include the lateral ligamentous structures: the anterior and posterior talofibular ligaments (ATFL and PTFL) and the calcaneofibular ligament (CFL). The dynamic restraints include the peroneal muscles. If the foot is inverted more rapidly than reflex active contraction of the peroneal muscles, or if the peroneal muscles are too weak to overcome the inversion stress, then the inversion stress is transferred primarily to the lateral ligaments, and this may result in a tear of these structures. The typical pattern of tear involves the ATFL, the most commonly injured of the three ligaments. It is also the weakest of the lateral ligaments and is under tension at the time of the injury when the foot is plantarflexed. The CFL may also be injured with severe inversion injuries.

Another mechanism of injury about the ankle is eversion, which may result in injury to the deltoid ligament. However, eversion injuries may include more severe forces and a direction of application of force that often results in either ankle fracture or significant ankle instability. Therefore, isolated deltoid ligament injuries are not as commonly seen as those of the lateral ligaments (McConkey et al. 1991).

A third mechanism of injury occurs when the dorsiflexed ankle is subjected to external rotation. In the dorsiflexed position, the talus is locked in the mortise, and external rotation results in tension on the anterior ankle syndesmosis. In the adult, this may result in injury to the anterior tibiofibular (syndesmotic) ligament. However, in the young athlete with open physes, this mechanism may result in the juvenile Tillaux fracture (Griffin 1994; McManama 1998).

Examination and Treatment

In the growing child, the physical examination should attempt to pinpoint the exact area of tenderness. A physeal injury may frequently be the result of these types of force application. Therefore, it is important to rule out tenderness at the distal fibular physis. This tenderness is a sign of a Salter-Harris type I fracture of this growth plate.

Ankle sprains are graded by severity into three categories. A grade I sprain involves pain in the supporting structures but no actual instability or stretching of the fibers. There may be minimal or no accompanying swelling with this type of injury. A grade II injury involves a partial tear through the ligaments and is often accompanied by swelling. A grade III injury, or complete tear of the ligamentous structures in the ankle, is often accompanied by severe swelling and a marked amount of pain. A physical examination may help a practitioner to assess the grade of injury by using the anterior drawer sign and inversion stress on the ankle, but usually an accurate examination cannot be performed acutely because of the patient's pain and apprehension. In some instances, it may be helpful to infiltrate the lateral aspect of the ankle with local anesthetic in order to complete the stability examination.

Treatment for most ankle sprains can be based on three phases;

■ **The first phase** involves protective bracing of the ankle to prevent further injury to the ligamentous structures and to reduce swelling and inflammation in the injured area. With a removable ankle stirrup brace that prevents varus and valgus stress on the ankle, active weight bearing can be started as pain allows. Depending on the severity of the sprain, this process can take anywhere from 1 to 8 weeks. Immobilization in a removable cast boot may allow the anterior talofibular ligament to heal in a physiologic, stable position and allow early weight bearing.

■ **The second phase** of active rehabilitation may begin once the swelling and pain have subsided. This includes both passive and active assisted range-of-motion exercises for the ankle and subtalar joint, as well as early peroneal strengthening exercises. This process is continued, with ongoing protective bracing if needed, until normal range of motion and strength are attained. Functional rehabilitation, including proprioceptive retraining, may be accomplished with tilt board exercises and active balance exercises

■ **The third phase** of treatment, when pain has completely resolved and passive stability has been regained, involves more active functional rehabilitation. This may include straight running and figure-of-eight pivoting. Depending on the severity of the ankle sprain, protective bracing may need to be continued during this time.

Ankle sprains result in altered sensation and muscle function, leading to a proprioception deficit (Bullock-Saxton 1994). Regaining effective proprioceptive function is therefore a key goal of the rehabilitation program.

Most grade I ankle sprains will have progressed through the full rehabilitation process within 6 to 8 weeks. Grade II sprains may require ongoing protective bracing or taping once participation in sport resumes at approximately 8 to 12 weeks after injury. Grade III sprains may require ongoing protective bracing for 3 to 6 months, depending on their severity. Surgical treatment for acute ankle sprains is controversial.

Many practitioners and patients regard the ankle sprain as a rather innocuous injury, and a thorough functional rehabilitation program is seldom used in the general population or in many athletic participants. In one study, 55% of patients who had a history of ankle sprain had not sought medical attention (Smith & Reischl 1986). However, it is not uncommon to see many long-term sequelae from ankle sprains (Vahvanen et al. 1983; Verhagen et al. 1995; Yeung et al. 1994). In one review of 577 patients 6.5 years after sustaining an ankle sprain, 39% were found to have residual complaints of pain, swelling, or fear of instability, and 36% of the follow-up group of patients were under 20 years of age (Verhagen et al. 1995). In addition, conditions such as anterolateral ankle impingement syndrome, osteochondral fracture of the talar dome, recurrent ankle instability, or unrecognized subtalar joint instability may result from foot and ankle injury. Inversion injury of the foot and ankle may also result in other injuries, such as fracture of the base of the fifth metatarsal, lateral process of the talus, or anterior process of the calcaneus.

Recurrent Ankle Instability Resulting From Ligamentous Insufficiency

Recurrent ankle instability in the pediatric and adolescent age group is uncommon. It is less common in the pediatric age group before physeal closure than it is in the adolescent group. Recurrent ankle instability can be classified as structural (i.e., lack of intact ligament or bony support) or functional instability (i.e., inadequate proprioception or muscle function, pain inhibition of muscle function in the presence of intact structural supports). The majority of cases of recurrent ankle instability are associated with inadequate immobilization or rehabilitation after an initial ankle sprain injury. The history is typically one of an initial inversion ankle sprain that has been inadequately treated, usually with a short period of immobilization followed by no rehabilitation. The instability may be a result of the failure to regain adequate protective proprioception about the ankle joint (Bullock-Saxton 1994). Furthermore, peroneal weakness may contribute to poor dynamic lateral support. In addition, structural factors may

include a torn ATFL or CFL that has not healed properly.

The presence of ankle pain, or mechanical symptoms such as clicks or giving way, may indicate an osteochondral lesion. In addition, recurrent subluxation of the peroneal tendons can also produce recurrent ankle instability or apprehension.

The initial management of an adolescent with recurrent ankle instability, depending on the cause, usually includes a directed rehabilitation program. This includes a period of rest and immobilization to allow swelling and inflammation to settle down, if necessary, followed by a strengthening program including the peroneal muscles, and functional proprioceptive rehabilitation.

The imaging modalities utilized to evaluate joint instability include standard radiographs of the ankle to rule out structural deficiencies (fracture, osteochondral talar dome lesions), and stress views to evaluate the integrity of the ATFL and CFL.

Surgical indications for this problem include lack of response to an adequate physiotherapy and rehabilitation program, or demonstration of increased talar tilt or translation on the stress views of the ankle.

Reconstructive procedures for recurrent instability include direct, anatomic repair of the torn ATFL (Broström 1966). The lateral ligaments are either imbricated in midsubstance or are shortened and reinserted onto the lateral malleolus. Both the ATFL and CFL can be reconstructed using this type of procedure.

Other types of reconstructive procedures involve the creation of a soft tissue sling to replace the ATFL and CFL. The Evans procedure uses the entire peroneus brevis tendon, brought through a tunnel in the distal fibula (Evans 1953). The Watson-Jones procedure (see chapter 26) also uses the peroneus brevis tendon, looping it through drill holes in the neck of the talus and the distal fibula. The Chrisman-Snook procedure (see chapter 27), which uses a split portion of the peroneus brevis tendon brought through drill holes in the distal fibula and calcaneus, reconstructs both the ATFL and CFL (Chrisman & Snook 1969). These procedures, however, are not used in children or adolescents with open growth plates, as they create a very high risk of growth plate abnormalities in the distal fibular physis. Young, skeletally immature patients who require surgical stabilization are usually treated by an anatomic reconstruction that imbricates the ATFL and CFL directly and has less risk to the distal fibular physis.

The result of these different procedures is that approximately 90% of cases will have satisfactory clinical results. Postoperatively, the foot is immobilized in a below-knee cast for 8 weeks and then is slowly mobilized with a protective ankle brace that allows dorsiflexion and plantarflexion with minimal inversion and eversion of the ankle. Risk factors for surgical failure may include generalized excessive ligamentous laxity and collagen disorders.

Osteochondral Defect

Osteochondral lesions of the talar dome may be observed as a sequela of ankle trauma. Although these lesions are not common, a typical history is that of undiagnosed ankle pain as the long-term sequela of a past inversion injury (Anderson et al. 1989). These lesions may be referred to as *osteochondritis dissecans* or *osteochondral defects* and may be a result of ankle injury, usually inversion sprain. These lesions can be found on both the medial and lateral sides of the talar dome.

The original classification of osteochondral defects (Berndt & Harty 1959) has recently been expanded to include five different types (Loomer et al. 1993). Type I is a pure compression injury; type II is partially detached but undisplaced; type III is completely detached but undisplaced; type IV is a displaced fragment; and type V is a radiolucent defect.

Diagnosis

Common symptoms may include pain, and in the case of displaced lesions, mechanical symptoms such as locking, clicking, or catching may occur. Physical examination with the foot fully plantarflexed may reveal a tender area that coincides with the location of the lesion on the dome of the talus, or may be unremarkable for talar dome tenderness.

Plain radiographs may be unremarkable, but occasionally these lesions are evident. If plain radiographs are negative, then a technetium-99 bone scan may reveal a focus of increased uptake localized to the talar dome. If the bone scan is positive, the practitioner may proceed to a CT scan for exact localization of the lesion. Alternatively, an MRI scan may help to confirm the diagnosis as well as aid in localization of the lesion. If imaging is negative, other causes of ankle pain and instability may be considered, including lateral impingement syndrome, recurrent subluxation of the peroneal tendons, or recurrent subluxation of the ankle joint from a chronically torn ATFL or CFL. In some cases in which imaging is negative, an isolated chondral injury may be identified with arthroscopy.

Treatment

Early type I, II, and III osteochondral lesions may be treated initially by immobilization and nonweightbearing. Persistent symptoms after nonoperative treatment of type I, II, and III lesions

may be treated with excision and curettage. The majority of lower grade lesions can be treated arthroscopically, but some osteochondral lesions may require an anterior or posterior arthrotomy for visualization and treatment. The displaced type IV fragment may be treated by arthroscopy or arthrotomy and excision. Depending on symptoms, the radiolucent defect may be either observed or treated with surgical curettage and drilling (Loomer et al. 1993). If the osteochondral fragment is large, the surgeon may consider reduction, cancellous bone grafting, and absorbable pin fixation. Cartilage grafting is currently being investigated, but long-term results are unavailable.

After swelling and pain have decreased following arthroscopic excision and curettage, the patient is mobilized. A therapy program, consisting of strengthening, stretching, and eventual functional rehabilitation, may be started as soon as symptoms will allow. Six to 8 weeks of nonweightbearing activity may be necessary, with a return to full activities by 3 to 6 months postoperatively.

Long-term sequelae of osteochondral injuries include ankle synovitis, impingement, and post-traumatic arthritis.

Dislocation or Subluxation of the Peroneal Tendons

Peroneal tendon subluxation and dislocation is not uncommon in the pediatric population. It is often either overlooked or confused with ankle sprain. Differentiation can be made according to the area of maximum tenderness, which in recurrent or acute subluxation of the peroneal tendons is usually just posterior to the lateral malleolus and the posterior border of the distal fibula (Jones 1993).

This injury is usually seen with sports that involve pivoting, jumping, or rapid acceleration and deceleration, such as basketball and tennis. It has also been observed in alpine skiing. The mechanism of injury is usually forced dorsiflexion with peroneal contraction and foot eversion (Micheli et al. 1989). It may also occur after inversion injury to the foot and ankle.

There are congenital causes for this problem, in addition to the acute traumatic causes. Congenital factors that contribute to this injury include a flat or convex posterior surface to the distal fibula and lateral malleolus, instead of the concave groove that is usually present.

Diagnosis

The physical findings in the acute setting involve lateral ankle swelling and tenderness about the distal posterior aspect of the lateral malleolus. With passive or active eversion and dorsiflexion of the foot, the actual subluxation may be demonstrable. This test can be quite painful in the acute traumatic situation, but with chronic peroneal subluxation this may be demonstrated with minimal pain.

Normally, the peroneal tendons are held in the posterior lateral malleolar groove by the superior and inferior peroneal retinacula. The pathologic findings associated with acute or chronic peroneal subluxation include retinacular separation from the dense fibrous lip of the lateral malleolus, elevation of the retinaculum, or avulsion of the lateral malleolus itself (Eckert & Davis 1976).

Plain radiographs are advised for two reasons. First, plain radiographs help to rule out other conditions that may be difficult to clinically distinguish from peroneal subluxation. Second, an avulsion fracture from the posterolateral rim of the lateral malleolus can sometimes be observed on a radiograph.

In addition to the acute traumatic injury or the chronic recurrent injury, occasionally a young athlete with an asymptomatic ankle may have incidental subluxation of the peroneal tendons. In this case the subluxation is seen in the absence of symptoms or compromised athletic performance.

Treatment

Treatment is based on the clinical situation. In situations of incidental finding with no symptoms or functional disability, no treatment other than strengthening the peroneal muscles in the nonsubluxed position is indicated. In the case of acute traumatic injury, initial treatment may include either operative or nonoperative methods. Nonoperative treatment can consist of a compression dressing fabricated with a U-shaped felt pad strapped around the lateral malleolus. This is placed under a plaster splint until swelling subsides. The patient is then placed in a well-molded cast or removable cast boot for 4 to 8 weeks. When the cast is removed, a rehabilitation program is started to help the patient regain range of motion and strength (Jones 1993).

In the acute traumatic setting, operative treatment is also a reasonable option. Either bone or soft tissue procedures may be considered. In the acute setting, soft tissue procedures are usually adequate and involve the attachment of the superior peroneal retinaculum to periosteum and, therefore, reconstitution of the fibro-osseous tunnel for the peroneal tendons (Eckert & Davis 1976). The retinaculum can be attached directly to bone, either by placing sutures directly through bone with the help of drill holes, or by using suture anchors. The repair is then protected in a well-molded cast for 4 to 8 weeks before commencing a rehabilitation program.

In the case of chronic recurrent subluxation of the peroneal tendons, either soft tissue or bony procedures are indicated. Soft tissue procedures are similar to those described previously for acute traumatic injury. Bony procedures can include either a posterior bone block (Jones 1932) or a distal bone block, both of which are designed to create a deeper fibro-osseous tunnel and bony shelf to contain the peroneal tendons (Micheli et al. 1989). The success rate for these sliding fibular grafts is approximately 90% for return to athletic activities after appropriate healing and rehabilitation (Micheli et al. 1989).

Anterolateral Ankle Impingement Syndrome

Another long-term sequela that may follow inversion foot and ankle injury is chronic anterolateral ankle pain secondary to impingement of synovitis, a capsular tear, or meniscoid lesion. The history usually includes previous acute injury, such as an inversion sprain. Some patients develop ankle impingement after a previous ankle fracture. Furthermore, repetitive ankle dorsiflexion activity, such as the demi-plié in dancers, may cause anterior ankle bony impingement and secondary impinging osteophytes between the anterior lip of the tibial plafond and the dorsal talar neck.

Chronic anterolateral ankle joint pain, with or without intermittent localized swelling in this area, is usually the chief complaint. Anterolateral joint line tenderness and an audible click with dorsiflexion-plantarflexion of the ankle may be present (Meislin et al. 1993). Plain radiographs and bone scans may be negative for osteochondral lesions or chronic mechanical lateral ankle instability. However, in cases with bony impingement, a lateral radiograph may reveal osteophytes at the anterior tibial plafond and dorsal talar neck, and the bone scan might show increased radiotracer uptake in this region.

The differential diagnosis in a patient with symptoms of anterolateral ankle pain includes osteochondral lesions of the talus and fractures of the anterior process of the calcaneus, anterior talar beak, base of the fifth metatarsal, and lateral process of the talus. Peroneal tendinitis, subluxating peroneal tendons, sinus tarsi syndrome, chronic ankle instability, and syndesmotic ligament injury may also be considered.

The initial treatment of anterolateral soft tissue and bony impingement is nonoperative. This can include a period of immobilization and physiotherapy, which may include local modalities such as ultrasound as well as range-of-motion exercises, strengthening, and functional rehabilitation. Persistent pain despite 3 months of nonoperative treatment is an indication for arthroscopic debridement of this area

(Meislin et al. 1993). Arthroscopic findings may include hypertrophic synovial thickening and scar tissue anterolaterally, and a flap-like meniscoid lesion may be present. Impingement may be demonstrated with dorsiflexion of the ankle. Chondromalacia of the talar dome and distal tibia may also be identified. Impinging osteophytes may be removed with arthroscopic visualization and bone instruments such as osteotomes and rotary burrs.

Arthroscopic debridement of the scar tissue from the anterolateral aspect of the ankle, using a mechanical shaver, can result in up to 90% satisfactory results (Meislin et al. 1993). Arthroscopic excision of osteophytes for bony impingement appears to be similarly successful. However, recurrent synovitis or osteophytes and persistent or recurrent pain may occur despite surgery.

Postoperatively, these patients are allowed to bear weight as soon as symptoms allow. Functional rehabilitation, strengthening, and range of motion may be helpful. With a successful resolution of these symptoms, many patients may be able to return to progressive sport activity within 6 to 12 weeks of surgery.

Ankle Fractures

The same mechanisms of injury that produce ankle sprains and ligament injuries in the adult may result in ankle fractures in the skeletally immature athlete. The most common of these is a Salter-Harris type I fracture through the distal fibular physis. The mechanism of inversion and plantarflexion, similar to that of the ankle sprain in the adult, can produce this injury. This may be an incomplete fracture with the epiphysis undisplaced. Differentiation between this fracture and an ankle sprain is often difficult and is usually based on the specific and most dominant area of tenderness. In the Salter-Harris type I fracture, the area of maximum tenderness is directly over the physis. In the ankle sprain, the maximum area of tenderness is over the anterior talofibular ligament. Inversion stress placed on the ankle can produce pain with both of these entities.

Findings on the plain radiographs might not be helpful in differentiating these two injuries. In the case of a fracture, there may be an area of increased soft tissue swelling opposite the distal fibular physis, but this is not always the case. The diagnosis is primarily based on strong clinical suspicion and a diagnostic area of localized tenderness.

Fracture types and their treatments include the following:

■ For **undisplaced fractures**, 3 to 4 weeks of cast immobilization, followed by range-of-motion exer-

cises, strengthening, and eventual functional rehabilitation, are usually satisfactory. In the rare case when a displaced fracture occurs in an adolescent just prior to physeal closure, open reduction and internal fixation with tension band wiring can be an effective technique. This allows early range-of-motion exercises at the ankle and may limit ankle stiffness and muscle atrophy.

■ Another fracture that may be seen in the adolescent during physeal closure is the **juvenile Tillaux fracture**. This is an avulsion fracture of the anterolateral aspect of the distal tibial epiphysis and is a Salter-Harris type III fracture. During development, the physis first closes centrally, then progresses to closing at the posteromedial and medial aspects, and finally closes anterolaterally (McManama 1998; Rang 1983). At 13 to 14 years of age, when the only area of the physis that remains open is the anterolateral portion, an avulsion fracture may occur when the anterior tibiofibular ligament pulls this fragment of bone off the distal tibia (Rang 1983). A typical mechanism of injury involves external rotation of the fibula about the tibia. With this fracture, it is essential to accurately assess displacement. In addition to plain radiographs, tomography or CT scan may be useful in determining the degree of gap and step deformity within the joint surface. This fracture is often displaced proximally and laterally. In most cases in which the step deformity or gap in the joint surface exceeds 2 mm, an open reduction and internal fixation is suggested (Ertl et al. 1988; Kling 1990). This can be done through an anterolateral arthrotomy, using an image intensifier and small cannulated screws.

■ A third and more complex fracture is the **triplane fracture involving the distal tibia.** This consists of fracture in three planes: a coronal split in the distal tibia down to the distal tibial physis, a horizontal fracture through the physis itself, and a sagittal split through the epiphysis (Ertl et al. 1988; Rang 1983). As is the case with the Tillaux fracture, this can occur during the period of physeal closure when the middle and medial portions of the distal tibial physis have closed. The tibia plus the fused medial physis rotate away from the remainder of the distal tibial physis. Accurate imaging to judge displacement is important. The most effective modality for this is high resolution CT scanning, with or without three-dimensional reconstruction. This can clearly show the degree of step deformity and gap within the joint. The criteria for open reduction and internal fixation are the same as for the Tillaux fracture. If there is more than a 2-mm gap or step deformity in the joint surface, treatment includes anatomic reduction and fixation with cannulated screws or Kirschner wires (Ertl et al. 1988; Kling 1990). Because this fracture occurs at a period of development so close to physeal closure, the physis may be traversed with internal fixation devices.

■ In both the athletic and nonathletic preadolescent and adolescent patient, a variety of other complex fractures can occur. A **Salter-Harris type II fracture** through the distal tibial physis can be seen in patients participating in sports that involve jumping and landing, such as gymnastics, figure skating, or ballet (McManama 1998), or the twisting and pivoting sports, such as soccer and alpine skiing (Krueger-Franke et al. 1992). The principles involved in the assessment and treatment of physeal fractures must be applied. In the case of **Salter-Harris type III and IV fractures**, anatomic reduction and fixation is important to ensure a minimum risk of post-traumatic arthritis, growth arrest, or angular deformity. Salter-Harris type II fractures, if in acceptable anatomic position, can be treated by closed means of reduction and fixation (Kling 1990).

Tarsal Coalition

Any young patient who presents with chronic ankle pain should be assessed to rule out the possibility of tarsal coalition. Tarsal coalition is an entity in which at least two of the tarsal bones are connected by an initially fibro-osseous bridge that, during the typical period of closure of the physes, may become bony, more rigid, and symptomatic with pain. The most common of these tarsal coalitions is the calcaneonavicular, and the second most common is the talocalcaneal. The incidence of tarsal coalition is approximately 1-3% in the general population (Olney & Asher 1984). The calcaneonavicular coalitions can be bilateral in up to 60% of cases, and talocalcaneal coalitions can be bilateral in up to 50% of cases (Cowell 1975).

Diagnosis

During early adolescence, when the coalition is ossifying, vague hindfoot pain may be experienced by the patient. This may be aggravated by running activities, or by any type of weightbearing activities on uneven ground.

Physical findings may include an antalgic gait, pes planus deformity, increased ankle or hindfoot valgus malalignment, tight peroneal muscles that resist inversion, and a stiff, immobile subtalar joint.

Radiographic studies include anteroposterior, lateral, and oblique views of the foot. A calcaneonavicular coalition may be evident on the oblique view of the foot. A talocalcaneal coalition can be more difficult to visualize on plain radiographs. The Harris axial view of the calcaneus may occasionally reveal a talocalcaneal coalition; a prominent medial bony mass may be observed, and a sloping middle facet of the subtalar joint is also noted. Secondary radiographic changes, including beaking and shortening of the talar neck, a ball-and-socket ankle joint, or elongation of the lateral process of the calcaneus, may be noted. With a strong clinical suspicion and suggestive findings on the plain radiographs, CT scan evaluation is warranted, and may clearly define the bony anatomy of a talocalcaneal coalition.

Treatment

Initial treatment includes immobilization, orthotic insoles, and modification of activities. Failure of nonoperative treatment is the main indication for surgical treatment (O'Neill & Micheli 1989).

The calcaneonavicular coalition can be removed through a dorsolateral approach with excision of the fibro-osseous or osseous coalition and interposition of a soft tissue spacer, such as the extensor digitorum brevis muscle or a fat graft, into the space (Cowell 1975). Up to 88% of patients treated in this manner may return to sport with satisfactory motion and no symptoms (Cowell 1975).

Excision of the talocalcaneal coalition is done through a medial approach, with protection of the neurovascular bundle. Although the results of these procedures may be satisfactory in terms of pain relief, there is often very little increase in the degree of subtalar motion after these coalitions have been excised. However, talocalcaneal coalitions involving greater than 25% of the joint space may be less amenable to excision.

The age range for tarsal coalition in symptomatic adolescent athletes is 9-17 years (O'Neill & Micheli 1989). In a follow-up of 20 patients operated on for this condition, either with resection of the bar or subtalar arthrodesis, 95% had excellent or good results by objective scoring and 85% had excellent or good subjective results.

In patients with severe malalignment of the foot, simple excision of the coalition might not be adequate. In these cases, bracing or hindfoot (subtalar or triple) arthrodesis may be an effective means of maintaining stability in the hindfoot and relieving the painful symptoms.

Accessory Navicular Bone

A variety of accessory ossicles can be encountered in the foot and ankle. The most common of these is the accessory navicular. This is a prominent, massive bone over the medial aspect of the navicular that is often part of the tibialis posterior tendon insertion. It usually forms as an accessory center of ossification of the navicular. It may cause symptoms because of its prominence over the medial side of the foot. Furthermore, a synchondrosis may form between the accessory navicular and the body of the navicular, and motion of the site can cause ongoing irritation, especially in the athletic individual. In athletes who wear tight boots, such as figure skaters, the prominence associated with this condition can be quite painful.

In patients with persistent pain, simple excision of the ossicle may be effective in relieving painful symptoms. In the young patient, the ossicle may be removed from around the fibers of the tibialis posterior tendon, and the tendon may then be sutured to the navicular bone. However, excision of the medial navicular prominence may also be required, because the prominent medial navicular may cause ongoing pain.

■ References

Anderson IF, Crichton KJ, Grattan-Smith T, Cooper RA, Brazier D. 1989. Osteochondral fractures of the dome of the talus. J Bone Joint Surg Am 71:1143-1152.

Berndt AL, Harty M. 1959. Transchondral fractures (osteochondritis dissecans) of the talus. J Bone Joint Surg Am 41:988-1020.

Boruta PM, Bishop JO, Braly WG, Tullos HS. 1990. Foot fellows review: acute lateral ankle ligament injuries: a literature review. Foot Ankle 11:107-113.

Broström L. 1966. Sprained ankles: Part V. Treatment and prognosis in recent ligament ruptures. Acta Chir Scand 132:537-550.

Bullock-Saxton JE. 1994. Local sensation changes and altered hip muscle function following severe ankle sprain. Phys Ther 74:17-28.

Canale ST, Williams KD. 1992. Iselin's disease. J Pediatr Orthop 12:90-93.

Chrisman OD, Snook GA. 1969. Reconstruction of lateral ligament tears of the ankle. J Bone Joint Surg Am 51:904.

Churchill JA, Mazur JM. 1995. Ankle pain in children: Diagnostic evaluation and clinical decision making. J Am Acad Orthop Surg 3:183-93.

Cowell HR. 1975. Diagnosis and management of peroneal spastic flatfoot. Instr Course Lect 24:94-102.

Eckert WR, Davis EA. 1976. Acute rupture of the peroneal tendons. J Bone Joint Surg Am 58:670-673.

Ertl JP, Barrack RL, Alexander AH, VanBuecken K. 1988. Triplane fracture of the distal tibial epiphysis: Long-term follow-up. J Bone Joint Surg Am 70:967-976.

Evans DL. 1953. Recurrent instability of the ankle: a method of surgical treatment. Proceedings of the Royal Society of Medicine 46:343.

Griffin LY. 1994. Common sports injuries of the foot and ankle seen in children and adolescents. Orthop Clin North Am 25:83-93.

Hergenroeder AC. 1990. Diagnosis and treatment of ankle sprains: a review. Am J Dis Child 144:809-814.

Jones DC. 1993. Tendon disorders of the foot and ankle. J Am Acad Orthop Surg 1:87-94.

Jones E. 1932. Posterior bone block for peroneal tendon subluxation. J Bone Joint Surg 14:574-576.

Kling TF. 1990. Operative treatment of ankle fractures in children. Orthop Clin North Am 21:381-392.

Krueger-Franke M, Siebert CH, Pfoerringer W. 1992. Sports-related epiphyseal injuries of the lower extremity. J Sports Med Phys Fit 32:106-111.

Loomer R, Fisher C, Lloyd-Smith R, Sisler J, Cooney T. 1993. Osteochondral lesions of the talus. Am J Sports Med 21:13-19.

Maehlum S, Daljord AO. 1984. Acute sports injuries in Oslo: a one-year study. Br J Sports Med 18:181-185.

McConkey JP, Lloyd-Smith R, Li D. 1991. Complete rupture of the deltoid ligament of the ankle. Clin J Sport Med 1:133-137.

McManama GB. 1998. Ankle injuries in the young athlete. Clin Sports Med 7:547-562.

Meislin RJ, Rose DJ, Parisen JS, Springer S. 1993. Arthroscopic treatment of synovial impingement of the ankle. Am J Sports Med 21:186-189.

Micheli, LJ. 1983. Overuse injuries in children's sports: the growth factor. Orthop Clin North Am 14:337-360.

Micheli, LJ, Ireland, ML. 1987. Prevention and management of calcaneal apophysitis in children and adolescents. J Pediatr Orthop 7:34-38.

Micheli LJ, Waters PM, Sanders DP. 1989. Sliding fibular graft repair for chronic dislocation of the peroneal tendons. Am J Sports Med 17:68-71.

Olney BW, Asher MA. 1984. Tarsal coalition and peroneal spastic flatfoot: a review. J Bone Joint Surg Am 66:976-984.

O'Neill DB, Micheli LJ. 1989. Tarsal coalition; a follow-up of adolescent athletes. Am J Sports Med 17:544-549.

Outerbridge AR, Micheli, LJ. 1995. Overuse injuries in the young athlete. Clin Sports Med 14(3):503-516.

Rang, M. 1983. Children's fractures. Philadelphia: Lippincott. p. 312.

Schmidt-Olsen S, Jorgensen U, Kaalund S, Sorensen J. 1991. Injuries among young soccer players. Am J Sports Med 19:273-275.

Smith RW, Reischl SF. 1986. Treatment of ankle sprains in young athletes. Am J Sports Med 14:465-471.

Stanitski CL, Micheli LJ. 1993. Observations on symptomatic medial malleolar ossification centers. J Pediatr Orthop 13:164-168.

Trott AW. 1983. Foot and ankle problems in children and adolescents: sports aspects. In: Kiene RH, Johnson KA, editors. American Academy of Orthopaedic Surgeons symposium on the foot and ankle. St. Louis: Mosby. p. 34-49.

Vahvanen V, Westerlund M, Kajanti M. 1983. Sprained ankle in children: a clinical follow-up study of 90 children treated conservatively and by surgery. Ann Chir Gynaecol 72(2):71-75.

Verhagen RAW, de Keizer G, van Dijk CN. 1995. Long-term follow up of inversion trauma of the ankle. Arch Orthop Trauma Surg 114:92-96.

Yeung MS, Chan Kai-Ming, So CH, Yuan WY. 1994. An epidemiological survey on ankle sprain. Br J Sports Med 28(2):112-116.

Chapter 33

Prevention of Acute Ankle Ligament Sprains in Sport

Martin P. Schwellnus, MBBCh, MSc (Med), MD, PhD, FACSM

The key to the successful management of acute ankle sprains in sport is prevention. In this chapter, strategies for the prevention of acute ankle sprains in sport will be discussed. The review notes will, for the most part, be confined to a discussion on the prevention of lateral ligament sprains, because they are so common, and therefore most studies have focused on this injury. Where applicable, specific prevention strategies for medial ligament complex and syndesmotic sprains will be discussed.

A strategy for the prevention of acute ankle sprains in sport has to start with the identification of the known risk factors for ankle sprains. Risk factors can be classified as extrinsic (factors outside the body) and intrinsic (factors within the body) (Barker et al. 1997; Garrick 1977). The postulated extrinsic and intrinsic risk factors for ankle sprains are listed in table 33.1. A distinction between modifiable and nonmodifiable risk factors can be made. A strategy for preventing ankle sprains in different sports must focus on minimizing or removing the modifiable risk factors for acute ankle sprains.

In this chapter, strategies for reducing the extrinsic and intrinsic risk factors for acute ankle sprains will be discussed. Reference to the role of each risk factor in the prevention of primary (first injury) and secondary (recurrent injury) ankle sprains, as well as the proposed mechanism by which each risk factor affects the risk for an acute ankle sprain, will also be examined.

■ Extrinsic Risk Factors for Ankle Sprains in Sport

The extrinsic factors affecting risk for an acute ankle sprain include type of footwear, use of strapping or taping, use of orthoses, playing surface, match play, and player position. The scientific evidence obtained from laboratory-based studies, as well as epidemiological studies linking each of these factors to the risk

Table 33.1 Extrinsic and Intrinsic Risk Factors for Acute Ankle Sprains in Sport

Extrinsic risk factors	Intrinsic risk factors
Poor footwear*	Previous ankle sprain
No strapping/taping*	Poor proprioceptive function*
No orthoses*	Ankle eversion/inversion muscle strength*
Playing surface*	Ankle dorsiflexion/plantarflexion muscle strength*
Match play	Foot type and alignment
Player position	Ankle joint range of motion* Dominance Gender

* Indicates a modifiable risk factor.

of sustaining an acute ankle sprain, will now be discussed.

Footwear

It has been suggested that the type of footwear worn by athletes is a risk factor for acute ankle sprains (Barker et al. 1997). It has been postulated that footwear may be protective (Bonstingl et al. 1975; Garrick & Requa 1973), as well as causative (Robbins & Gouw 1991; Robbins & Waked 1998), in acute ankle sprains. In the last two to three decades, a number of biomechanical and clinical studies have been performed to define the role of footwear in the prevention of acute ankle sprains (Barrett & Bilisko 1995).

Biomechanical Studies

A number of biomechanical studies have tested different hypotheses relating footwear to ankle injuries.

In particular, questions have been asked regarding whether footwear affects the external stresses on the ankle joint, the proprioceptive function of the foot, or the torque related to the shoe-surface interface. The hypotheses, main findings, and limitations of these studies are summarized in table 33.2.

It appears that high-top shoes can improve the stability of the ankle joint. However, this has not been tested without excluding the dynamic stabilizer function of the ankle joint.

The design of the cleats of a shoe appears to be important in the transmission of forces to the lower limb. Multi-cleated shoes result in a reduced torque to the lower limb, thereby reducing the risk of injury to the lower limb generally, but not the ankle specifically. There is also some evidence to suggest that the foot contact with the shoe can reduce proprioceptive input. Although not tested in a clinical study, this reduction in proprioceptive input could potentially result in an increased incidence of ankle sprains.

Table 33.2 Footwear in the Prevention of Acute Ankle Sprains: Biomechanical Studies

Hypothesis	Main finding(s)	Limitations of the studies
High-top shoes improve the stability of the ankle joint.	High-top sports shoes provide more stability to the ankle than low-top sports shoes (cadaver study) (Shapiro et al. 1994).	Limitation: Dynamic stabilizer function has been excluded.
	High-top soccer shoes transmit a lower load to the ankle compared with low-top shoes (mathematical modeling) (Johnson et al. 1976).	Limitations: Minimum shoe height not defined, and model not adequately validated.
Stiff low-top shoes increase loads on the ankle joint by reducing mobility of the subtalar joint.	Stiff low-top shoes can reduce subtalar joint mobility, thereby increasing stresses on the ankle joint (mathematical modeling) (Johnson et al. 1976).	Limitation: Mathematical modeling study with no other laboratory data to support the hypothesis
Footwear can decrease the proprioceptive input to the ankle and increase the risk of injury.	A smooth, firm foot contact surface has a lower plantar discomfort rating (proprioceptive input) compared with a rigid irregular surface (Robbins & Gouw 1991).	Limitation: The results of this single experiment cannot be translated to the role of footwear in increasing the risk of ankle sprains without further studies.
High-top shoes can increase the proprioceptive input and therefore reduce the risk of ankle sprains.	This hypothesis has not been tested in a laboratory but has been suggested (Petrov et al. 1988).	Limitation: No data available
Shoes with smaller multiple cleats reduce the torque at the shoe-turf interface	Multi-cleated shoes had significantly lower torque at the shoe-turf interface on natural grass compared to shoes with fewer cleats (Bonstingl et al. 1975).	Limitation: This study linked knee, not ankle, injuries to the shoe design.
The forces generated in the lower leg differ when different shoes are tested on different surfaces.	The moment of rotation of different shoes on the same surface varied considerably. The moment of rotation of the same shoe on different surfaces varied (Heidt et al. 1996).	Limitations: Test-retest reliability of measure of moment of rotation was low. Testing speed lower than physiological speeds.

Clinical Studies

A limited number of clinical studies have examined the relationship between footwear and the risk of ankle sprains in basketball and soccer. The hypotheses, some parameters of some studies, main findings, and conclusions of three studies are presented in table 33.3.

The factor in footwear design that has most frequently been investigated is the possible role of high-top shoes in reducing the risk of ankle sprains (Petrov 1988). The results from three studies indicate that, in the absence of additional taping or external support, wearing high-top shoes does not reduce the risk of ankle sprains. Indeed, in one study, the wearing of low-top shoes resulted in a lower incidence of ankle sprains compared with high-top shoes (Rovere et al. 1988). In two recently published meta-analyses, it was also concluded that the role of footwear in the prevention of ankle sprains is not clear (Quinn et al. 2000; Verhagen et al. 2000).

In summary, although a protective influence of footwear is suggested from the results of biomechanical studies, footwear without additional support from taping or bracing does not appear to have a strong influence on the risk of ankle sprains in sport. The potential negative effect that footwear may have on the proprioceptive function of the foot requires further investigation.

Strapping (Taping)

Strapping (often called "taping") is one of the oldest methods of preventing ankle sprains in sport. The earliest report indicating that strapping reduces the risk of ankle sprains was published in 1946 (Quigley et al. 1946). In this study, a 50% reduction in the incidence of ankle sprains in taped ankles was reported. In the last three to four decades, a number of biomechanical and clinical studies have been performed to examine the role of strapping on the risk of ankle sprains in sport (Čallaghan 1997). In addition, the role of strapping on exercise performance has also been investigated.

Biomechanical Studies

The results of studies examining the role of strapping in the prevention of ankle sprains are listed in table 33.4. A number of hypotheses have been tested, including the role of ankle strapping on mechanical stability of the ankle, the ability of strapping to resist an inversion moment that is applied to the ankle, the effect of strapping on ankle range of motion before and after an exercise session, and the effect of ankle strapping on proprioceptive function of the ankle before and after an exercise session. A final, as yet poorly investigated, factor is the influence different materials and strapping techniques have on prevention of ankle sprains.

Table 33.3 Footwear in the Prevention of Acute Ankle Sprains: Clinical Studies

Hypothesis	Some parameters and main findings	Conclusion(s)
High-top shoes decrease the incidence of ankle sprains in basketball players.	2,562 basketball players (nonrandomized) 4 groups of exposures (high top, no tape; high top, taped; low top, no tape; low top, taped) Incidence of ankle sprains (injuries/1,000 games)—high top, no tape: 30.4; high top, taped: 6.5; low top, no tape: 33.4; low top, taped: 17.6 (Garrick & Requa 1973)	In untaped ankles, high-top shoes do not reduce ankle sprains significantly (high top 30.4/1,000 games, low top 33.4/1,000 games). High-top shoes together with taping reduce the incidence of ankle sprains.
High-top shoes together with taping or wearing an ankle stabilizer decrease the relative risk of ankle sprains in football players.	297 college football players (retrospective study, nonrandomized) The incidence of injury (injuries/1,000 exposures) in games was: high top and tape (13.5), low top and tape (9.5), high top and stabilizer (7.0), low top and stabilizer (1.6) (Rovere et al. 1988).	Low-top shoes were associated with lower injury rates than high-top shoes regardless of wearing a stabilizer or taping.
High-top shoes decrease the incidence of ankle sprains in basketball players.	622 college basketball players (randomized, prospective study) The incidence of injury (injuries/10,000 player minutes) for three types of footwear was: high top with inflatable air chambers (2.69), high top (4.80), low top (4.06) (nonsignificant difference between groups) (Barrett et al. 1993).	No significant difference between groups, indicating that there is no strong relationship between shoe type and ankle sprains.

Table 33.4 Strapping in the Prevention of Acute Ankle Sprains: Biomechanical Studies

Hypothesis	Main finding(s)	Conclusion(s)
Ankle strapping reduces the mechanical instability of the ankle joint in the frontal plane (talar tilt, internal/external rotation).	There was a significant reduction in talar tilt after strapping (Larsen 1984; Karlsson et al. 1993; Vaes et al. 1985, 1998; Yamamoto et al. 1993). Talar tilt was not reduced significantly after strapping (using stress radiography) (Karlsson 1992). Ankle strapping reduced internal and external rotation of the ankle joint (Bruns et al. 1996).	Ankle strapping does, in most studies, improve mechanical instability in the frontal plane.
Ankle strapping reduces the mechanical instability of the ankle joint in the saggital plane (anterior talar translation).	There was a significant reduction in anterior talar translation after strapping (Karlsson 1989; Vaes et al. 1984; Bruns et al. 1996). Anterior talar translation was not reduced significantly after strapping (using stress radiography) (Karlsson 1992).	Ankle strapping does not restore mechanical instability in the saggital plane, but possibly reduces it (some studies)..
Ankle strapping that is applied before exercise resists an inversion moment that is applied to an ankle.	The inversion moment required to invert the ankle to 30° was increased in taped cadaver ankles (Shapiro et al. 1994). Maximal resistance to an inversion moment before exercise was increased by 10% using ankle strapping, irrespective of application of pre-wrap (Manfroy et al. 1997).	Ankle strapping provides a mechanical resistance to inversion (in the absence of dynamic control function). Ankle strapping provides a mechanical resistance to inversion (in the presence of dynamic control function).
Ankle strapping that is applied before exercise resists an inversion moment that is applied to an ankle after an exercise session.	Maximal resistance to an inversion moment applied after exercise was not altered by ankle strapping applied before a vigorous 40-min exercise session (Manfroy et al. 1997).	Ankle strapping does not provide mechanical resistance to inversion after vigorous exercise (in the presence of dynamic control function).
Different methods of ankle strapping can affect the range of motion of the ankle joint.	Standard strapping with an additional subtalar sling decreased ankle range of motion more than standard strapping alone (Wilkerson 1991).	Strapping technique can alter the effects of strapping on ankle range of motion.
Ankle strapping that is applied before exercise decreases ankle range of motion before exercise.	Ankle strapping significantly decreased ankle range of motion before exercise (Fumich et al. 1981; Greene & Wright 1990; McCluskey et al. 1976).	Ankle strapping is effective in restricting ankle range of motion before exercise.
Ankle strapping that is applied before exercise decreases ankle range of motion after an exercise session.	Ankle strapping loosens after exercise and only restricts range of motion in extremes of motion (Fumich et al. 1981; McCluskey et al. 1976; Myburgh et al. 1984). Ankle strapping maximally reduced inversion and eversion range of motion 20 min into exercise (Greene & Wright 1990).	Ankle strapping is only effective in restricting extremes of ankle range of motion after short-duration exercise.
Ankle strapping that is applied before exercise improves the proprioceptive function of the ankle joint.	Ankle strapping has a stimulating effect on the peroneus brevis muscle in mechanically unstable ankles (Glick et al. 1976). Reaction time of the peroneus brevis muscle was significantly improved, but not normalized in taped mechanically unstable ankles (Karlsson 1992). Ankle strapping did not alter peroneal reaction time in unstable ankles (Konradsen & Bohsen Ravin 1991).	Most but not all studies show that ankle strapping improves parameters of proprioceptive function (peroneus brevis activation, mean and maximum postural sway, single-leg stance and jump tests, foot position error) in unstable ankles before exercise. Ankle strapping also appears to improve proprioceptive function (foot position error) in stable ankles before exercise.

(continued)

Table 33.4 *(continued)*

Hypothesis	Main finding(s)	Conclusion(s)
Ankle strapping that is applied before exercise improves the proprioceptive function of the ankle joint. *(continued)*	Maximum and mean postural sway decreased in functionally unstable taped ankles of football players before a practice session (Leanderson et al. 1996). Ankle strapping improved proprioceptive function (single leg stance test, single leg jump test, angle-reproduction test) (Jerosch et al. 1995). Foot position error on different sloped surfaces was significantly less in noninjured taped vs. untaped ankles before exercise (Robbins et al. 1995). There was no significant difference in movement perception between a control vs ankle sprain group in taped and. untaped conditions (Refshauge et al. 2000)	
Ankle strapping that is applied before exercise improves proprioceptive function of the ankle joint after an exercise session.	Foot position error on different sloped surfaces after exercise was significantly more than before exercise (Robbins et al. 1995). Maximum and mean postural sway decreased in functionally unstable untaped ankles of football players after vs before a practice session (Leanderson et al. 1996). Foot position error on different sloped surfaces after exercise was significantly less in noninjured taped vs untaped ankles (Robbins et al. 1995). Maximum and mean postural sway decreased in functionally unstable taped ankles of football players before a practice session (Leanderson et al. 1996).	Proprioceptive function (foot position error) of the normal joint decreases after exercise. Proprioceptive function (mean and maximum postural sway) of the unstable ankle joint increases after exercise. Ankle strapping improves proprioceptive function (foot position error) of the normal ankle joint after exercise. Ankle strapping does not improve proprioceptive function (mean and maximum postural sway) of the unstable ankle joint after exercise.

The results of most studies indicate that ankle strapping improves mechanical stability in the frontal plane. However, ankle strapping does not appear to restore mechanical stability in the sagittal plane to the same extent. It is possible that this may be related to the strapping technique that is used. Strapping techniques vary considerably among different studies.

The ability of strapping to resist an inversion moment applied to the ankle before an exercise session is well documented. This function of strapping is independent of the normal dynamic control function of the ankle joint. However, once an exercise session has been completed (in most instances more than 40 minutes of vigorous exercise), the ability of strapping to resist an inversion moment applied to the ankle is diminished. Similarly, strapping is effective in restricting ankle range of motion before an exercise session, but after exercise, strapping can only limit extremes of range of motion.

Biomechanical studies show that one of the most important benefits of strapping is its ability to improve parameters of proprioceptive function (peroneus brevis activation, mean and maximum postural sway, single-leg stance and jump tests, foot position error). This benefit is mainly demonstrated in previously injured unstable ankles and is particularly evident before an exercise session. However, it has been documented that ankle strapping also appears to reduce ankle dorsiflexion range of motion (Cordova et al. 2000) and improve one parameter of proprioceptive function (foot position error) in noninjured stable ankles before exercise.

It has been shown that after an exercise session, two parameters of proprioceptive function, namely mean and maximum postural sway, improve in unstable ankle joints, whereas foot position error in a normal ankle joint deteriorates. However, it has been shown that after exercise, ankle strapping improves proprioceptive function (foot position error) of the normal ankle joint, but does not improve proprioceptive function (mean and maximum postural sway) of the unstable ankle joint. The precise reasons for these findings are not clear, and require further investigation.

Clinical Studies

A number of studies have been conducted to determine the effects of ankle strapping on the incidence of ankle sprains in a variety of sports (table 33.5). In a recently published meta-analysis, it was concluded that strapping can reduce the incidence of ankle sprains (Verhagen et al. 2000).

It is, however, very important to draw a distinction between the potential benefit of strapping in noninjured ankles (primary prevention) and in previously injured ankles (secondary prevention). From the clinical studies, there is limited evidence that ankle strapping reduces the risk (incidence) of ankle sprains in normal (noninjured) ankles. These findings would indicate that, despite providing mechanical support to the normal ankle, strapping does not protect the ankle from sprains. The results from biomechanical studies indicate that the possible reasons for this may be that either the mechanical support offered by strapping in a normal ankle is only temporary (due to loss of support during the exercise session), or that there are no additional positive effects of strapping on the proprioceptive control of the normal ankle.

However, there is stronger evidence that ankle strapping can reduce the incidence of ankle sprains in previously injured ankles. The results from the bio-

mechanical studies indicate that the main reason for this is probably improved proprioceptive function throughout the exercise session, rather than mechanical support, which diminishes throughout the exercise session.

An important consideration for any athlete or coach is whether strapping could negatively affect exercise performance. A number of studies have been conducted to examine this question. Studies differ considerably with respect to the type of performance tests used. In table 33.6, the results and conclusions from studies examining the effects of taping on a variety of performance parameters are summarized.

The results of studies examining the effects of ankle strapping on exercise performance show that strapping can negatively affect a number of performance parameters. These include muscle strength, reaction time, fine motor coordination of the foot, and submaximal endurance. Performance parameters for which there is some, but not strong, evidence that strapping reduces performance are vertical jump ability and sprinting ability.

In summary, ankle strapping can reduce the incidence of acute ankle sprains in those individuals who previously sustained an ankle injury. The mechanism for the reduction in injury appears to involve improved proprioceptive function, rather than mechanical support. However, there is also some evidence that ankle strapping can negatively affect certain performance parameters, and this has to be taken into consideration when applying ankle strapping. There are insufficient studies to indicate which material or strapping technique should be employed.

Table 33.5 Strapping in the Prevention of Acute Ankle Sprains: Clinical Studies

Hypothesis	Some parameters and main finding(s)	Conclusion(s)
Strapping decreases the incidence of ankle sprains in noninjured players.	297 college football players (retrospective study, nonrandomized, no control group with no stabilizer or tape). The incidence of injury (injuries/1,000 exposures) in games was: high top and tape (13.5), low top and tape (9.5), high top and stabilizer (7.0), low top and stabilizer (1.6) (Rovere et al. 1988). 6 handball teams were studied over 2 years. Untaped players had a significantly greater incidence of ankle sprains compared with untaped players (Lindenberger et al. 1985 in Renström & Konradson 1997).	Ankle strapping may reduce the incidence of ankle sprains in previously noninjured ankles.
Strapping decreases the incidence of ankle sprains in previously injured players.	2,563 players with previous ankle sprains using ankle strapping with high support shoes. Incidence of ankle sprains in taped players (6.5/1,000 games) was less than untaped players (30.4/1,000 games) (Garrick & Requa 1973).	Ankle strapping in basketball players reduced the incidence of ankle sprains in previously injured ankles.

Table 33.6 The Effects of Strapping of the Ankle Joint on Exercise Performance

Performance parameter	Main finding(s)	Conclusion(s)
Explosive power	Ankle strapping did not affect vertical jump ability (Greene & Wright 1990; Verbrugge 1996). Ankle strapping did not affect broad jump ability (Burks et al. 1991). Ankle strapping reduced vertical jump ability (MacKean et al. 1995; Burks et al.1991).	There is some evidence that strapping can reduce explosive power as measured by vertical or broad jump tests.
Muscle strength	Ankle strapping reduced ankle strength in plantarflexion (14-22%) and in inversion (15-28%) (Kauranen et al. 1997).	Ankle strapping reduces plantarflexion and inversion muscle strength.
Sprinting/running	Ankle strapping did not affect 40 m sprint time (Verbrugge 1996). Ankle strapping reduced 40 m sprint performance (3.5%) (Burks et al. 1991). Ankle strapping did not affect agility running performance (Verbrugge 1996). Ankle strapping reduced 10 m shuttle run performance (1.6%) (Burks et al. 1991).	There is some evidence suggesting that strapping can reduce sprinting performance and shuttle run performance.
Reaction time	Ankle strapping reduced reaction time by 9-12% (Kauranen et al. 1997).	Ankle strapping reduces reaction time.
Fine motor coordination	Ankle strapping reduced foot tapping speed by 14% (Kauranen et al. 1997).	Ankle strapping reduces foot tapping speed.
Motor skill	Ankle strapping did not affect jump shot accuracy (basketball) (MacKean et al. 1995).	Ankle strapping does not affect jump shot accuracy in basketball.
Endurance	Ankle strapping reduced submaximal running performance (MacKean et al. 1995).	Ankle strapping reduces submaximal running performance.

Ankle Orthoses

The use of ankle orthoses to reduce the risk of ankle sprains has increased over the last two decades. There are a large variety of commercial braces available, each incorporating different design properties. It therefore becomes difficult to interpret the biomechanical and clinical studies that have been performed to determine the possible protective role of ankle orthoses in both noninjured (normal) and previously injured ankles.

Biomechanical Studies

A number of studies have been conducted to examine the biomechanical effects of ankle braces on the ankle joint. Studies have been designed to test a number of hypotheses. These include the effect of ankle orthoses on mechanical stability of the ankle in the frontal and sagittal planes, the ability of ankle orthoses to resist an inversion moment that is applied to the ankle joint, the ability of an ankle orthosis to restrict ankle range of motion before and after exercise, and the effect of orthoses on proprioceptive function of the ankle (table 33.7).

Biomechanical studies show that ankle braces are effective in providing mechanical stability to the ankle joint in both the frontal and the sagittal planes (Cordova et al. 2000). Furthermore, ankle braces effectively resist the application of an inversion moment that is applied to the ankle joint. However, there is no evidence that this property is still present after an exercise session. Ankle braces are also effective in reducing inversion ankle range of motion, both before and after an exercise session. This indicates that ankle braces appear to retain their properties after an exercise session better than strapping does.

Finally, biomechanical studies also indicate that ankle orthoses improve proprioceptive function of unstable ankle joints before an exercise session. The ability of orthoses to retain this effect after an exercise session has not been tested.

Table 33.7 Ankle Bracing With Orthoses in the Prevention of Acute Ankle Sprains: Biomechanical Studies

Hypothesis	Main finding(s)	Conclusion
Ankle bracing reduces the mechanical instability of the ankle joint in the frontal plane (talar tilt, internal/external rotation).	Ankle bracing (Push) reduced subtalar eversion but not plantar/dorsiflexion during running (De Clercq 1997). Ankle orthoses reduced but did not prevent talar tilt during running and sudden inversion (Scheuffelen et al. 1993). Ankle bracing (Adimed Stabil 2, Basko Camp, Cliagamed, Malleocast, Malleo-Med, Mikros OV, Push, Talocrur) reduced internal and external rotation of the ankle joint (Bruns et al. 1996).	Ankle bracing reduces the mechanical instability of the ankle in the frontal plane.
Ankle bracing reduces the mechanical instability of the ankle joint in the saggital plane (anterior talar translation).	Ankle bracing (Malleoloc) minimally reduced anterior translation of the ankle joint (Wiley & Nigg 1996). Ankle bracing (Adimed Stabil 2, Basko Camp, Cliagamed, Malleocast, Malleo-Med, Mikros OV, Push, Talocrur) reduced anterior translation of the ankle joint (Bruns et al. 1996).	Most ankle braces appear to reduce the mechanical instability of the ankle joint in the saggital plane.
Ankle bracing that is applied before exercise resists an inversion moment that is applied to an ankle.	Ankle bracing (McDavid Ankle-Guard, Air-Stirrup, Gelcast, Super-8, Donjoy FG-062, Eclipse Excel Ankle Support, Ankle Stabilizer, High Top Ankle Support) resists an inversion moment that is applied to the ankle (Shapiro et al. 1994). Ankle bracing (Axini, Push) applied to the ankle before exercise reduced the inversion ankle torque during static and dynamic conditions (Thonnard et al. 1996).	Ankle braces applied before an exercise session resist an inversion moment that is applied to the ankle.
Ankle bracing that is applied before exercise decreases ankle range of motion before exercise.	Ankle bracing (nonrigid subtalar stabilizer [STS]) reduced ankle inversion range of motion during vertical loading (Anderson et al. 1995). Ankle bracing (Leuko, Nessa, Donjoy ALP, Malleoloc) reduced ankle inversion range of motion (Gross et al. 1994; Tweedy et al. 1994).	Ankle braces applied before an exercise session reduce inversion range of motion of the ankle joint.
Ankle bracing that is applied before exercise decreases ankle range of motion after an exercise session.	Ankle bracing (Leuko, Nessa, Donjoy ALP, Malleoloc) reduced ankle inversion range of motion after 20-40 min exercise session (Tweedy et al. 1994; Gross et al. 1994).	Ankle braces applied before an exercise session reduce inversion range of motion of the ankle joint after an exercise session.
Ankle bracing that is applied before exercise improves the proprioceptive function of the ankle joint.	Ankle bracing (Mikros, Aircast) improved proprioceptive function in unstable ankle joints (single-leg stance test, single-leg jump test, angle-reproduction test) (Jerosch et al. 1995). Rigid and flexible ankle orthoses improved postural sway in unstable ankles (Baier & Hopf et al. 1998). Custom-made foot orthotics improved postural sway in sprained ankles (Guskiewicz & Perrin 1996).	Ankle braces improve proprioceptive function of the ankle joint before an exercise session.

Clinical Studies

A number of clinical studies have tested the hypotheses that ankle bracing reduces the incidence of ankle sprains in normal ankles (primary prevention) and previously injured ankles (secondary prevention) (table 33.8).

The results from studies examining the role of an ankle orthosis in the primary prevention of ankle sprains are conflicting (Callaghan 1997). In some studies, the incidence of ankle sprains in previously noninjured ankles is reduced by wearing an ankle orthosis (Rovere et al. 1988; Sitler et al. 1994). However, in other studies, this finding could not be confirmed (Surve et al. 1994; Tropp et al. 1985). In two studies (Sitler et al. 1994; Surve et al. 1994), subjects were randomly allocated to treatment groups, and followed in a prospective manner. At best, it can be concluded that there is some, but weak, evidence that prophylactic bracing with an ankle orthosis could reduce the risk of first-time ankle sprains.

The value of an ankle brace in the secondary prevention of ankle sprains is clear (Verhagen et al. 2000). There is particularly strong evidence to indicate that previously injured players will reduce their risk of recurrent ankle sprains by wearing an ankle orthosis (Quinn et al. 2000). However, this has not been tested for all the different types of ankle orthoses. Finally, in one study, it was shown that the incidence of recurrent, severe ankle sprains is reduced by wearing an ankle orthosis (Surve et al. 1994).

A concern that can be raised if ankle orthoses are worn is that an orthosis can transmit high forces to the knee joint, and thereby increase the incidence of knee injuries. This hypothesis has been tested in two studies. In both these studies, the wearing of ankle braces did not result in an increase in the incidence of knee injuries in soccer players (Surve et al. 1994) or basketball players (Sitler et al. 1994).

The possible negative effect of wearing an ankle orthosis on exercise performance has also been investigated in a number of studies (table 33.9).

The results of studies that are available indicate that, in most instances, ankle braces do not decrease explosive power, sprint performance, or agility running performance. However, the effect of ankle

Table 33.8 Ankle Bracing With Orthoses in the Prevention of Acute Ankle Sprains: Clinical Studies

Hypothesis	Some parameters and main finding(s)	Conclusion(s)
Ankle orthoses decrease the incidence of ankle sprains in normal (noninjured) ankles.	111 soccer players with no previous ankle problems were allocated nonrandomly to either an ankle orthosis (Step 1) group or control group. The seasonal incidence (%) of ankle sprains in the orthosis group (6.7%) was similar to the control group (11.5%) (values calculated from data in tables) (Tropp et al. 1985). 297 college football players (retrospective study, nonrandomized, no control group with no stabilizer or tape). The incidence of injury (injuries/1,000 exposures) in games was: high top and tape (13.5), low top and tape (9.5), high top and stabilizer (7.0), low top and stabilizer (1.6) (Rovere et al. 1988). 1,601 recreational basketball players with normal ankles wearing either an ankle brace (Aircast Sports Stirrup) or no brace. The incidence of ankle sprains (per 1,000 exposures) was lower in the brace group (1.6/1,000) compared with the control group (5.2/1,000) (Sitler et al. 1994). 629 soccer players were studied in different groups over a season. In the players with normal ankles, there was no difference in the incidence of ankle sprains in players wearing a Sports Stirrup ankle brace (0.97/1,000 hrs) compared with players not wearing a brace (0.92/1,000 hrs) (Surve et al. 1994).	There is weak evidence that ankle orthoses worn by athletes on normal (noninjured) ankles decrease the risk of an ankle sprain. The incidence of ankle sprains in players wearing an ankle orthosis on a normal ankle may be affected by the shoe type worn by the player.

Hypothesis	Some parameters and main finding(s)	Conclusion(s)
Ankle orthoses decrease the incidence of ankle sprains in abnormal (previously injured) ankles.	120 soccer players with a previous ankle problem were allocated nonrandomly to either an ankle orthosis (Step 1) group or control group. The seasonal incidence (%) of ankle sprains in the orthosis group (2%) was lower than that in the control group (25%) (Tropp et al. 1985). 629 soccer players were studied in different groups over a season. In the players with previously injured ankles, there was a lower incidence of ankle sprains in players wearing a Sports Stirrup ankle brace (0.46/1,000 hrs) compared with players not wearing a brace (1.16/1,000 hrs) (Surve et al. 1994).	There is strong evidence that ankle orthoses decrease the incidence of ankle sprains in players who had a previous ankle sprain.
Ankle orthoses decrease the incidence of severe ankle sprains in abnormal (previously injured) ankles.	629 soccer players were studied in different groups over a season. In the players with previously injured ankles, there was a lower incidence of severe (Grade II and III) ankle sprains in players wearing a Sports Stirrup ankle brace (0.0.14/1,000 hrs) compared with players not wearing a brace (0.77/1,000 hrs) (Surve et al. 1994).	There is some evidence that the incidence of severe ankle injuries in previously injured ankles can be reduced by an ankle orthosis.

Table 33.9 The Effects of Ankle Orthoses on Exercise Performance

Performance parameter	Main finding(s)	Conclusion(s)
Explosive power	Ankle bracing (Donjoy ALP, Aircast, Malleoloc) did not affect vertical jump performance (Gross et al. 1994; Wiley & Nigg 1996; Gross et al. 1997). Ankle bracing decreased vertical jump performance (Swede-O-brace, 4%; Kallassy, 3.4%) (Burks et al. 1991). Ankle bracing (Kallassy) did not affect broad jump performance (Burks et al. 1991). Ankle bracing decreased broad jump performance (Swede-O-brace, 3.6%) (Burks et al. 1991).	In most instances, ankle bracing does not decrease vertical jump or broad jump performance.
Sprinting/running	Ankle bracing (Aircast, Kallassy, Donjoy ALP) did not affect 40 m sprint performance (Verbrugge 1996; Gross et al. 1996; Burks et al. 1991; Gross et al. 1997). Ankle bracing (Swede-O-brace, Kallassy) did not affect 10 m shuttle run performance (Burks et al. 1991). Ankle bracing (Swede-O-brace, 3.2%) reduced 40 m sprint performance (Burks et al. 1991). Ankle bracing (Aircast, Malleoloc, Donjoy ALP) did not affect agility running performance (Verbrugge 1996; Gross et al. 1996; Wiley & Nigg 1996; Gross et al. 1997).	In most instances, ankle bracing does not affect running or sprinting performance.

orthoses on muscle strength, reaction time, fine motor coordination, motor skill, and endurance has not been investigated. It must be pointed out that not all the types of braces have been assessed, and preliminary data show that different braces have different effects on exercise performance.

Other Extrinsic Risk Factors

The last three extrinsic risk factors in acute ankle sprains are the playing surface, role of match play vs. training, and player position. These three risk factors have not been well studied. The scientific evidence for these extrinsic factors as risk factors for acute ankle sprains will now be discussed.

■ **Playing surface.** It is commonly suggested that the playing field surface can be a risk factor for sport injuries, including ankle sprains (Levy et al. 1990; Skovron et al. 1990). In particular, artificial turf or wet playing fields have been suggested as risk factors for ankle injuries (Ekstrand & Nigg 1989; Skovron et al. 1990). A number of biomechanical studies have shown that the interaction between playing surface and footwear is important and can affect the forces that are applied to the ankle and the lower limb (Ekstrand & Nigg 1989; Heidt et al.

1996). There is, however, very little evidence from clinical epidemiological studies that playing surface is a cause for ankle injuries. In one prospective study, which was conducted over a soccer season, no relationship between wet playing field conditions and ankle sprains could be established (Schwellnus et al. 1992).

■ **Match play.** A number of studies have shown that the incidence of ankle injuries is higher during match play than during practices. This holds true for a number of different sports including volleyball (Bahr et al. 1994; Yde & Nielsen 1988) and soccer (Surve 1991).

■ **Player position.** It has been well documented that in a number of different sports, the incidence of ankle sprains is higher in certain player positions (Rovere et al. 1988; Surve 1991) or court positions (Bahr et al. 1994).

■ Intrinsic Risk Factors

A number of intrinsic risk factors for ankle sprains have been suggested (table 33.10). These include a previous ankle sprain, poor proprioceptive function, ankle eversion/inversion muscle strength, ankle

Table 33.10 Intrinsic Risk Factors for Acute Ankle Sprains in Sport

Hypotheses	Some parameters and main findings	Conclusion(s)
Previous ankle sprain	The seasonal incidence (%) of ankle sprains in soccer players with a previous ankle sprain was 47% compared with the noninjured players (25%) (Ekstrand & Gillquist 1983).	There is strong evidence to suggest that a previous ankle sprain is a significant risk factor for an ankle sprain.
	The incidence of ankle sprains in military recruits that were previously injured was higher than in noninjured recruits (Milgrom et al. 1991).	
	The seasonal incidence (%) of ankle sprains in 117 soccer players was higher in the group with a previous ankle "problem" (25%) compared with the group with "no previous problem" (11%) (Tropp et al. 1985).	
	Recreational basketball players with a previous ankle injury had a 1.4 times greater risk to suffer from a repeat injury (Sitler et al. 1994).	
	Soccer players with a history of a previous ankle sprain had a higher incidence (0.86/1,000 hrs play) of ankle sprains (0.46/1,000 hrs) (Surve et al. 1994).	
	There was no evidence that a previous ankle injury increased the risk of ankle sprains in studies on basketball (Barret et al. 1993; Sitler et al. 1994), field hockey, or lacrosse (Baumhauer et al. 1995a and b).	

Hypotheses	Some parameters and main findings	Conclusion(s)
Poor proprioceptive function or balance	The seasonal incidence of ankle sprains in soccer players with a previous ankle problem was higher in a group not performing ankle disk training compared with a group performing ankle disk training (Tropp et al. 1985). There was no evidence that a positive Romberg's test preseason is associated with an increased risk of ankle sprains in soccer players (Schwellnus et al. 1992). Subjects with high sway scores (poor balance) had 7 times as many ankle sprains compared with a control group (low sway scores) (McGuine et al. 2000).	There are only a few studies that have studied the role of proprioception or poor balance in the prevention of ankle sprains. At present there is only weak epidemiological evidence that decreased proprioceptive function or poor balance is a risk factor for ankle sprains.
Ankle eversion and inversion muscle strength	A prospective study on 145 college athletes showed that the ankle eversion to inversion muscle strength ratio was greater in the injured (ankle inversion sprains) vs noninjured group (Baumhauer et al. 1995a). A supervised rehabilitation program, including muscle strength, resulted in a reduced incidence of ankle sprains (control 29%, rehabilitation group 7%) (Holme et al. 1999).	Weak ankle inversion (lower inversion to eversion strength ratio) has been identified as a significant risk factor for ankle sprains.
Ankle dorsiflexion and plantarflexion muscle strength	A prospective study on 145 college athletes showed that the ankle plantarflexion strength as well as plantar- to dorsiflexion muscle strength ratio was greater in the injured (ankle inversion sprains) vs non-injured group (Baumhauer et al. 1995a).	Weak ankle dorsiflexion strength (in cluding lower dorsiflexion to eversion strength ratio) has been identified as a significant risk factor for ankle sprains.
Foot type and alignment	A prospective study on 145 college athletes showed that the ankle eversion to inversion muscle strength ratio was greater in the injured (ankle inversion sprains) vs. non-injured group (Baumhauer et al. 1995a)	Specific anatomical foot types have not been identified as risk factors for ankle injuries.
Ankle joint range of motion	Ankle range of motion did not predict ankle injuries in ballet dancers (Wiesler et al. 1996). A prospective study on 145 college athletes showed that subtalar inversion range of motion, but not generalized laxity (Beighton score), was greater in the injured (ankle inversion sprains) vs noninjured group (Baumhauer et al. 1995a). In a prospective study, decreased dorsiflexion range of motion was not associated with an increased incidence of ankle sprains in soccer players (Schwellnus et al. 1992).	Generalized laxity and ankle dorsi-range of motion are not associated with increased risk of ankle sprains, but increased subtalar joint range of motion may be a risk factor.
Dominance	The dominant leg of soccer players sustained more ankle injuries than the nondominant leg (Ekstrand & Gillquist 1983). In a prospective study on 145 college athletes, left leg dominance was identified as a risk factor for ankle sprains (Baumhauer et al. 1995a).	There is some evidence to suggest that dominant ankles are more likely to be injured than the nondominant ankles.

(continued)

Table 33.10 *(continued)*

Hypotheses	Some parameters and main findings	Conclusion(s)
Dominance (continued)	629 soccer players were studied in different groups over a season. There was a higher incidence of ankle sprains in dominant (0.64/1,000 hrs) compared with nondominant ankles (0.28/1,000 hrs) (not statistically significant) (Surve et al. 1994).	
Gender	In a prospective study of 4,940 female and 6,840 male collegiate basketball players, females had a 25% greater risk of sustaining a grade I ankle sprain (Hosea et al. 2000).	Female athletes may have a higher risk of sustaining an acute ankle sprain when paricipating in the same sport as males

dorsiflexion/plantarflexion muscle strength, foot type and alignment, ankle joint range of motion, dominance, and gender. The scientific evidence that all these factors are indeed risk factors for ankle sprains is not clear in all instances. In table 33.10, the main findings of some of the important studies, and the conclusions that can be drawn from these studies regarding the relationship between the postulated risk factors and ankle sprains, are depicted.

A previous ankle sprain is a significant risk factor for a repeat ankle sprain. This is suggested by the findings of most of the prospective studies that have been conducted to determine the relationship between the risk of ankle sprains and previous ankle injury. Evidence that poor proprioceptive function is a risk factor for an ankle sprain is less convincing. This risk factor is commonly postulated as the mechanism by which a previous injury predisposes to a repeat injury. However, more clinical studies are required to confirm that poor proprioception is a risk factor for ankle sprains.

It has recently been shown, in a prospective clinical study, that both weak ankle eversion and dorsiflexion muscle strength are associated with ankle sprains. The findings of this study need to be confirmed by others. However, current evidence suggests that ankle muscle weakness is a risk factor for ankle sprains. In two recently published reviews, it was concluded that rehabilitation, in particular proprioceptive training, could reduce the incidence of ankle sprains in athletes with recurrent ankle sprains (Thacker et al. 1999; Verhagen et al. 2000).

Foot type and lower limb alignment do not appear to be risk factors for ankle injuries, and only excessive subtalar joint range of motion, rather than generalized laxity, is a risk factor for ankle sprains. Finally, there is some, but not strong, evidence that the dominant limb is more at risk for sustaining an ankle sprain than the nondominant limb.

■ Summary and Practical Application

In this chapter, the prevention of ankle sprains has been reviewed by considering the scientific evidence that supports specific extrinsic and intrinsic risk factors for ankle sprains. Any ankle injury prevention program should follow a stepwise approach by first considering which proposed extrinsic and intrinsic risk factors for ankle sprains have strong or reasonable scientific evidence to support their role as risk factors. In addition, modifiable risk factors need to be identified in a specific athlete or group of athletes, preferably in the preseason period. A suitable preventive program can then be implemented to correct the modifiable risk factors that have been identified.

Three Steps in Prevention

Step 1: What are the "true" risk factors for ankle sprains in sports?

Extrinsic risk factors

- Poor footwear
- Lack of external ankle support in previously injured ankles
- Match play
- Player position

Intrinsic risk factors

- Previous ankle sprain
- Poor proprioceptive function
- Ankle muscle weakness
- Dominance
- Gender

Step 2: Assessment of the athlete(s)

History

- Previous ankle injury
- Feeling of weakness or instability
- Footwear use
- Player position
- Dominance
- Use of external ankle support

Clinical examination

- Ankle muscle strength
- Subtalar joint range of motion
- Mechanical and functional instability
- Proprioception

Special investigations

- Isokinetic muscle strength (plantar-/dorsiflexion and inversion/eversion)
- Proprioception (stabilometry, postural sway)

Step 3: Preventive measures

- Attend to footwear
- Provide external support (previously injured ankles)
- Muscle strength training
- Proprioceptive training
- Sport-specific conditioning

■ References

Anderson DL, Sanderson DJ, Henning EM. 1995. The role of external nonrigid ankle bracing in limiting ankle inversion. Clin J Sports Med 5(1):18-24.

Bahr R, Karlsen R, Lian O, Ovrebo R. 1994. Incidence and mechanisms of acute ankle inversion injuries in volleyball. A retrospective cohort study. Am J Sports Med 22:595-600.

Baier M, Hopf T. 1998. Ankle orthoses effect on single-limb standing balance in athletes with functional ankle instability. Arch Phys Med Rehabil 79 (8):939-944.

Barker HB, Beynnon BD, Renström PAFH. 1977. Ankle injury risk factors in sports. Sports Med 23 (2):69-74.

Barrett J, Bilisko T. 1995. The role of shoes in the prevention of ankle sprains. Sports Med 20(4):277-280.

Barrett JR, Tanji JL, Drake C, Fuller D, Kawasaki RI, Fenton RM. 1993. High- versus low-top shoes for the prevention of ankle sprains in basketball players. A prospective randomized study. Am J Sports Med 21(4):582-585.

Baumhauer JF, Alosa DM, Renström PAFH, Trevino S, Beynnon B. 1995a. A prospective study of ankle injury risk factors. Am J Sports Med 5:564-570.

Baumhauer JF, Alosa DM, Renström PAFH, Trevino S, Beynnon B. 1995b. Test re-test reliability of ankle injury risk factors. Am J Sports Med 23:571-574.

Bonstingl RW, Morehouse CA, Niebel BW. 1975. Torques developed by different types of shoes on various playing surfaces. Med Sci Sports 7(2):127-131.

Bruns J, Scherlitz J, Luessenhop S. 1996. The stabilizing effect of orthotic devices on plantar flexion/dorsal extension and horizontal rotation of the ankle joint. Int J Sports Med 17:614-618.

Burks RT, Bill BG, Marcus R, Barker HB. 1991. Analysis of athletic performance with prophylactic ankle devices. Am J Sports Med 19:104-106.

Callaghan MJ. 1997. Role of ankle taping and bracing in the athlete. Br J Sports Med 31:102-108.

Cordova ML, Ingersoll CD, LeBlanc MJ. 2000. Influence of ankle support on joint range of motion before and after exercise: a meta-analysis. J Orthop Sports Phys Ther 30(4):170-177.

De Clercq DL. 1997. Ankle bracing in running: the effect of a Push type medium ankle brace upon movements of the foot and ankle during the stance phase. Int J Sports Med 18 (3):222-228.

Ekstrand J, Gillquist J. 1983. Soccer injuries and their mechanisms: a prospective study. Med Sci Sports Exerc 15(3):267-270.

Ekstrand J, Nigg BM. 1989. Surface-related injuries in soccer. Sports Med 8(1):56-62.

Fumich RM, Ellsion AE, Guerin GJ, Grace PD. 1981. The measured effect of taping on combined foot and ankle motion before and after exercise. Am J Sports Med 9(3):165-170.

Garrick JG. 1977. The frequency of injury, mechanism of injury and epidemiology of ankle sprains. Am J Sports Med 5:241-242.

Garrick JG, Requa RK. 1973. Role of external support in the prevention of ankle sprains. Med Sci Sports 5:200-203.

Glick JM, Gordon RB, Nishimoto D. 1976. The prevention and treatment of ankle injuries. Am J Sports Med 4:136-141.

Greene TA, Wright CR. 1990. A comparative support evaluation of three ankle orthosis before, during and after exercise. J Orthop Sports Phys 11:453-456.

Gross MT, Batten AM, Lamm AL, Lorren JL, Stevens JJ, Davis JM, Wilerson GB. 1994a. Comparison of Donjoy ankle ligament protector and subtalar sling ankle taping in restricting foot and ankle motion before and after exercise. J Orthop Sports Phys Ther 19(1):33-41.

Gross MT, Clemence LM, Cox BD, McMillan HP, Meadows AF, Piland CS, Powers WS. 1997. Effect of lateral orthoses on functional performance of individuals with recurrent lateral ankle sprains. J Orthop Sports Phys Ther 25(4):245-252.

Gross MT, Everts JR, Roberson SE, Roskin DS, Young KD. 1994b. Effect of Donjoy ankle ligament protector and Aircast Sport-Stirrup orthoses on functional performance. J Orthop Sports Phys Ther 19(3):150-156.

Guskiewicz KM, Perrin DH. 1996. Effect of orthotics on postural sway following inversion ankle sprain. J Orthop Sports Phys Ther 23(5):326-331.

Heidt RS, Dormer SG, Cawley PW, Scranton PE, Losse G, Howard M. 1996. Differences in friction and torsional resistance in athletic shoe-turf surface interfaces. Am J Sports Med 24(6):834-842.

Holme E, Magnusson SP, Becher K, Bieler T, Aagaard P, Kjaer M. 1999. The effect of supervised rehabilitation on strength, postural sway, position sense and re-injury risk after acute ankle ligament sprain. Scand J Med Sci Sports 9(2):104-109.

Hosea TM, Carey CC, Harrer MF. 2000. The gender issue: epidemiology of ankle injuries in athletes who participate in basketball. Clin Orthop 372:45-49.

Jerosch J, Hoffstetter I, Bork H, Bischof M. 1995. The influence of orthoses on the proprioception of the ankle joint. Knee Surg Sports Traumatol Arthrosc 3(1):39-46.

Karlsson J. 1989. Chronic lateral instability of the ankle joint: a clinical radiological and experimental study [dissertation]. University of Goteborg, Goteborg, Sweden.

Karlsson J. 1992. The effect of external ankle support in chronic lateral ankle joint instability: an electromyographic study. Am J Sports Med 20:257-261.

Karlsson J, Sward L, Andreasson GO. 1993. The effect of taping on ankle stability. Practical implications. Sports Med 16:210-215.

Kauranen K, Sira P, Vanharanta H. 1997. The effect of strapping on the motor performance of the ankle and wrist joints. Scan J Med Sci Sports 7(4):238-243.

Konradsen L, Bohsen Ravin J. 1991. Prolonged peroneal reaction time in ankle instability. Int J Sports Med 12:290-292.

Larsen E. 1984. Taping the ankle for chronic instability. Acta Orthop Scand 55:551-553.

Leanderson J, Eriksson E, Nilsson C, Wykman A. 1996. Proprioception in classical ballet dancers: a prospective study of the influence of an ankle sprain on proprioception in the ankle joint. Am J Sports Med 24:370-374.

Levy IM, Skovron ML, Agel J. 1990. Living with artificial grass: a knowledge update. Part 1: basic science. Am J Sports Med 18(4):406-412.

Lindenberger U, Resse D, Andreasson G et al. 1985. The effect of prophylactic taping of ankles. Gothenburg, Sweden: Chalmers Technical University.

MacKean LC, Bell G, Burnham RS. 1995. Prophylactic ankle bracing vs. taping: effects on functional performance in female basketball players. J Orthop Sports Phys Ther 22(2):77-81.

Manfroy PP, Ashton-Miller JA, Wojtys EM. 1997. The effect of exercise, prewrap, and athletic tape on the maximal active and passive ankle resistance to ankle inversion. Am J Sports Med 25(2):156-163.

McCluskey GM, Blackburn TA, Lewis T. 1976. Prevention of ankle sprains. Am J Sports Med 4:151-157.

McGuine TA, Greene JJ, Best T, Leverson G. 2000. Balance as a predictor of ankle injuries in high school basketball players. Clin J Sports Med 10(4):239-244.

Milgrom C, Shlamkovitch N, Finestone A, Eldad A, Laor A, Danon YL, Lavie O, Wosk J, Simkin A. 1991. Risk factors for the lateral ankle sprain: A prospective study among military recruits. Foot Ankle 12(1):26-30.

Myburgh KH, Vaughan CL, Isaacs SK. 1984. The effects of ankle guards and taping on joint motion before, during and after a squash match. Am J Sports Med 12(6):441-446.

Petrov O, Blocker K, Bradbury R, Saxena A, Toy ML. 1988. Footwear and ankle stability in the basketball player. Clin Podiatr Med Surg 5(2):275-290.

Quigley TB, Cox J, Murphy J. 1946. Protective device for the ankle. J Am Med Assoc 123:924.

Quinn K, Parker P, de Bie R, Rowe B, Handoll H. 2000. Interventions for preventing ankle ligament injuries. Cochrane Database Syst Rev 2:CD000018.

Refshauge KM, Kilbreath SL, Raymond J. 2000. The effect of recurrent ankle inversion sprain and taping on proprioception at the ankle. Med Sci Sports 32(1):10-15.

Renström PAF, Konradson L. 1997. Ankle ligament injuries. Br J Sports Med 31:11-20.

Robbins SE, Gouw GJ. 1991. Athletic footwear: unsafe due to perceptual illusions. Med Sci Sports Exerc 22(2):217-224.

Robbins S, Waked E. 1998. Factors associated with ankle injuries: preventive measures. Sports Med 25(1):63-72.

Robbins S, Waked E, Rappel R. 1995. Ankle taping improves proprioception before and after exercise in young men. Br J Sports Med 29(4):242-247.

Rovere GD, Clarke TJ, Yates CS, Burley K. 1988. Retrospective comparison of taping and ankle stabilizers in preventing ankle injuries. Am J Sports Med 16(3):228-233.

Scheuffelen C, Rapp W, Golhoer A, Lohrer H. 1993. Orthotic devices in functional treatment of ankle sprain. Stabilizing effects during real movements. Int J Sports Med 14(3):140-149.

Schwellnus MP, Surve IN, Noakes TD. 1992. Does heel cord stretching prevent ankle injuries in soccer players? Am J Sports Med 24(5):S145.

Shapiro MS, Kabo M, Mitchell PW, Loren G, Tsenter M. 1994. Ankle sprain prophylaxis: an analysis of the stabilizing effects of braces and tape. Am J Sports Med 22:71-82.

Sitler M, Ryan J, Wheeler B, McBride J, Arciero R, Anderson J, Horodyski M. 1994. The efficacy of a semirigid ankle stabilizer to reduce acute ankle injuries in basketball. Am J Sports Med 22(4):454-461.

Skovron ML, Levy IM, Agel J. 1990. Living with artificial grass: a knowledge update. Part 2: epidemiology. Am J Sports Med 18(5):510-513.

Surve I. 1991. BSc (Hon) Sports Medicine thesis, Univeristy of Cape Town Medical School, South Africa.

Surve I, Schwellnus MP, Noakes TD. 1994. A fivefold reduction in the incidence of recurrent ankle sprains in soccer players using the Sport-Stirrup orthosis. Am J Sports Med 22(5):601-606.

Thacker SB, Stroup DF, Branche CM, Gilchrist J, Goodman RA, Weitman EA. 1999. The prevention of ankle sprains in sports. A systematic review of the literature. Am J Sports Med 27(6):753-760.

Thonnard JL, Bragard D, Willems PA, Plaghki L. 1996. Stability of the braced ankle. A biomechanical investigation. Am J Sports Med 24(3):356-361.

Tropp H, Askling C, Gillquist J. 1985. Prevention of ankle sprains. Am J Sports Med 13:259-262.

Tweedy R, Carson T, Vicenzino B. 1994. Leuko and Nessa ankle braces: effectiveness before and after exercise. Aust J Sci Med Sport 26(3-4):62-66.

Vaes P, De Boeck H, Handelberg F, Opdecam P. 1984. Comparative radiologic study of the influence of ankle joint bandages on ankle stability. Acta Orthop Belgique 50:636-644.

Vaes P, De Boeck H, Handelberg F, Opdecam P. 1985. Comparative radiologic study of the influence of ankle joint bandages on ankle stability. Am J Sports Med 13(1):46-50.

Vaes P, Duquet W, Handelberg F, Casteleyn PP, Van Tiggelen R, Opdecam P. 1998. Objective roetgenologic measurements of the influence of ankle braces on pathologic joint mobility. A comparison of 9 braces. Acta Orthop Belgique 64(2):201-209.

Verbrugge JD. 1996. The effects of semirigid Air-Stirrup bracing vs. adhesive ankle taping on motor performance. J Orthop Sports Phys Ther 23(5):320-325.

Verhagen EA, van Mechelen W, de Vente W. 2000. The effect of preventive measures on the incidence of ankle sprains. Clin J Sports Med 10(4):291-296.

Wiesler ER, Hunter DM, Martin DF, Curl WW, Hoen H. 1996. Ankle flexibility and injury patterns in dancers. Am J Sports Med 24(6):754-757.

Wiley JP, Nigg BM. 1996. The effect of an ankle orthosis on ankle range of motion and performance. J Orthop Sports Phys Ther 23(6):362-369.

Wilkerson GB. 1991. Comparative biomechanical effects of the standard method of ankle taping and a taping method designed to enhance subtalar instability. Am J Sports Med 19 (6):588-595.

Yamamoto T, Kigawa A, Xu T. 1993. Effectiveness of functional ankle taping for judo athletes: a comparison between judo bandaging and taping. Br J Sports Med 27(2):110-112.

Yde J, Nielsen AB. 1988. Epidemiological and traumatological analyses of injuries in a Danish Volleyball club. Ugeskr Laeger 150:1022-1023.

Chapter 34

Preventing Ankle Injuries in Parachuting

John B. Ryan, MD, FACS

A parachute (French: para = "preventing"; chute = "fall") is a large umbrella-shaped fabric canopy used to reduce the speed of a person or object falling from the air. Leonardo daVinci was the first to suggest, in 1514, the idea of a human falling in a controlled fashion to the ground, suspended underneath a canopy sail. In 1785, Jean Pierre Blanchard demonstrated the practicality of parachutes by dropping animals attached to small parachutes from balloons. In 1793, Blanchard broke his leg on landing while parachuting himself, and he thus became the first documented case of a parachute injury. In 1797, Andre Jack Garnevin became the first man to jump from a balloon, which he did at the height of 3,000 feet over Paris. His first parachute resembled a beach umbrella with a basket suspended beneath it. Captain Tom Baldwin advanced the art of parachuting by using a body harness connected to the parachute canopy by shroud lines, thus replacing the under slung basket used by Garnevin. Captain Albert Berry became the first man to jump from an aircraft in March of 1912, at St. Louis, Missouri. Parachutes became standard equipment for crew members of balloons and planes, and eventually became standard equipment for early passenger airplanes. Later, parachutes became an integral part of the ejection seat utilized in high-performance military aircraft.

Claire Lee Schennault, an American army officer, developed the idea of using aircraft and infantry soldiers with parachutes (paratroopers). In the late 1930s and early 1940s, several centers were developed to train military personnel in airborne operations. These specialized soldiers are frequently flown behind enemy lines to perform commando missions, secure airfields for routine troop landings, and provide flexibility for large-scale airborne invasions.

Although first developed to protect balloonists and airplane crew personnel, parachuting is a popular recreational event practiced by civilians. In 1983, it was reported that as many as 20 million people in the United States had made a parachute jump at one time in their life (Petras & Hoffman 1983).

■ Parachuting Apparatus and Technique

Parachutes have evolved over the years, but Leonardo daVinci's basic design is recognizable today—an object to be slowed in descent is attached to a large, minimally permeable cloth canopy by thin cords (risers).

How Parachutes Work

Although there are many different designs for parachutes, the basic principle is that the parachute canopy fills and traps air, which creates drag and slows the object that the canopy is attached to. There is a small hole in the apex of the canopy that allows air to escape slowly, preventing oscillation and providing some additional maneuverability. The design of the standard round parachute reduces the free-fall speed of a body in air from 54 m per second to a landing speed of approximately 5 to 6 m per second. This is the equivalent of jumping off a wall approximately 10 or 12 feet high. The parachute not only has a vertical speed component of 5 to 6 meters per second, but also has a linear velocity that is affected principally by prevailing ground winds.

Preparing to land in a parachute is similar to landing an airplane. Under ideal conditions, the jumper attempts to create a forward velocity, with respect to the ground, in the direction of the prevailing winds. Ideally, a front attitude or side attitude landing is preferable to a backward landing. The arms, hands, and elbows are tucked close to the side and in front of the face. The hips and knees are slightly flexed. The toes are plantigrade and are the initial point of preferred contact with the ground. As contact occurs, the parachutist rotates so that the side of the leg makes second contact, followed by the thigh, buttocks, and lateral back; the parachutist tucks the chin to the chest to avoid head contact. This maneuver (the parachute landing fall) has been studied and found to markedly reduce the peak loads experienced during any fall from a height by distributing the forces over a large portion of a surface area of the body. Rearward landings cause heel contact first, followed by buttocks, followed by posterior cervical and head region. Although not preferable, continuing to roll with the rearward parachute landing fall allows the jumper to basically perform a rear somersault and again distribute large forces over a greater portion of the body. However, rearward falls are best avoided because of the potential for head and neck injury.

Initially, parachute landing instructors suggested that keeping the feet at shoulder-distance apart was the preferred method. Further study showed, however, that this broad-based landing caused significant leg, ankle, and lower extremity injuries secondary to preferential landing on one extremity. The present doctrine is to keep both feet and legs together and roll off the balls of both feet onto the right or left lateral leg and thigh, then to the buttocks and the large muscles of the posterolateral chest wall. Once on the ground, the parachutist detaches the canopy by release pins in order to avoid being dragged along as the canopy is refilled by ground winds and begins acting like a sail.

Influence of Equipment, Technique, and Environment on Parachute Landings

There are several different types of parachutes. Canopy parachutes differ in size, shape, and material composition. Standard military parachutes allow for a prelanding velocity of 17 feet per second, which is the equivalent of jumping off a 12-foot wall (Department of the Army 1991). Other parachutes are able to reduce this vertical descent significantly more, thus providing for a much softer landing. These parachutes are utilized in training to avoid injuries, but not in combat situations because they expose the unprotected soldiers to enemy fire for longer periods of time as they slowly float toward the ground (Bagian 1992). There is a rectangular, maneuverable parachute used by high altitude, low opening parachutists that is quite maneuverable and which allows for significant longitudinal velocity, almost making the parachutist a one-person sailing machine. Depending on the altitude at opening, these parachutes can provide traversing distances of several miles. When landing in a parasail, the parachutist begins a running maneuver just above

ground contact in the direction of longitudinal velocity, and does a stand-up landing. If this is not possible, a standard parachute landing fall is performed.

Military parachutists are occasionally required to land on very hard surfaces (Kragh et al. 1996; Kragh & Taylor 1996; Pirson & Verbiest 1985). In attempting to gain control of military airports, Army Rangers are frequently required to land on hard tarmac or concrete. These surfaces frequently increase contusion injuries. Landings on the sides of hills and on rugged terrain frequently increase lower extremity injuries. Nighttime maneuvers, especially when there is no moon illumination, prevent soldiers from seeing the ground they will land on. The most difficult landings probably occur with excessive wind gusts. These gusts cause sudden oscillations in parachutes, placing the jumpers at increased risk of high velocity landings. Injuries significantly increase when ground wind speeds are recorded at greater than 14 to 15 knots (Cugnoni & Whitworth 1992; Pirson & Verbiest 1985). During combat, troops are dropped from altitudes of 500 to 1,200 feet. This is done to minimize their exposure in the air as nondefensible targets. Low altitude drops limit the amount of maneuvering needed to clear obstacles and to correct malfunctions.

■ Incidence and Mechanism of Injuries

The U.S. Army Safety Center collects data on all military injuries requiring a visit to health care facilities and admissions to hospitals (Bricknell et al. 1999). In addition, the medical literature has many articles about the mechanism of injuries in military training and sport parachuting.

Incidence of Injuries

Military parachute death rates are 1.7 per 100,000 military jumps, as reported from the U.S. Army Safety Center and averaged over the years 1980 to 1990 (Mellen & Sohn 1990). Annually, there are between 200,000 and 300,000 Army parachute deployments. Almost 100,000 military personnel of nearly 800,000 active duty United States Army men and women had successfully completed airborne training and were on active duty as of January 31, 1991. Injury rates range from 3.1 to 14 per 1,000 jumps in published reports; however, the definition of an injury was not consistent throughout these articles (Amoroso et al. 1997; Bar-Dayan et al. 1998; Craig & Morgan 1997; Cugnoni & Whitworth 1992; Davison 1990; Ekeland 1997; Farrow 1992; Gill & Hopkins 1988; Kragh et al. 1996; Miser et al. 1995; Murray-Leslie et al. 1977; Schneider et al. 2000; Craig et al. 1996;

Bagian 1992). In 1971, the United States Army Research Institute of Environmental Medicine conducted a study during basic airborne training and documented an injury rate as high as 14% among soldiers making five jumps over a 1-week period. Ankle injuries in this study accounted for 25.5% of all injuries. Lower extremity injuries accounted for 60% of all injuries.

Ankle injuries represent the predominant injury in both civilian and military parachuting. In a study of civilian parachute injuries, 37% (65 of 176) were ankle injuries (Ellitsgaard 1987). Davison (1990) found that ankle injuries accounted for 30% to 60% of all parachute injuries. Kirby (1974) documented that 30% of 520 injuries were ankle fractures or sprains. Petras and Hoffman (1983) reported that 58% (41 of 71) of serious injuries confirmed by radiography were ankle injuries. During the carefully controlled conditions of airborne school, 4.7% (23 of 490) of students sustained ankle injuries while completing qualifying jumps. During Operation Just Cause in Panama, 8.2% of U.S. Army Rangers (51 of 624) sustained ankle injuries: 39% of these soldiers had to be evacuated, and 27% were nonambulatory (Miser et al. 1995). These injuries occurred during a night jump under fire.

In a review of 344 injured men and women reported to the U.S. Army Safety Center database between the years 1980 and 1990, injuries occurred 65% of the time during landing, 12% of the time as a result of ground obstacles. The remainder of injuries occurred while parachutists were exiting the aircraft, during collisions with other jumpers, during times when jumpers had difficulties in gaining control of the canopy that were associated with malfunctions of the equipment, and after landing (Bricknell et al. 1999).

Mechanism of Ankle Injuries During Parachute Landing Falls

The ankle is most stable in a neutral or slight dorsiflexion. This is because the talus is broader anteriorly, thus filling the space between the medial and lateral malleolus (the mortise), taking maximum benefit of the anatomic stability of the distal tibia, fibula, and proximal talus and surrounding ligaments. With plantarflexion, the narrow part of the talus rotates into the ankle mortise, and there is potential increased mediolateral laxity. Occasionally, the jumper lands on either side of the foot, thus twisting the ankle. The most frequent mechanism of ankle injury is inversion, landing on the lateral side of the foot, which causes the talus to rotate inwardly in the ankle mortise, stressing the lateral ligament complex. If the medial side of the foot and the great toe contact the ground

first, the foot rotates outward, causing increased stress to the medial ligaments and to the syndesmosis. With the foot and ankle in a plantarflexed position if the jumper comes down too fast, ground contact can force the talus superiorly through the posterior, central, or anterior aspect of the distal tibia, creating a fracture. Whether the ligaments fail or the bone is fractured is determined primarily by the position of the foot at the time of ground contact and the rate of descent. Direct axial loading usually causes a fracture of the distal tibia either anteriorly, posteriorly, or both (Pilon fracture). Twisting injuries to the ankle can create ligamentous injuries, fractures, or both.

The vast majority of ankle injuries are sprains, and the most common sprains are inversion sprains. This is most likely due to the fact that the foot is slightly inward in the plantarflexed position at ground contact. Similar injury patterns have been seen in other training and sporting events (Chapman 1975; Hopkinson et al. 1990; Israeli et al. 1981; Mack 1982; Murray-Leslie et al. 1977; Saunders 1980).

■ Prevention of Ankle Injuries

Ankle injuries have been reduced in sport. Applying similar devices in military parachuting seems to be reasonable.

Preventive Measures

Ankle injuries are the most common ligamentous injuries in sport. Taping of the ankle, lace-up ankle braces, and semirigid ankle orthoses have been successful in reducing ankle sprains (Rovere et al. 1988; Sitler et al. 1994). Lace-up ankle braces inside the combat boot have been used over the years to prevent recurrent injuries in soldiers with chronic instability. In 1991, the Aircast Corporation in Summit, New Jersey, developed an outside-the-boot ankle orthosis that prevented inversion and eversion while applied over the military combat boot, and which allowed the physiologic dorsiflexion and plantarflexion of the ankle joint that are necessary for a well-executed parachute landing fall (figure 34.1). This brace was tested on cadavers and was found to be more supportive than lace-up ankle braces or inside-the-boot ankle braces. The brace provided adequate mobility to allow for normal jumping, walking, and running.

Airborne School Testing of an Outside-the-Boot Orthosis

In order to demonstrate a benefit of this brace in preventing ankle injuries, a study team was assembled from the U.S. Army Medical Research and Development Command (Letterman Army Institute of Research and the

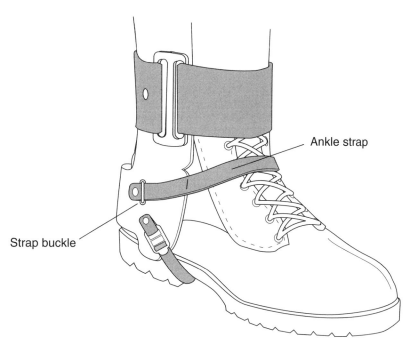

■ Figure 34.1 The outside-the-boot ankle orthosis.

Institute of Environmental Medicine). The airborne training school at Fort Benning, Georgia, was chosen as the test site because of the interest of the command in preventing injuries, the logistics of monitoring the study, the number of predictable jumps over time, and the controlled conditions of basic airborne training.

The Initial Study

After approval of the protocol by a human use review board, volunteers were sought from four consecutive classes at the U.S. Army Airborne School at Fort Benning, Georgia to participate in a test to evaluate the efficacy of the outside-the-boot airborne ankle brace (Amoroso et al. 1998). Fourteen hundred and fourteen students were briefed, and 777 volunteered and gave written consent to participate in this study. Of the participants, 745 completed all study requirements. Of these, 369 wore the brace, and 376 did not wear the brace. Volunteers made five static line parachute jumps, with a total of 3,674 jumps. A jump-related injury was defined as any musculoskeletal or traumatic condition that occurred while exiting the aircraft, performing a parachute landing fall, or running off the drop zone, and that resulted in a visit to the health care provider. All injuries were evaluated and verified by an orthopedic surgeon. The outside-the-boot brace consists of two hard plastic, lateral shells lined with air cells, joined distally by a 4-inch plastic connector around the heel. The brace is secured to the ankle and foot by Velcro straps and allows physiologic dorsiflexion/plantarflexion motion, but prevents the extremes of ankle motion in inversion and eversion.

Overall, 5.1% of the nonbrace group and 4.3% of the brace group experienced at least one injury. The incidence of ankle sprains was 1.9% in nonbrace wearers and .3% in brace wearers. Both groups were equal in regard to height, weight, sex, and physical fitness. This study group was a young, physically fit population. Approximately one-fifth of the participants were smokers and half had a history of previous ankle sprains. In the nonbrace group, there were seven lateral ankle sprains, no medial ankle sprains, two syndesmosis sprains, and one ankle fracture. In the brace group, there was one lateral ankle sprain, no medial ankle sprains, two syndesmosis sprains, and two ankle fractures. Syndesmosis injuries result from external rotation of the foot and ankle. There is no known device that adequately protects against this mechanism of injury. One fracture in the brace group was a posterior malleolar fracture secondary to axial loading and, probably, a too-rapid descent or increased plantarflexion (incorrect landing attitude) of the foot and ankle at the time of ground contact. The other fracture in the brace group resulted from an external rotation of the foot and ankle that caused a medial malleolus fracture, a syndesmosis sprain, and a high fibular fracture. The mechanism of this injury is catching the great toe and/or the medial part of the foot on the ground and externally rotating the ankle. Again, this mechanism is similar to that of the syndesmosis sprain, which is not preventable by any device presently marketed. The fracture in the nonbrace group was a bimalleolar fracture resulting from inversion of the ankle, with fracture of the lateral malleolus (distal fibula) and the medial malleolus. There were no increased injuries associated with brace wear. There were occasional subjective complaints arising from use of the brace. These related to contusions caused by the top of the brace extending above the leather or canvas boot worn by the soldiers. However, no one missed any training because of contusions.

In this study, there was a statistically significant decrease in the incidence of inversion ankle injuries in the braced group, as compared to the nonbraced group. Assuming an incidence rate of 4% for disabling inversion ankle injuries, the expected number of such injuries on an annual basis would be 800 to 1,200, if 20,000 to 30,000 airborne operational jumps per year are assumed. If the ankle brace is only 50% effective, the potential reduction in ankle injuries would be as many as 600 per year across the U.S. Army.

Follow-Up to the Initial Study

In a follow-up evaluation, consecutive classes of airborne students all wearing the braces were compared to historical controls during the same months in previous years before the braces were used. There was a 50% reduction in ankle sprains and an 80% reduction in ankle fractures in this review. During the same year, evaluation of data indicated that there was a slight increase in the incidence of ankle injuries when compared to the study group. Further evaluation by the staff at the airborne school uncovered the fact the some students were loosely applying the brace or not using the under-the-heel strap, which is a component of the brace for stability. The students were advised and checked for proper wear of ankle braces and over the next several months, the rate of ankle injuries returned to rates similar to the braced group in the prospective randomized study. This indicates that the protective nature of the brace requires appropriate attention to detail in regard to wearing the brace according to manufacturer's specifications and keeping it snug but not too tight.

This outside-the-boot ankle brace has been shown to be effective in controlling inversion ankle sprains in airborne students. The brace has obvious application in civilian parachuting when jumpers are using canopy parachutes similar to those used by the study group. In addition, rectangular/parasail jumpers would most likely benefit from the protective aspects of this brace in preventing inversion ankle injuries, as they land in a running step and frequently land on uneven terrain.

■ References

Amoroso PJ, Bell NS, Jones BH. 1997. Injury among female and male army parachutists. Aviat Space Environ Med 68(11):1006-1011.

Amoroso PJ, Ryan JB, Bickley B, Leitschuh P, Taylor DC, Jones BH. 1998. Braced for impact: reducing military paratroopers' ankle sprains using outside-the-boot braces. J Trauma 45(3):575-580.

Bagian JP. 1992. Comparison of parachute landing injury incidence between standard and low porosity parachutes. Aviat Space Environ Med 63(9):802-804.

Bar-Dayan Y, Bar-Dayan Y, Shemer J. 1998. Parachuting injuries. A retrospective study of 43,542 military jumps. Mil Med 163(1):1-2.

Bricknell MC, Amoroso PJ, Yore MN. 1999. What is the risk associated with being a qualified military parachutist? Occup Med (Lond) 49(3):139-145.

Chapman M. 1975. Sprains of the Ankle. In American Academy of Orthopaedic Surgeons Instructional Course Lectures 24:294-308. Rosemont, Illinois.

Craig SC, Morgan J. 1997. Parachuting injury surveillance, Fort Bragg, North Carolina, May 1993 to December 1994. Mil Med 162(3):162-164.

Cugnoni HL, Whitworth I. 1992. Injuries related to wind speed. Ann R Coll Surg Engl 74(4):294-296.

Davison D. 1990. A review of parachuting injuries. Injury 21:314-316.

Department of the Army. 1991. Basic Parachuting Techniques and Training. Washington, DC: Department of the Army.

Ekeland A. 1997. Injuries in military parachuting: a prospective study of 4499 jumps. Injury 28(3):219-222.

Ellitsgaard N. 1987. Parachuting injuries: a study of 110,000 sports jumps. Br J Sports Med 21(1):13-17.

Farrow GB. 1992. Military static line parachute injuries. Aust N Z J Surg 62(3):209-214.

Gill RM, Hopkins GO. 1988. Stress fracture in parachute regiment recruits. J R Army Med Corps 134(2):91-93.

Hopkinson WJ, St. Pierre P, Ryan JB, Wheeler JH. 1990. Syndesmosis sprains of the ankle. Foot Ankle 10(6):325-330.

Israeli A, Horoszowski H, Chechick A, Farine I. 1981. Beware the "simple" fibular fracture (a clue for severe unstable ankle injury). Br J Sports Med 15(4):269-271.

Kirby N. 1974. Parachuting injuries. Proc Royal Soc Med 67:17.

Kragh JF Jr, Taylor DC. 1996. Parachuting injuries: a medical analysis of an airborne operation. Mil Med 161(2):67-69.

Kragh JF Jr, Jones BH, Amaroso PJ, Heekin RD. 1996. Parachuting injuries among Army Rangers: a prospective survey of an elite airborne battalion. Mil Med 161(7):416-419.

Mack RP. 1982. Ankle injuries in athletics. Clin Sports Med 1(1):71-84.

Mellen PF, Sohn SS. 1990. Military parachute mishap fatalities: a retrospective study. Aviat Space Environ Med 61(12):1149-1152.

Miser WF, Doukas WC, Lillegard WA. 1995. Injuries and illnesses incurred by an army ranger unit during Operation Just Cause. Mil Med 160(8):373-380.

Murray-Leslie CF, Lintott DJ, Wright V. 1977. The knees and ankles in sport and veteran military parachutists. Ann Rheum Dis 36(4):327-331.

Petras AF, Hoffman EP. 1983. Roentgenographic skeletal injury patterns in parachute jumping. Am J Sports Med 11(5):325-328.

Pirson J, Verbiest E. 1985. A study of some factors influencing military parachute landing injuries. Aviat Space Environ Med 56(6):564-567.

Rovere G.D, et al. 1988. Retrospective comparison of taping and ankle stabilizers in preventing ankle injuries. Am J Sports Med 16(3):228-233.

Saunders EA. 1980. Ligamentous injuries of the ankle. Am Fam Physician 22(2):132-138.

Schneider GA, Bigelow C, Amoroso PJ. 2000. Evaluating risk of re-injury among 1214 army airborne soldiers using a stratified survival model. Am J Prev Med 18(3 Suppl):156-163.

Sitler M, Ryan J, Wheeler B, McBride J, Arciero R, Anderson J, Horodyski M. 1994. The efficacy of a semirigid ankle stabilizer to reduce acute ankle injuries in basketball. A randomized clinical study at West Point. Am J Sports Med 22(4):454-461.

Chapter 35

Preventive Effects of an On-Shoe Brace on Ankle Sprains in Infantry

Gideon Mann, MD; Gadi Kahn, MD; M. Suderer, MD; A. Zeev, PhD; Naama Constantini, MD; and Meir Nyska, MD

Ankle sprain is the most common injury in athletes and in people performing sports activities (Frey et al. 1996; Mann et al. 1994). Epidemiology and incidence is widely discussed in chapters 1, 5, 20, 32, and 33. Of patients sustaining an acute ankle sprain, 20% to 40% will have residual complaints, depending on the severity of the initial trauma (Klenerman et al. 1996, 1998; Leanderson et al. 1996; Milgrom et al. 1991).

Because of the high incidence and cost of ankle sprains, programs to prevent them are being introduced. The main measures include conditioning and training activities and various external ankle supports. Strengthening, stretching, and proprioception activities have been shown in limited studies to reduce the risk of ankle sprains (Ashton-Miller et al. 1996; MacPherson et al. 1995; Mann et al. 1994; Rifat & McKeag 1996; Shapiro et al. 1994; Wester et al. 1996). External supports, such as various techniques of taping, have been the traditional methods used to prevent these injuries. These improve proprioception, prevent eversion injuries, and limit the range of motion (Ashton-Miller et al. 1996; Bennell & Goldie 1994; Klenerman 1998; Leanderson et al. 1996; MacPherson et al. 1995; Mann et al. 1994; Rifat & McKeag 1996; Shapiro et al. 1994; Thonnard et al. 1996). An alternative to prophylactic taping is the use of an ankle stabilizer. Ranging from semirigid to cloth lace-on braces, they increase resistance to inversion, do not limit jumping or running ability, and do not increase the risk for other injuries (Bennell & Goldie 1994; Bruce et al. 1996; Guskiewicz & Perrin 1996; Leanderson et al. 1996; Mann et al. 1994; MacPherson et al. 1995; Myburgh 1984; Putukian et al. 1996; Rifat & McKeag 1996; Shapiro et al. 1994; Sitler et al. 1994; Surve et al. 1994; U.S. Army;

Wiley & Nigg 1996). Most of these studies were performed in athletes who experienced at least one ankle injury in the past. Studies in the military population are limited mainly to sports activity (Sitler et al. 1994). Further details on prophylaxis and prevention can be found in chapter 5.

All the braces in use at present are designed for in-shoe use and are therefore inconvenient for infantry units in which regular activity takes place in army boots. The development of the "Jump Brace," which is an on-shoe brace, planned originally to prevent ankle sprains in parachuting, has led to trials of its efficacy in prevention of acute ankle sprains in infantry units during their regular and advanced training activities.

■ Materials and Methods

One hundred and three Israeli border police fighters took part in an advanced commanding course. Prior to commencing training, all participants were given a detailed explanation of the study and signed a consent form. Participants were then divided into two groups: one group consisted of participants already suffering from recurrent ankle sprains (33 fighters), and the other consisted of participants not suffering from recurrent ankle sprains (70 fighters). The two groups were further randomly divided into two subgroups: One of 50 fighters who received an overshoe brace ("Jump Brace," Aircast Company, 1995), and the other of 53 fighters who did not receive the brace. Fighters who received the brace constituted the research group, whereas those who did not receive the brace constituted the control group (figure 35.1).

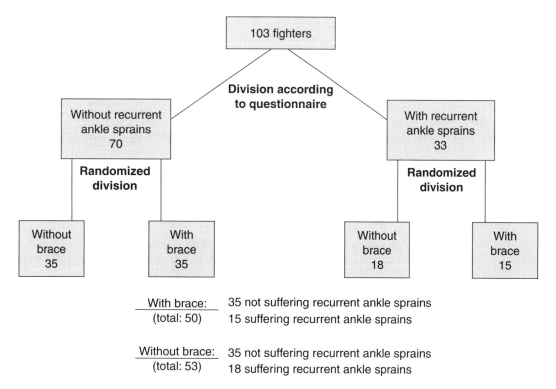

Figure 35.1 Division into research (with brace) and control (without brace) groups.

Participants were examined regularly as needed by the unit's medical officer and the organic medical team who took part in the research. The course continued for 3 months, during which the fighters performed various military activities, such as walking, running, sport activities, and navigation by day and by night while carrying 15-30 kg of arms and equipment.

Description of the Brace

The brace is constructed by the Aircast Company primarily for use in parachuting (figure 35.2). It is a semirigid orthotic that has semirigid plastic side supports connected by a posterior semicircular bar covering the heel. The sidewalls are tightened using two wide Velcro straps and a narrow anterior ankle stabilizer Velcro strap, devised to enable the use of the brace in the infantry. Another strap holds the heel of the boot and is connected to the sidewalls. This strap has also been reinforced to enable infantry use.

Protocol of the Study

At commencement of the course, the fighters were examined by two orthopedic surgeons, with all measurements being taken by one examiner (G.M.). All participants had the following data recorded: height, weight, body mass index (BMI), presence of scoliosis

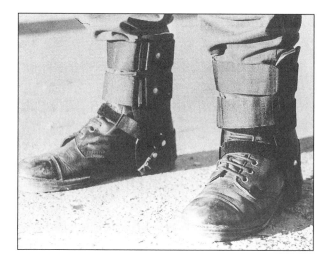

Figure 35.2 The on-shoe brace.

or spine deformity, leg length, joint laxity, ankle motion, subtalar motion, foot motion, ankle stability, heel valgus, and footprint. Sensitivity and swelling of the ankle were looked for and recorded. Parameters were graded as normal (0), mild (1), or severe (2). Joint laxity was evaluated by thumb-to-forearm and back flexion (Bird 1979; Durkan et al. 1988; Wynne-Davies 1971). Footprint was evaluated as normal, mild, or obvious high arch, or mild or obvious flat foot (Simon & Claustre 1982; Goldcher 1987). Figure 35.3 shows the ankle evaluation section of the physical examination form.

Details were recorded concerning ethnic origin, past physical activity, and previous ankle or other injuries (figure 35.4). All participants signed an informed consent form and the experimental group received the brace.

During the course, all the fighters were closely followed up by the medical staff. Every ankle sprain was documented and evaluated concerning mecha-

nism of injury, whether it occurred with or without the brace, and the severity of the sprain. Three grades were used according to swelling, walking ability, and pain (figure 35.5) (Mann et al. 1994; Peri 1993). The medical staff included four integral paramedics and a physician who was part of the investigator group.

At the end of the study, a questionnaire was filled out by the experimental group concerning comfort, durability, ability of the brace to prevent ankle sprains, satisfaction with the brace, and general remarks (figure 35.6). Any broken brace was immediately replaced and the broken braces were analyzed to verify

Border Police Research: Prevention of Ankle Sprains

Date: _____   Weight: _____

Family name: _____   Height: _____

First name: _____   Year of birth: _____

Personal army #: _____   Identity card #: _____

	Right	Left
1. Swelling		
none	O	O
slight	O	O
moderate	O	O
severe	O	O
2. Lateral sensitivity		
none	O	O
slight	O	O
moderate	O	O
severe	O	O
3. Medial sensitivity		
none	O	O
slight	O	O
moderate	O	O
severe	O	O
4. Dorsiflexion		
normal	O	O
slightly reduced	O	O
moderately reduced	O	O
severely reduced	O	O
5. Plantarflexion		
normal	O	O
slightly reduced	O	O
moderately reduced	O	O
severely reduced	O	O
6. Subtalar motion		
normal	O	O
slightly reduced	O	O
moderately reduced	O	O
severely reduced	O	O

7. Foot motion

normal	O	O
slightly reduced	O	O
moderately reduced	O	O
severely reduced	O	O

8. Crepitation

none	O	O
mild	O	O
moderate	O	O
obvious	O	O

9. Stability

Tilt

normal	O	O
+1	O	O
+2	O	O
+3	O	O

Drawer

normal	O	O
+1	O	O
+2	O	O
+3	O	O

10. Heel position

normal	O	O
slight valgus	O	O
obvious valgus	O	O
slight varus	O	O
obvious varus	O	O

11. Arch of foot

normal	O	O
slightly flattened	O	O
obviously flattened	O	O
slightly high arched	O	O
obviously high arched	O	O

12. Joint laxity (thumb to forearm)

normal	O	O
borderline	O	O
obvious	O	O

13. Joint laxity (hand to floor)

normal	O	O
borderline	O	O
obvious	O	O

Doctor's name: _____

Doctor's signature: _____

■ **Figure 35.3** The ankle evaluation section of the physical examination form.

Border Police Research: Prevention of Ankle Sprains

Date: _____   Weight: _____

Family name: _____   Height: _____

First name: _____   Year of birth: _____

Personal army #: _____   Identity card #: _____

Ethnic origin:
- O Ashkenazi
- O Sephardic
- O Druse
- O Russian
- O Caucasian
- O Ethiopian
- O Other (specify): _____

Have you suffered from a previous ankle sprain?

If "yes," complete the following form. If "no," stop here.

- O no
- O yes   O right   O left

What year? _____

What month? _____

In what circumstances?
- O soccer
- O basketball
- O volleyball
- O army training
- O physical education lesson
- O other (specify):

The pain caused was:
- O minor
- O moderate
- O severe

Walking ability:
- O easy
- O difficult
- O impossible

Swelling occurring was:
- O slight
- O moderate
- O severe

Did pain continue after the sprain?
- O yes
- O no

Pain severity:
- O slight
- O medium
- O severe

Location of pain:
- O medial side of ankle
- O lateral side of ankle

After the injury did an ankle sprain occur?
- O yes
- O no

If yes, what was its frequency?
- O once a week or on any activity
- O once in one or two months
- O once in three months or more

Signature: _____

■ **Figure 35.4** Personal data form and data concerning previous ankle sprains.

Border Police Research: Prevention of Ankle Sprains

Date: _____

Family name: _____

First name: _____

Personal army #: _____

Identity card #: _____

Received a brace:

○ yes
○ no

Did you have an ankle sprain since the previous form you filled out?

○ yes
○ no

If "yes," how many sprains did you have?

○ one
○ two
○ three
○ four
○ five
○ more than five (specify): _____

First sprain	Second sprain	Third sprain	Fourth sprain
Pain on the first occasion was	**Pain on the second occasion was**	**Pain on the third occasion was**	**Pain on the fourth occasion was**
○ mild ○ moderate ○ severe	○ mild ○ moderate ○ severe	○ mild ○ moderate ○ severe	○ mild ○ moderate ○ severe
Walking ability ○ with no difficulty ○ with difficulty ○ impossible	○ with no difficulty ○ with difficulty ○ impossible	○ with no difficulty ○ with difficulty ○ impossible	○ with no difficulty ○ with difficulty ○ impossible
Swelling was ○ slight ○ moderate ○ severe	○ slight ○ moderate ○ severe	○ slight ○ moderate ○ severe	○ slight ○ moderate ○ severe
Were you using a brace when the ankle sprain occurred? ○ yes ○ no	○ yes ○ no	○ yes ○ no	○ yes ○ no

Doctor's name: _____

Doctor's signature: _____

For the medical team: If more than four sprains occurred, hand out another form.

■ **Figure 35.5** Follow-up form for the occurrence of ankle sprains during the course.

Border Police Research: Prevention of Ankle Sprains

Date: _____

Family name: _____

First name: _____

Personal army #: _____

Identity card #: _____

A. Comfort

very uncomfortable	1
uncomfortable	2
reasonable	3
comfortable	4
very comfortable	5

B. Durability

very bad	1
not durable enough	2
reasonable	3
durable	4
very durable	5

How many weeks until brace needed repairing? _____ weeks

How many weeks until brace needed replacement? _____ weeks

C. Ability to prevent ankle sprain

does not prevent	1
prevents a little	2
prevents about 50%	3
usually prevents	4
always prevents	5

D. Evaluation and suggestions for improvement

_____

_____

_____

_____

Signature: _____

■ **Figure 35.6** Personal evaluation form for the on-shoe brace.

common mechanical problems. It should be noted that fighters were requested to evaluate various components of compliance and brace evaluation on a scale of 1 to 5, while results were summarized in this text on a scale of 1 to 10.

■ Statistical Analysis

Statistical evaluation was done by the Department of Statistics of the Zinman College of Physical Education at the Wingate Institute, which had not originally been involved in the research program. The incidence of acute ankle sprains was calculated using the chi-square test and $p < .05$ was selected as statistically significant. Pearson correlation coefficient was calculated for physical body parameters and the physical examination. They were compared using the t-test and $p < .05$ was selected as statistically significant. One-way ANOVA was used for comparing the physical parameters, the parameters of physical examination, and the incidence of ankle sprains in the different groups.

■ Results

The weight and height in the experimental group were somewhat higher, but the BMI was the same for both groups (table 35.1). The "stability factor of the ankle" was calculated as a summation of the scoring of the drawer and inversion tests. Statistically significant negative correlation was found between stability factor and the age of the fighters. As the age increased, the stability factor was lower ($p = .025$). A statistically significant correlation was found between height, weight, and decreased range of motion of the ankle (plantarflexion and dorsiflexion).

Comparisons Between the Experimental and the Control Groups

Our basic assumption was that the brace would reduce the incidence of ankle sprains if it were comfortable enough to be used regularly. Thus, comparison of the two groups was the central part of this research.

Previous Ankle Sprains

In evaluation of the history, 59% (61/103) of the fighters reported at least one significant ankle sprain in the past, and 32% (33 fighters) reported previous recurrent sprains. In the experimental group of 50 soldiers, 15 suffered from previous recurrent ankle sprains and in the control group, 18 suffered from previous recurrent ankle sprains. No statistical difference was found between the groups concerning previous sprains.

Sprains During the Course

In the control group, 31 of the fighters had ankle sprains during the course (58.5%), and in the experi-

mental group, 9 fighters (18%) had sprains during the course. The difference was significant (figure 35.7 and table 35.2). Four fighters out of the nine in the experimental group who sprained their ankles during the course reported that the sprain occurred while not using the brace. The difference between the groups in the grade I sprain was significant, as was the difference in grade II sprains. In grade III sprains there was no difference. The number of sprains during the course in the experimental group was 23 and in the control group it was 92. The difference between the groups (using chi-square) was highly significant ($p = .014$). There was no difference between fighters who suffered an ankle sprain and those who did not concerning the different physical parameters and body measurements.

Injury Factor

The "injury factor" was calculated as the summation of the number of sprains and their severity (tables 35.3a and 35.3b). Each grade I sprain received one point, grade II received four points, and grade III received six points. The higher values for grades II and III were given because of the higher clinical significance (Jackson et al. 1974) and the occurrence of late complications in these groups and not in the group with grade I ankle sprains (Peri 1993). The injury factor in the group that used the brace was 1.64 and in the control group it was 5.53. This difference was found to be significant ($p = .005$). However, there was no difference when the injury factor was compared for the fighters who

Table 35.1 Height, Weight, BMI, and Parameters of Physical Examination

	Research group (with brace)	Control group (without brace)	Significance (*p*-value)
Fighters	50	53	-
BMI	23.76 ± 2.24	23.17 ± 2.00	0.168
Height	178.62 ± 6.40	175.90 ± 6.47	0.018
Weight	75.85 ± 8.37	71.80 ± 8.36	0.039
Plantarflexion	43.72 ± 7.85	42.92 ± 7.61	0.618
Subtalar motion	0.18 ± 0.53	0.37 ± 0.81	0.194
Foot motion	0.22 ± 0.59	0.26 ± 0.50	0.746
Tilt	0.22 ± 0.55	0.30 ± 0.65	0.533
Draw	0.27 ± 0.57	0.36 ± 0.52	0.391
Heel position (valgus or varus)	0.54 ± 0.79	0.75 ± 0.97	0.256
Joint laxity (thumb to forearm)	0.53 ± 0.83	0.42 ± 0.76	0.527
Joint laxity (hand to floor)	0.64 ± 0.69	0.69 ± 0.68	0.733

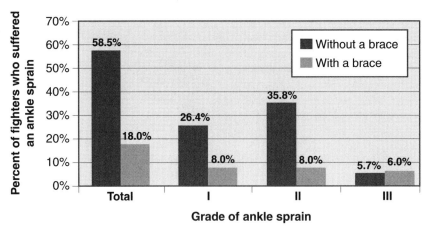

■ **Figure 35.7** Percent of fighters who sustained an ankle sprain during the course in both groups according to the grade of injury.

Table 35.2 Incidence of Ankle Sprains During the Course in Control and Experimental Groups According to the Grade of Sprain

	Fighters	Fighters with ankle sprains	Ankle sprains grade I	Ankle sprains grade II	Ankle sprains grade III
Research group (with brace)	50	9 (18%)	4 (8%)	4 (8%)	3 (6%)
		*	*	*	
Control group (without brace)	53	31 (58.5%)	14 (26.4%)	19 (35.8%)	3 (5.7%)

* Statistically significant difference between the groups.

Table 35.3a The Injury Factor in the Various Groups

Group	Fighters	Injury factor
Without brace (without recurrent sprains)	35	4.94
Without brace (with recurrent sprains)	18	6.66
With brace (without recurrent sprains)	35	0.74
With brace (with recurrent sprains)	15	3.73

Table 35.3b The Injury Factor When Divided Into Two Groups Only

Group	Injury factor
Experimental group (with the brace)	1.64
Control group (without the brace)	5.53

Significance: $p = .005$.

eventually did suffer an ankle sprain in the experimental group (9.11) to the injury factor of those who sprained their ankles in the control group (9.45) (table 35.3c)

In the experimental group, 10% suffered other injuries, compared to 15% in the control group.

The small difference was not significant. The injuries included anterior knee pain with or without acute trauma, metatarsalgia, plantar fasciitis, Achilles tendinitis, and calf pain. It should be emphasized that no rise in knee injuries was noted.

Comparison of the Subgroups

The subgroups, namely those suffering or not suffering from recurrent ankle sprains prior to the course, would affect the incidence of injury and thus were separately compared.

Previous Ankle Sprains

Within the experimental group (the group using the brace), there were 35 fighters who did not have repeated ankle sprains before the course (figure 35.1), and of these, 3 fighters (8.6%) had one or more ankle sprains during the course. Within the group of 15 soldiers with a history of repeated ankle sprains before the course who were wearing the brace, 6 (40%) had ankle sprains during the course. In the control group, 35 soldiers did not suffer repeated ankle sprains before the course, and 18 (51.4%) of them sustained a sprain during the course. The highest incidence of sprains during the course was in the subgroup of fighters with previous recurrent sprains and not using a brace. Thirteen out of 18, or 72.2%, of this subgroup had at least one acute ankle sprain during the course (figure 35.8 and table 35.4).

All the preceding differences between the groups were statistically significant using the chi-square test ($p < .001$). There was no significant difference between the two subgroups of the control group (those not using the brace).

Injury Factor

There was a significant difference between all the subgroups concerning the "injury factor" using one-way ANOVA (tables 35.3a and 35.3b). The "injury factor" was significantly different between the subgroup with the brace and without history of recurrent sprains and the two subgroups without the brace, using post hoc test. There was no difference between the subgroups concerning associated injuries.

Physical Parameters and Physical Examination

No difference was found among the subgroups in physical examination parameters using one-way ANOVA (table 35.1). The BMI was significantly higher in the subgroup with the brace and with a history of recurrent ankle sprains when compared

Table 35.3.c. The Injury Factor in Fighters Who Eventually Sustained an Ankle Sprain in the Experimental Group Compared to Those Who Sprained Their Ankle in the Control Group

Group	Injury factor
Experimental group who sustained an ankle sprain	9.11
Control group who sustained an ankle sprain	9.45

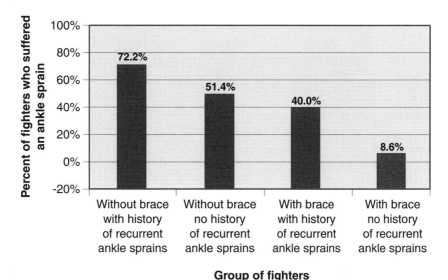

■ **Figure 35.8** Percent of fighters who sustained an ankle sprain during the course according to history of recurrent ankle sprain.

Table 35.4 Occurrence of Ankle Sprains During the Course With Reference to the Previous History of Recurrent Ankle Sprains

Group	Fighters	Fighters with ankle sprains	Frequency of ankle sprains (%)
Without brace (without recurrent ankle sprains)	35	18	51.4
Without brace (with recurrent ankle sprains)	18	13	72.2
With brace (without recurrent ankle sprains)	35	3	8.6
With brace (with recurrent ankle sprains)	15	6	40.0

Significance (chi^2) $p < .001$.

with the subgroup with the brace and without a history of recurrent ankle sprains ($p = .023$), and also when compared with the subgroup without brace and without history of recurrent ankle sprains ($p = .008$) using the post hoc test. Comparison, using the t-test, of the average BMI of both subgroups who had a history of recurrent ankle sprains (24.08) showed that the BMI was significantly higher in both the groups suffering from recurrent ankle sprains when compared with both groups who did not give a history of recurrent ankle sprains (23.16), showing a p-value of 0.045.

Evaluation of the Brace

The evaluation was done using a standardized questionnaire (figure 35.6). The compliance of the fighters to the brace was good. Most of them wore the brace all the time, including during navigations and marching. Only two fighters used the brace once and stopped using it. The comfort of the brace received a score of 6.66 on a scale of 1 to 10, the durability of the brace received a score of 6.52 out of 10, and subjective estimation of the ability of the brace to prevent ankle sprains received a score of 8.46 out of 10.

General Remarks

Remarks concerning the brace that were repeatedly noted were that the brace could be broken easily and the frame should be stronger. The straps were not strong enough, and tightening them strongly caused pressure on the ankle. If the straps were not tightened enough, the brace would rub the malleoli on both sides of the ankle and cause blisters in the areas of pressure. During walking on uneven terrain, the brace held the ankle tightly and comfortably as long as the distance was not too long. In running, it was less comfortable because it caused a certain limitation of motion. Except for three fighters who recommended not using the brace, all the rest highly recommended its use.

Broken Braces

Altogether, 19 broken braces were replaced, and in 10 of them there were only minor problems. In 12 braces there was a broken lateral inferior extension (ear). In seven braces the metal buckle of the ankle strap was bent. In five braces a partial break of the lateral column was noted and in four braces the lateral column was totally broken (figure 35.9). In another two braces the ankle strap was torn and in two the cushioning pads were lost.

■ Discussion

1. **Selection of research groups** (figure 35.4). Prior to randomized selection to experimental (using brace) and control (not using brace) groups, the total group was divided (according to a questionnaire) into those already suffering from recurrent ankle sprains and those not suffering from recurrent ankle sprains (figure 35.4). After the selection of the groups at random, both groups were comparable concerning history of ankle sprain before the course and in the parameters of physical examination (table 35.1).

2. **BMI—The Body Mass Index** (table 35.1). The body mass index (BMI) of the two groups was similar, but the height and weight were higher in the experimental group. Lavi (1990) and Milgrom et al. (1991) suggested that body moment of inertia correlates with the incidence of ankle sprains. We found that the BMI had a correlation with the incidence of ankle sprains, as reported by questionnaire before the course. In the experimental group, the weight and height were somewhat higher than in the control group and, therefore, according to Lavi and Milgrom, this group should have had a higher risk for ankle sprains. Accordingly, a higher incidence of ankle sprains should have occurred in the experimental group. This would further emphasize the preventive effect of the on-shoe brace.

3. **Sprains before the course.** Fifty-nine percent of the fighters had at least one sprain before the course.

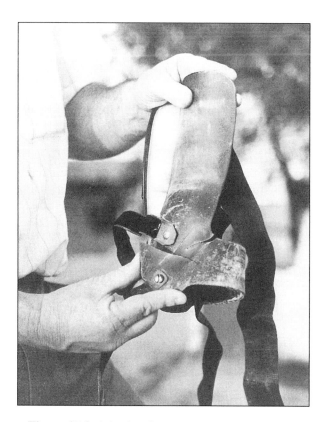

■ **Figure 35.9** A broken brace.

This does not differ significantly from similar data previously reported (Mann et al. 1994; Rifat & McKeag 1996; Surve et al. 1994). However, 32% of the fighters reported they had recurrent ankle sprains, an incidence that is far higher than in the general population. Our group of fighters had already served 1 year in active police infantry service, in which they were exposed to high levels of physical and sports activities. The great majority of the unit was also actively involved in soccer or basketball. The incidence of ankle sprains in such sport activities is known to be as high as 40% (Renström & Konradsen 1997; Rifat & McKeag 1996; Sitler et al. 1994; Surve et al. 1994). While evaluating cadets due to be included in a study similar to the present study, Sitler et al. (1994) found only 177 subjects with previously injured ankles and 1,424 subjects without previous injury. The reason for this difference is unclear, because their study group was of a similar age group to our own and was chosen from a young, healthy population serving in the army.

4. **Body measurements and physical examination parameters** (table 35.1 and figure 35.3). There was a correlation between the age of the fighters and the "stability factor." The age range of the fighters was rather small (19-21) years, and it is difficult to assume that 3 years of difference, even in active service, can have an effect on the stability of the ankle. One explanation might be that the older fighters had spent more time in police or army service, commencing at the age of 18. The longer exposure to army service conditions may have increased the incidence of ankle sprains. Decreased range of motion has been suggested as a risk factor for ankle sprains (Surve et al. 1994). Increased height and weight may also be risk factors for ankle sprains (Milgrom et al. 1991; Lavi 1990). In our study, there was a correlation between height and weight and decreased range of ankle motion. This combination may have added to the incidence of ankle sprains before the course.

5. **Ankle sprains during the course** (figure 35.7 and table 35.2). The incidence of ankle sprains in sports activities is 20-45% (Garrik 1977a, 1977b). The incidence of ankle sprains in the control group was 58.5%, which is higher than expected. One of the reasons for the high incidence is that in our study there was a continuous presence of medical staff, which documented all occasions and all degrees of ankle sprains. In most of the studies performed on athletes, there was no continuous presence of medical staff, so that it is possible that minor ankle sprains were not reported and that the true incidence of ankle sprains was higher.

■ Recently, Konradsen et al. (1998) found that acute ankle inversion injuries result in marked changes in the patient's ability to assess ankle inversion position. These changes lasted for at least 12 weeks after the injury. A reduction in eversion strength was noted 3 weeks after injury. Injured personnel who are not dismissed from their duty for more than a few days still have these deficits and are therefore prone to recurrent injury. It may be concluded that using the brace is especially important in soldiers who had a recent sprain, thus preventing its recurrence.

■ The brace reduced the incidence of an ankle sprain significantly. This was mainly in the less severe grade I and II sprains. No difference was found in the prevention of grade III sprains, most probably because of the small number. The clinically important sprains are grades II and III. These cause inability to return to full activity for at least 2 weeks when compared with less severe sprains (grade I), where absence from work is less than a week (Jackson et al. 1974). Later complications also occur mainly in grades II and III (Peri 1993). When combining our grade II and III groups, there was a significant reduction of the incidence of ankle sprains in the braced group (table 35.2 and figure 35.7). These findings are in agreement with similar studies in the U.S. Army (Report No. T95-I). Surve et al. (1994)

found that a brace prevented mainly the severe sprains and not the minor ones. However, their study was performed on soccer players during the game itself, and no trained medical staff was present on the field. Therefore, it is probable that most minor sprains were missed.

■ In the present study, the reduction of ankle sprains in fighters without a history of recurrent ankle sprains was higher than the reduction of sprains in fighters with a history of recurrent ankle sprains. The efficacy of the brace, therefore, is highest in preventing the first sprain (figure 35.8 and table 35.4). This finding is in contrast with others who found that a brace prevented ankle sprains better in athletes with a history of recurrent ankle sprains (Shapiro et al. 1994; Sitler et al. 1994; Surve et al. 1994). Sitler et al. (1994) found that an ankle brace prevented mainly sprains occurring in contact activity. In our study design we did not differentiate between these parameters. There are no data in Sitler's study concerning the group of subjects with previous ankle injury.

6. **The injury factor** (tables 35.3a and 35.3b). In the braced group, the injury factor was significantly lower than in the unbraced group. When calculating the injury factor concerning only fighters suffering from an ankle sprain during the course, there was no difference between the groups, thus leading to the conclusion that the brace reduced the number of sprains but did not affect the severity of the sprain when it eventually occurred. Sitler et al. (1994) also found that a brace did not reduce the severity of sprains. Ashton-Miller et al. (1996) evaluated evertor muscle strength when the ankle was in 15° of inversion while using different orthoses and shoes. They concluded that fully activated and strong ankle evertor muscles are the best protection for a near maximally inverted ankle at footstrike. At 15° of inversion, the evertor muscles can develop roughly three times larger moments than any of the present combinations of three-quarter-top shoes and tape or orthosis, and up to six times more resistance to moments than the baseline resistance developed by the unprotected ankle. Three-quarter-top shoes and tape or orthosis increased the baseline resistance by a factor of 1.42 and 1.77, respectively. These data explain our finding that in mild and moderate injury, when the evertor muscles (which make up the most important defense mechanism) are not activated, orthoses take a significant part in stabilizing the ankle. However, in severe trauma it is beyond the ability of an orthosis to prevent an injury.

7. **Subgroups.** Fighters with a history of recurrent ankle sprains had a higher incidence of ankle sprains during the course (figure 35.8 and table 35.4). It was significant in the experimental group and borderline in the control group. Therefore, history of recurrent ankle sprains is a major risk factor, and such fighters during military activity are at a higher risk of spraining their ankles and should probably protect their ankles during high-risk activities. Wearing an orthosis very clearly lowered the incidence of acute sprains when no history of recurrent ankle sprain was noted, but also when there was a history of recurrent ankle sprains, although the incidence of acute ankle sprains was still relatively high. It might be that the combination of orthoses with evertor muscle strengthening will further reduce this incidence.

8. **Evaluation of the brace** (figure 35.6). The overall compliance of the fighters for wearing the brace was good, satisfaction was high, efficacy evaluation was very good, and most of them recommended its use. It was comfortable for wearing, but mainly in walking and less so in running. Similar results were observed in players wearing semirigid orthotics in basketball (Sitler et al. 1994). The players liked the brace and of 48% of them receiving the orthosis at the beginning of the study, 70% reported positive or indifferent attitude to the orthosis.

The durability of the orthosis has to be improved. In most of the damaged braces, the supporting area around the ankle was broken. This area probably takes most of the supportive forces and needs to be reinforced.

■ Conclusions

1. An on-shoe brace significantly reduced (by two-thirds) the incidence of acute ankle sprains in fighters taking a military infantry advanced course.

2. The efficiency of the brace is significant in primary and secondary prevention of acute ankle sprains.

3. The fighters in our study had a higher previous incidence of recurrent ankle sprains than expected.

4. Fighters with a history of recurrent ankle sprains had a higher risk for acute sprain.

5. The on-shoe brace is comfortable, has good user compliance especially in long-distance walking, and does not increase the incidence of other injuries.

6. There is room for improvement of the durability of the brace.

This study was presented to the Sackler Tel Aviv University Medical School as an MD thesis by Dr. Gadi Kahn upon conclusion of his studies.

This study was supported by a research grant of Aircast Company, USA.

■ References

Ashton-Miller JA, Ottaviani RA, Hutchinson C, Wojtys EM. What best protects the inverted weightbearing ankle against further inversion? Am J Sports Med 24:800-809 (1996).

Bennell KL, Goldie PA. The differential effects of external ankle support on postural control. J Orthop Sports Phys Ther 20:287-295 (1994).

Bird HA. Joint laxity. Rep Rheum Dis Jan (67-68):[no pagination]. (1979)

Bruce J, Scherlitz J, Luessenhop S. The stabilizing effect of orthotic devices on plantar flexion/dorsal extension and horizontal rotation of the ankle joint. An experimental cadaveric investigation. Int J Sports Med 17:614-618 (1996).

Durkan JA, Wynne GF, Haggerty JF. Extraarticular reconstruction of the anterior cruciate ligament insufficient knee. A long-term analysis of the Ellison procedure. Am J Sports Med 17:112-17 (1988).

Ekstrand J. The First Hellenic Congress for Prevention of Injury in Athletes, Athens, Greece, 6-9 October, 1988.

Frey C, Bell J, Teresi L, Kerr R, Feder K. A Comparison of MRI and clinical examination of acute lateral ankle sprains. Foot Ankle Int 17:533-537 (1996).

Garrik JG, Requa RK. Role of external support in the prevention of ankle sprains. Med Sci Sports 5:200-203 (1977a).

Garrik JG. The frequency of injury, mechanism of injury and epidemiology of ankle sprains. Am J Sports Med 5:241-242 (1977b).

Goldcher A. Podologie. Paris: Masson. (1987).

Guskiewicz KM, Perrin DH. Effect of orthotics on postural sway following inversion ankle sprain. J Orthop Sports Phys Ther 23:326-331 (1996).

Jackson DW, Ashley RL, Powell JW. Ankle sprains in young athletes. Clin Orthop Rel Res 101:201-215 (1974).

Klenerman L. The management of sprained ankles. J Bone Joint Surg Br 80:11-12 (1998).

Klenerman L, van Dijk CN, Bossuyt PM, Marti RK. Medial ankle pain after lateral ligament rupture. J Bone Joint Surg Br 78:526-527 (1996).

Konradsen L, Olesen S, Hansen HM. Ankle sensorimotor control and eversion strength after acute ankle inversion injuries. Am J Sports Med. Jan-Feb;26(1):72-7 (1998).

Lavi O. A prospective study of risk factors for lateral ankle sprains in infantry recruits. M.D. thesis. Hadassah-Hebrew University Medical School (1990).

Leanderson J, Ekstam S, Salomonsson C. Taping of the ankle—the effect on postural sway during perturbation before and after a training session. Knee Surg Sports Traumatology Arthroscopy 4:53-56 (1996).

Leanderson J, Erikson E, Nilson C, Wykman A. Proprioception in classical ballet dancers. Am J Sports Med 24:370-374 (1996).

MacPherson K, Sitler M, Kimura I, Horodyski M. Effect of a semi-rigid and soft-shell prophylactic ankle stabilizer on selected performance tests among high school football players. J Orthop Sports Phys Ther 21:147-152 (1995).

Mann G, Peri C, Finsterbush A, Frankl U, Nyska M, Matan Y. Recurrent ankle sprain: literature review. Isr J Sports Med Jan:104-113 (1994).

Milgrom C, Shlamkowitch N, Finestone A, Eldad A, Laor A, Danon Y, Lavi O, Wosk J, Simkin A. Risk factors for lateral ankle sprains: prospective study among military recruits. Foot Ankle 12:26-30 (1991).

Myburgh KH, Vaughan CL, Isaacs SK. The effect of ankle guards and taping on joint motion before, during and after a squash match. Am J Sports Med 6:354-446 (1984).

Peri C. Recurrent ankle sprain: mechanical stability vs. functional stability. M.D. thesis. Hadassah Hebrew University Medical School (1993), Jerusalem, Israel.

Putukian M, Knowles WK, Swere S, Castle NG. Injuries in indoor soccer. The Lake Placid Dawn to Dark Soccer tournament. Am J Sports Med 24:317-322 (1996).

Renstrom Per AFH, Konradsen L. Chronic ankle instability. Isr J Sports Med Oct:1-6 (1997).

Rifat SF, McKeag DB. Practical methods of preventing ankle injuries. Am Fam Phys 53:2491-2498, 2501-2503 (1996).

Shapiro MS, Kabo M, Mitchell PW, Loren G, Tsenter M. Ankle sprain prophylaxis: an analysis of the stabilizing effects of brace and tape. Am J Sports Med 22:78-82 (1994).

Simon L, Claustre J. Troubles congenitaux et statiques du pied. Otheses plantaires. Paris: Masson (1982).

Sitler M, Ryan J, Wheeler B, McBride J, Arciero R, Anderson J, Horodyski M. The efficacy of a semi-rigid ankle stabilizer to reduce acute ankle injuries in basketball. Am J Sports Med 22:454-461 (1994).

Surve I, Schwellnus MP, Noakes T, Lombard C. A fivefold reduction in the incidence of recurrent ankle sprains in soccer players using the Sport-Stirrup orthosis. Am J Sports Med 22:601-606 (1994).

Thonnard JL, Bragard D, Willems PA, Plaghki L. Stability of the braced ankle. A biomechanical investigation. Am J Sports Med 24:356-361 (1996).

U.S. Army Research Institute of Environmental Medicine. Impact of an outside-the-boot ankle brace on sprains associated with military airborne training. Natick MA. Report No. T95-1.

van Galen WCC, Diederiks J. Sportsblessures breed uitgemeneten (sports injuries in a wider perspective), De Vries-Gorch, Haarlem, 1990 In de Bie RA, de Vet HCW, Kripschild PG, et al. The prognosis of ankle sprains. Int J Sports Med 18:285-289 (1997).

Wester JU, Jespersen SM, Nielsen KD, Neumann L. Wobble board training after partial sprains of the lateral ligaments of the ankle: a prospective randomized study. J Orthop Sports Phys Ther 23:332-336 (1996).

Wiley JP, Nigg BM. The effect of an ankle orthosis on ankle range of motion and performance. J Orthop Sports Phys Ther 23:362-369 (1996).

Wynne-Davies R. Familial joint laxity. Proc R Soc Med 64:689-690 (1971).

Credits

Figures 2.1a, 2.1b: Reprinted, by permission, from R. Behnke, 2001, *Kinetic anatomy* (Champaign, IL: Human Kinetics), 231, 230.

Figures 2.2a, 2.5, 2.7, 2.9: Adapted, by permission, from R. Behnke, 2001, *Kinetic anatomy* (Champaign, IL: Human Kinetics), 227, 235, 232.

Figures 2.2b, 2.3: Reprinted, by permission, from J. Watkins, 2001, *Structure and function of the musculoskeletal system* (Champaign, IL: Human Kinetics), 207, 208.

Figure 2.4: Reprinted, by permission, from J. Watkins, 1999, *Structure and function of the musculoskeletal system* (Champaign, IL: Human Kinetics), 210.

Figure 24.2: Reprinted, by permission, from G.J. Davies, 1994, *A compendium of isokinetics in clinical usage and rehabilitation techniques,* 4th ed. (Onalaska, WI: S&S Publishers), 88.

Figure 28.1a-d: Reprinted, by permission, from T.O. Clanton and L.C. Schon, 1999, Athletic injuries to the soft tissues of the foot and ankle. In *Surgery of the foot and ankle,* vol. II, 7th ed., edited by R.A. Mann and M.J. Couglin (St. Louis, MO: Mosby), 1137.

Figure 30.2, 30.4, 30.6, 30.10, 30.12: Adapted, by permission, from R.O. Lundeen, 1992, *Manual of ankle and foot arthroscopy* (New York: Churchill Livingstone).

Tables 24.2 and 24.3: From G.J. Davies, 1994, *A compendium of isokinetics in clinical usage and rehabilitation techniques,* 4th ed. (Onalaska, WI: S&S Publishers).

Table 7.1: Reprinted, by permission, from G.K. Sefton et al., 1979, "Reconstruction of the anterior talofibular ligament for the treatment of the unstable ankle," *The Journal of Bone and Joint Surgery* 61:352-354.

Table 7.2: Adapted, by permission, from R. St. Pierre, F. Allman, F.H. Bassett III, J.L. Goldner, and L.L. Fleming, 1982, "A review of lateral ankle ligamentous reconstructions," *Foot & Ankle* (3):114-23

Table 7.3: Adapted, by permission, from J. Karlsson, and L. Peterson, 1991, "Evaluation of ankle joint function: the use of a scoring scale," *Foot Ankle International* 1:15-19.

Table 7.5: Adapted, by permission, from A. Kaikkonen, P. Kannus, and M. Jarvinen, 1994, "A performance test protocol and scoring scale for the evaluation of ankle injuries," *American Journal of Sports Medicine* 22 (4):462-469.

Table 7.6: Adapted, by permission, from R.A. de Bie et al., 1997, "The prognosis of ankle sprains," *International Journal of Sports Medicine* 18(4):285-289.

Tables 24.2 and 24.3: Reprinted, by permission, from G.J. Davies, 1994, *A compendium of isokinetics in clinical usage and rehabilitation techniques,* 4th ed. (Onalaska, WI: S&S Publishers), 88.

Figures 4.2a-b, 4.3, 8.1a-d, 8.2a-c, 8.3: Photos courtesy of Beat Hintermann

Figures 5.2, 5.15, 5.17: Photos courtesy of Rüidiger Reer

Figures 6.2, 6.3a-b, 19.1, 19.2a-b, 19.3: Photos courtesy of Gideon Mann and Meir Nyska

Figures 9.1, 9.2, 9.3, 9.4, 9.5, 9.6, 9.7: Photos courtesy of Ehud Rath

Figure 10.1a-b, 10.4a-b, 10.5, 10.7a-b, 10.9, 10.10a-b: Photos courtesy of Yaakov Applbaum

Figure 10.2a-b: Photos courtesy of R.A. Bloom

Figure 10.3: Photo courtesy of J.M. Gomori

Figure 10.6: Photo courtesy of Scott Fields

Figures 10.8a-b: Photos courtesy of R.A. Bloom

Figures 11.1, 31.1, 31.2a-b, 31.3, 31.4, 31.5a-b, 31.6a-b, 31.7, 31.8 a-c, 31.9: Photos courtesy of Wolf-Ruediger Dingels

Figure 12.1a-c, 12.2, 12.5, 35.2, 35.9: Photos courtesy of Gideon Mann

Figures 13.1, 13.2, 13.3, 13.4: Photos courtesy of Chaim Zinman

Figure 14.2: Photo courtesy of R. Kissling

Figures 15.1, 15.2, 15.3a-b, 15.6, 15.7, 15.9, 15.10 a-f, 15.12, 15.13a-b: Photos courtesy of Lew Schon

Figure 15.11: Photo courtesy of Aircast, Inc.

Figures 16.2, 16.3, 16.4, 16.5 a-d, 16.6, 16.7, 16.8 a-d, 16.9 a-d, 16.10a-b: Photos courtesy of C. Niek van Dijk

Figures 17.1, 17.4, 17.5, 17.6a-b, 17.8 a-c: Photos courtesy of Frank Spaas

Figures 21.1, 21.2, 21.3, 21.4, 21.5, 21.6, 21.7, 21.8: Photos courtesy of Deborah Mandis Cozen

Figures 22.1, 22.2, 22.3, 22.4, 22.5: Photos courtesy of David Mencher

Figures 27.1, 27.2, 27.3, 27.4: Photos courtesy of Alberto Macklin Vadell

Figures 30.3, 30.5a-b, 30.7, 30.8, 30.9, 30.11: Photos courtesy of Charles C. Southerland Jr.

Chapter 24 forms (Static Balance Test, Dynamic Balance Test, Functional Standing Long Jump and Hop Test Data Form, and Lower Extremity Functional Test): Courtesy of Gundersen-Lutheran Sports Medicine

Index

Note: Tables are represented by an italicized *t* following the page number; figures by an italicized *f.*

About the Editors

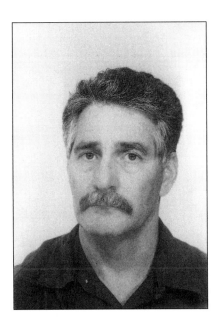

Meir Nyska, MD, has been a senior member in the department of orthopedic surgery at Hadassah University Medical Center in Jerusalem since 1992. He has lectured in medical schools since 1983. He earned his medical degree from the Hebrew University Hadassah Medical School. Dr. Nyska is a member of the Israeli Association of Orthopedic Surgery. He is a well-respected authority in the field and has been widely published. He is a founder and former president of the Israel Foot and Ankle Society, and he currently chairs the department of orthopedic surgery at the Meir University Hospital in Kfar Saba, Israel.

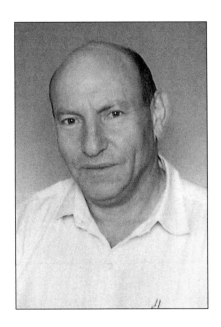

Gideon Mann, MD, is the director of the Sports Injuries Unit at Meir Hospital, Kfar Saba, Israel. He has been a senior orthopedic surgeon at Hadassah University Hospital since 1981 and at the Ribstein Center for Research and Sport Medicine at the Wingate Institute since 1990. He has lectured on arthroscopy, sport injuries, and related topics. Dr. Mann has published articles in international journals for more than 25 years. He earned his medical degree from Hebrew University Hadassah Medical School in Jerusalem in 1974. He is a former chair of the International Society of Arthroscopy, Knee Surgery and Orthopaedic Sports Medicine Committee, a former member of its board of directors, and president of the Israel Society of Sport Medicine from 1989 to 1999.

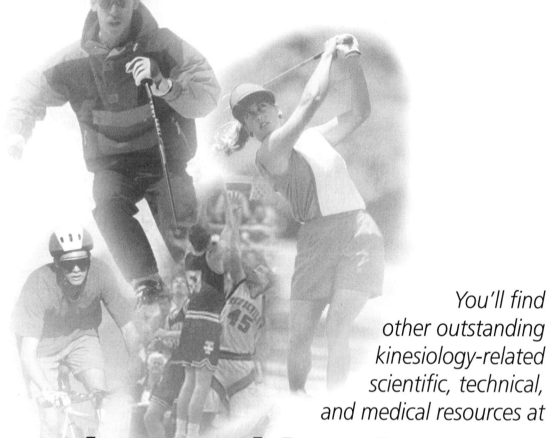